COSMETIC PROCEDURES in SKIN OF COLOR

PROCEDURES IN COSMETIC DERMATOLOGY

PROCEDURES IN COSMETIC DERMATOLOGY

Series Editors:
Jeffrey S. Dover MD, FRCPC and
Murad Alam, MD, MSCI, MBA

Recently published volumes:

2023
Surgical Lifting
First Edition
Hooman Khorasani, MD and Eyal Levit, MD
ISBN 978-0-323-67326-6

Soft Tissue Augmentation
Fifth edition
Jean Carruthers, MD, FRCS(C), FRC(Ophth),
Alastair Carruthers, MA, BM,
BCh, FRCPC, FRCP(Lon), Jeffrey S. Dover, MD, FRCPC,
Murad Alam, MD, MSCI, MBA and Omer Ibrahim, MD
ISBN 978-0-323-83075-1

Hair Restoration
First Edition
Murad Alam, MD, MSCI, MBA and Jeffrey S. Dover,
MD, FRCPC
ISBN 978-0-323-82921-2

Botulinum Toxin
Fifth edition
Alastair Carruthers,
MA, BM, BCh, FRCPC, FRCP(Lon),
Jean Carruthers, MD, FRCS(C), FRC(Ophth),
Jeffrey S. Dover, MD, FRCPC,
Murad Alam, MD, MSCI, MBA, and
Omer Ibrahim, MD
ISBN 978-0-323-83116-1

Forthcoming volumes:

2024
Cosmeceuticals
Fourth edition
Zoe Diana Draelos, MD
ISBN 978-0-443-11808-1

Photodynamic Therapy
Third edition
Macrene Alexiades, MD, PhD
ISBN 978-0-443-10689-7

Scar Management
Second Edition
Jessica G. Labadie, MD, Murad Alam, MD, MSCI, MBA, and
Jeffrey S. Dover, MD, FRCPC
ISBN 978-0-443-24590-9

Treatment of Leg Veins
Third Edition
Murad Alam, MD, MSCI, MBA, and Sirunya Silapunt, MD
ISBN 978-0-443-25011-8

PROCEDURES IN COSMETIC DERMATOLOGY

COSMETIC PROCEDURES
in SKIN OF COLOR

Edited by
Andrew F. Alexis, MD, MPH
Professor and Vice-Chair
Department of Dermatology
Weill Cornell Medicine
New York, New York
United States

Series Editors
Jeffrey S. Dover, MD, FRCPC, and
Murad Alam, MD, MSCI, MBA

ELSEVIER

Elsevier
1600 John F. Kennedy Blvd.
Ste 1800
Philadelphia, PA 19103-2899

Notice

Practitioners and researchers must always rely on their own experience and knowledge in evaluating and using any information, methods, compounds, or experiments described herein. Because of rapid advances in the medical sciences, in particular, independent verification of diagnoses and drug dosages should be made. To the fullest extent of the law, no responsibility is assumed by Elsevier, authors, editors, or contributors for any injury and/or damage to persons or property as a matter of products liability, negligence or otherwise, or from any use or operation of any methods, products, instructions, or ideas contained in the material herein.

Content Strategist: Jessica McCool
Content Development Specialist: Vaishali Singh
Content Development Manager: Somodatta Roy Choudhury
Publishing Services Manager: Shereen Jameel
Project Manager: Haritha Dharmarajan
Design Direction: Patrick Ferguson

Printed in India

Last digit is the print number: 9   8   7   6   5   4   3   2   1

 Working together to grow libraries in developing countries

www.elsevier.com • www.bookaid.org

Dedication

I dedicate this book to my late mother, Dr. Mercy Alexis, who was the first Black female dermatologist in Canada and my inspiration to become a dermatologist, as well as my wife, Dr. Ama Alexis, without whose support, this project would not have been possible.

CONTRIBUTORS

Oma N. Agbai, MD
Assistant Clinical Professor
Dermatology
University of California
Davis Health
Sacramento, California
United States

Crystal Aguh, MD
Assistant Professor
Department of Dermatology
Johns Hopkins University School of Medicine
Baltimore, Maryland
United States

Murad Alam, MD, MBA, MSCI
Professor and Vice-Chair
Department of Dermatology
Feinberg School of Medicine
Northwestern University
Chicago, Illinois
Professor
Departments of Surgery, Otolaryngology, and Medical
    Social Sciences
Feinberg School of Medicine
Northwestern University
Evanston, Illinois
United States

Andrew F. Alexis, MD, MPH
Professor and Vice-Chair
Department of Dermatology
Weill Cornell Medicine
New York, New York
United States

Sultan B. AlSalem, MD, MMSc, FAAD
Fellow
Dermatology
Weill Cornell Medicine
New York City, New York
United States

Eliot F. Battle Jr., MD
Clinical Instructor
Department of Dermatology
Howard University Hospital
Washington, District of Columbia
United States

Cheryl Marie Burgess, MD
Assistant Clinical Professor
Dermatology
Georgetown University
Washington, District of Columbia
Assistant Clinical Professor
Dermatology
The George Washington University
Washington, District of Columbia
United States

Valerie Dawn Callender, MD
Professor
Dermatology
Howard University College of Medicine
Washington, District of Columbia
Medical Director
Callender Dermatology & Cosmetic Center
Glenn Dale, Maryland
United States

Janeth R. Campbell, MS
N/A
N/A
Georgetown University School of Medicine
Washington, District of Columbia
United States

Henry H. L. Chan, MBBS, MD, PhD, FRCP
Honorary Clinical Professor
Division of Dermatology, Department of Medicine
The University of Hong Kong
Hong Kong
Visiting Scientist
Wellman Center for Photomedicine
Massachusetts General Hospital
Boston, Massachusetts
United States

Abigail Franco, MD
Assistant Professor
Dermatology
University of Rochester Medical Center
Rochester, New York
United States

Hassan Galadari, MD
Associate Professor
Medicine
College of Medicine and Health Sciences
UAE University
Al Ain
United Arab Emirates

Chee-Leok Goh, MD
Dermatology
National Skin Centre
Singapore

Pearl E. Grimes, Bachelor of Science, MD
Clinical Professor
Division of Dermatology
David Geffen School of Medicine University
Los Angeles, California
United States

Pearl E. Grimes, MD
Clinical Professor
Division of Dermatology
University of California
Director, Vitiligo and Pigmentation Institute
Los Angeles, California
United States

Sara Hogan, MD
Health Sciences Clinical Instructor
Dermatology
UCLA
Los Angeles, California
United States

Omer Ibrahim, MD
Associate
Dermatology
Chicago Cosmetic Surgery and Dermatology
Chicago, District of Illinois
United States

Sherrif F. Ibrahim, MD, PhD
Associate Professor
Dermatology
University of Rochester
Rochester, New York
United States

Jared Jagdeo, MD, MS
Associate Professor
Dermatology
SUNY Downstate
Brooklyn, New York
United States

Taylor A. Jamerson, BA
Medical Student
University of Michigan Medical School
Ann Arbor, Michigan
United States

Bianca Y. Kang, MD
Postdoctoral Research Fellow
Dermatology
Northwestern University Feinberg School of Medicine
Chicago, New York
Illinois
United States

Shilpi Khetarpal, MD
Assistant Professor of Dermatology
Dermatology
Cleveland Clinic Foundation
Cleveland, Ohio
United States

Alana Kurtti, MD, BS
Resident
EHMC
Englewood
United States

Malika A. Ladha, MD
Clinical Fellow (Aesthetic Dermatology)
Division of Dermatology
Department of Medicine
University of Toronto
Toronto
Canada

Melissa Laughter, MD, PhD
Medical Student
School of Medicine
University of Colorado
Aurora, Colorado
United States

Nicole Y. Lee, MD, MPH, FAAD
Physician
Dermatology
Wesson Dermatology
Great Neck, New York
United States

Elise D. Martin, MD
Resident
Department of Dermatology
Wake Forest
Winston-Salem, North Carolina
United States

Mayra B. C. Maymone, DDS, MD, DSc
Resident
Department of Dermatology
Brown University
Providence, Rhode Island
United States

Farah Moustafa, BS, MD
Attending Physician, Director, Laser & Cosmetic Center
Dermatology
Tufts Medical Center
Boston, Massachusetts
United States

Gilly Munavalli, MD, MHS, FAAD
Clinical Assistant Professor
Department of Dermatology
Wake Forest University
Winston-Salem, North Carolina
United States

Jasmine Onyeka Obioha, BA, MD
Attending
Dermatology
Cedars Sinai Medical Group
Beverly Hills, California
United States

Achiamah Osei-Tutu, MD
Dermatologist
University Hospital of Brooklyn
Brooklyn, New York
United States

Maritza Ivonne Perez, MD, FAAD
Professor
Dermatology
University of Connecticut School of Medicine
Farmington, Connecticut
Clinical Professor
Dermatology
Mount Sinai
New York City, New York
United States

Malcolm Pyles, MD, MBA
Resident Physician
Dermatology
Cleveland Clinic
Cleveland, Ohio
United States

Rebecca L. Quiñonez, MD, MS
Post Graduate Research Fellow
Dr. Phillip Frost Department of Dermatology and
    Cutaneous Surgery
University of Miami Miller School of Medicine
Miami, Florida
United States

Camille Robinson, BS
Medical Student
Dermatology
Duke School of Medicine
Durham, North Carolina
United States

Mona Sadeghpour, MD
Co-Founder, SkinMed Institute
Lone Tree
Colorado
United States

Nazanin Saedi, MD
Associate Professor, Director Laser Surgery and
**   Cosmetic Dermatology**
Dermatology
Thomas Jefferson University
Philadelphia, Pennsylvania
United States

Autumn Leslie Saizan, BS, MD
University of Rochester School of Medicine
University of Rochester School of Medicine and
    Dentistry
Rochester
Keck School of Medicine
Dermatology
Keck School of Medicine at University of Southern
    California
Los Angeles, California
United States

Sokhna Seck, MS
Medical Student
Cleveland Clinic Lerner College of Medicine
Case Western Reserve University
Cleveland, Ohio
United States

Susan C. Taylor, MD
Sandra Lazarus Professor of Dermatology
Department of Dermatology
Perelman School of Medicine
Philadelphia, Pennsylvania
United States

Neelam A. Vashi, MD
Associate Professor
Dermatology
Boston University
Boston, Massachusetts
United States

Rosannah Marie Velasquez, MD
Resident
Department of Dermatology and Cutaneous Biology
Thomas Jefferson University
Philadelphia, Pennsylvania
United States

Cindy Wassef, MD
Assistant Professor
Dermatology
Rutgers Robert Wood Johnson Medical School
Somerset
United States

Mara Weinstein Velez, MD, FAAD
Assistant Professor, Director, Cosmetic and Laser
**   Dermatology**
Dermatology
University of Rochester Medical Center
Rochester, New York
United States

Kiyanna Williams, MD
Section Head, Skin of Color Section
Dermatology
Cleveland Clinic
Cleveland, Ohio
United States

Heather Woolery-Lloyd, MD
Dr. Phillip Frost Department of Dermatology and
    Cutaneous Surgery
University of Miami Miller School of Medicine
Miami, Florida
United States

The term skin of color is used to describe the broad and diverse range of skin types that have in common increased epidermal melanin pigmentation, a tendency toward labile melanocyte responses to inflammation and injury, as well as distinct ethno-cultural nuances that are relevant to dermatologic care. Historically, the inclusion of populations with skin of color in educational materials, research studies, and care delivery related to cosmetic dermatologic procedures has been extremely limited. Lack of representation of the diverse racial, ethnic, and geographic populations with skin of color have contributed to disparities in access to safe and effective cosmetic therapies.

Over the past two decades, major shifts in global demographics, socioeconomic advancement, and cultural perceptions of beauty—coupled with remarkable advancements in available technologies and techniques that are suitable for darker skin phototypes—have set the stage for monumental increases in the range of cosmetic treatment options for patients with skin of color. This progress, which has translated into vast improvements in patient care, would not have been possible without the trailblazing work of visionary leaders in dermatology, many of whom are contributing authors to this text book.

The central aim of this book is to provide the reader with a comprehensive resource to help inform and guide the management of aesthetic concerns in diverse patient populations with skin of color. The book includes expert discussion of the leading cosmetic procedures using laser- or energy-based devices, injectables, and peeling agents, highlighting the nuances of performing them safely and effectively across the spectrum of skin of color. Recognizing that skin of color does not represent a homogenous or monolithic group, but rather a diverse range of phototypes and self-identified racial/ethnic groups, this textbook includes chapters on specific patient populations with skin of color, many of whom have not been represented in previous books on cosmetic procedures.

The publishing of this first edition comes at a time when the population seeking aesthetic procedures has evolved to include a sizable and increasing proportion of patients who have skin of color. In stark contrast, access to safe and effective cosmetic procedures has been hampered by knowledge gaps pertaining to best practices for skin of color. In this context, one of the goals of this book is to enhance the reader's knowledge of the depth and breadth of cosmetic procedures that can be individualized to effectively address the aesthetic concerns of diverse patients.

It has been a privilege to collaborate with some of the most renowned experts in the field of cosmetic dermatology who have generously shared their insights into performing safe, effective, and culturally aligned care for patients with skin of color. In many ways, this is a celebration of and testament to the advances made in our understanding of the diversity of approaches needed to expertly serve our global patient population.

ACKNOWLEDGMENT

I would like to acknowledge the mentors, pioneers, and leaders whose vision and dedication paved the way for advancing the care of patients with skin of color.

CONTENTS

VIDEO TABLE OF CONTENTS

Structural and Functional Differences and Their Relevance to Aesthetic Concerns and Approach to Treatment

Murad Alam, Bianca Y. Kang, Andrew Alexis

SUMMARY AND KEY FEATURES

- Successful treatment of aging requires awareness of racial and ethnic variations, as well as understanding of the differences in youthful ideals across racial and ethnic groups.
- Richly pigmented skin, compared to lightly pigmented skin, has more epidermal melanin, larger melanosomes that are singly dispersed, and labile melanocyte responses to injury and inflammation.
- Due to the photoprotective effect of increased melanin, features of intrinsic aging such as sagging due to fat redistribution and gravitational descent tend to be more prominent than, and appear before, extrinsic signs of facial aging.

- Volume correction and toxin injection should be targeted toward restoring a more youthful appearance based on the typical facial features of each patient's ethnicity, or multiple ethnicities, if they have mixed ethnicity.
- Skin tightening with energy-based devices, as well as more invasive procedures to correct excess skin and fat redistribution, may be considered to lessen the appearance of skin sagging.
- In all patients with skin of color, the risk of postinflammatory pigment alteration and scarring should be discussed. Treatment techniques should be adapted to help reduce this risk.

INTRODUCTION

Approaching the patient with skin of color patient requires both an understanding of patient-specific facial features as well as consideration of the patient's ethnicity and cultural values. In general, the baseline appearance of patients varies across self-identified racial categories and ethnic groups as well as Fitzpatrick skin phototype (SPT). Baseline contours may vary, and different anatomic subunits may be different in size and relation to one another (Figs. 1.1 and 1.2).

The aged contour can have a tendency to differ from one population to another, with, for instance, White (i.e., SPT I-III) patients having more wrinkles and folds, and African American patients (i.e., SPT IV-VI) having more lower face fullness and fat herniation.[1–3] While some generalizations can be made vis-à-vis typical anatomic and clinical differences between populations, it is paramount to appreciate individual variations in anatomy and skin characteristics as considerable diversity within population subcategories exists.

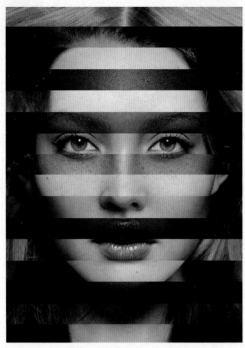

Fig. 1.1 Diversity of facial features. *(Art-collage No. 18 ("GRA-DIENT 99") of 99 portraits, from the project "The Ethnic Origins of Beauty"// "Les origines de la beauté." Used with permission from Natalia Ivanova.)*

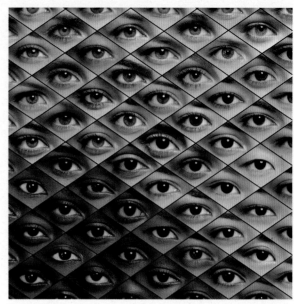

Fig. 1.2 Diversity of eye features. *(Art-collage No. 15 ("RHOM-BUS EYES") with elements of 48 different ethnic origins, from the project "The Ethnic Origins of Beauty"// "Les origines de la beauté." Used with permission from Natalia Ivanova.)*

Appreciating these baseline differences may be helpful for the physician to better understand patient expectations and thus develop an individualized treatment plan. Undoubtedly, successful practice of cosmetic surgery also requires insight into other cultural and social factors that may influence perceptions of beauty and treatment goals. Also, many patients of mixed ancestry are more complex than the generalizations described in this chapter. When available, looking at photos of the patient at a younger age may be useful in guiding cosmetic treatment.

CLASSIFICATIONS OF RACE AND ETHNICITY

There have been various attempts to classify people into distinct racial and ethnic categories. In 1961, anthropologist Stanley M. Garn defined nine geographical races based on relative genetic and geographic isolation: Amerindian, Polynesian, Micronesian, Melanesian-Papuan, Australian, Asiatic, Indian, European, and African.[4] Ethnicity, on the other hand, may refer to an individual's self-identification with a group or groups based on shared sociocultural beliefs, though this term is often used interchangeably with "race."[5,6] Many argue that racial and ethnic definitions are merely sociopolitical constructs and do not adequately embody the complexities of human diversity.[6,7] Indeed, the meaning of these terms are ever in flux and, even within a single race or ethnic group, skin color and anatomic structures may vary greatly.

Racial and ethnic categories used by the U.S. Census Bureau are often included in dermatology research studies. This includes five self-identified racial categories (White, Black or African American, American Indian or Alaska Native, Asian, and Native Hawaiian or Other Pacific Islander) and two ethnic groups ("Hispanic or Latino" and "Not Hispanic or Latino").[8] Despite their use in research studies, it is important to recognize that these categories are sociopolitical constructs that are not intended to be biologic or anthropological in nature. Notwithstanding the important limitations of racial/ethnic categorization, specific trends or shared characteristics relevant to dermatologists can be gleaned by data involving self-identified populations using U.S. Census Bureau definitions.

TABLE 1.1	Ethnic Groups That Comprise Persons Defined as Having Skin of Color
Black	African, Black persons of African descent, including African American, Caribbean American, and Latin American persons
Latino or Hispanic	Persons of Spanish and indigenous Central/South American descent, including Central Americans, South Americans, and Caribbean American persons of Spanish descent, including Cuban, Puerto Rican, and Dominican
East Asian	Chinese, Japanese, Korean
Southeast Asian and Pacific Islander	Filipino, Vietnamese, Cambodian, Thai, Malaysian, Laotian, Burmese, Hmong descent, Polynesian, Micronesian
Australoid	Australian aborigine, Melanesian descent (now the Republic of Guinea, Papua, Solomon Islands)
Native American	More than 560 recognized tribes, including Inuit
East Indian/South Asian	Indian, Pakistani, Bangladesh, Sri Lankan
Middle Eastern	Iranian, Iraqi, persons from Saudi Arabia and the Arabian Peninsula (including Kuwait, Bahrain, Oman, Qatar, the United Arab Emirates, Yemen), Lebanese, Afghani, Jordanian, Syrian, Israeli, Turkish, North African (Egypt, Morocco, Algeria, Libya)

Modified from Talakoub L, Wesley NO. Differences in perceptions of beauty and cosmetic procedures performed in ethnic patients. Semin Cutan Med Surg. 2009;28(2):115-129.

In dermatology, the Fitzpatrick skin phototype system is frequently used to categorize skin types based on color and propensity to burn.[7] However, limitations of this scale have been well described.[9,10] Later, the Lancer Ethnicity Scale was developed to also consider ethnicity and can be particularly useful in skin resurfacing in patients with skin of color and avoiding hyperpigmentation.[11] More recently, the terms "skin of color" and "ethnic skin" have been used to more broadly define darker skin, typically Fitzpatrick phototypes IV to VI (Table 1.1).[12,13]

Throughout this chapter, the terms "skin of color," "ethnic skin," and various descriptors of racial/ethnic groups will be discussed. These generalizations can help to guide the treating physician's approach to the aging patient with skin of color. Nevertheless, individual patient considerations, including cultural values, perceptions of beauty and aging, and treatment goals and expectations, are the most important factors. Each patient, regardless of race or ethnicity, is unique and must be treated as such.

AGING IN SKIN OF COLOR: CLOSE-UP DIFFERENCES IN TEXTURE AND FUNCTION

Ethnic Differences in Barrier Function
Barrier function of the stratum corneum differs between self-identified racial/ethnic groups. In 2010, Muizzuddin and colleagues collected tape strippings from the faces and forearms of 341 healthy adults of Black/African-American, White, and East Asian descent.[14] In this study, stratum corneum ceramide content was lowest in African Americans, consistent with the relatively high prevalence of xerosis in this group.[15] Barrier strength and maturation index were lowest in East Asian skin, possibly helping to explain increased skin sensitivity in this population.

Ethnic Differences in the Dermis
Structural differences in the dermis are also apparent across ethnicities. In a study of 388 African American, Mexican, White, and Chinese women, ages 18 to 78 and living in the same area for at least 2 years, Querleux et al. demonstrated that the sub-epidermal nonechogenic band, measured via optical coherence tomography, was a sensitive marker for aging, and was less pronounced in African Americans than other ethnicities.[16] By contrast, the thickness of the papillary dermis was stable over time and across ethnic groups.

Ethnic Differences in Photoaging
Ethnic differences in the skin often become more evident with photoaging. In general, the appearance of facial aging onsets at a later age and has a lower severity in individuals with darker skin or higher phototype.[17–20] Though overall sun exposure and ultraviolet (UV) radiation protection practices may vary between cultures

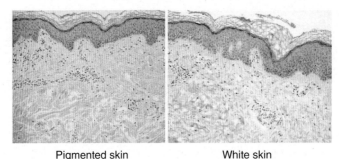

Pigmented skin   White skin

Fig. 1.3 Histology of epidermis and upper part of the dermis from pigmented skin and White skin, demonstrating concentration of pigment most notably along basal layer of the epidermis. *(From Jothishankar B, Stein SL. Impact of skin color and ethnicity. Clin Dermatol. 2019;37(5):418-429.)*

and geographic location, amount and distribution of melanin play a key role in explaining these differences (Fig. 1.3). Compared to lighter skin, darker skin contains larger and more numerous melanosomes, which are less aggregated, have a higher melanin content, and are more widely distributed in the epidermis (versus confined to the stratum basale).[17,21,22] As a result, darker skin is less penetrated by both UVA and UVB wavelengths.[23] Also due to increased melanin, however, darker skin is more prone to pigmentation disorders (e.g., melasma, postinflammatory hyperpigmentation, and dark infraorbital circles), which are a common treatment priority for patients with skin of color.[24] Additional structural differences in dark skin, such as dermal collagen bundles that are more tightly packed and closer to the epidermis, may also contribute to variations in photoaging.

Subjective Wrinkle Assessment Versus Quantitative Roughness Analysis

Though changes in the epidermis and dermis contribute to differences in aging between ethnicities, subtle facial changes due to aging may be difficult to appreciate with the naked eye. In certain circumstances, such as in research, it may be appropriate to consider more sensitive and objective measurements. In 2009, Fujimura and colleagues compared the utility of visual wrinkle assessment to objective measurement of skin roughness in characterizing ethnic differences in periorbital aging in 295 Japanese, Chinese, and German women, ages 16 to 76.[25] Skin roughness was measured with hydrophilic vinyl silicone molds of the periorbital region and the PRIMOS system (GFMessetechnik GmbH,

Tetlow, Germany), an instrument that quantifies three-dimensional skin microstructure. Compared to visual wrinkle assessments, roughness analysis was more sensitive and able to differentiate between ethnicities within the same age at the lateral corner of the eye. Below the eye, both visual assessments and roughness were comparably useful.

AGING IN SKIN OF COLOR: GROSS MORPHOLOGIC DIFFERENCES

There are, in general, similarities and differences in gross facial morphology across ethnic groups (Fig. 1.4). Of course, however, these are generalizations and there exists wide variation in appearance within ethnic groups. The physician should consider individual facial features, trends in morphology across ethnicities, as well as cultural and social influences on the patient's goals and expectations. Understanding these various factors may help to set the stage for developing a treatment plan with the patient while being respectful of their values and preferences.

Variations in fat distribution and skeletal structure contribute to differences in aging between ethnic groups. The thick skin-soft tissue envelope in skin of color patients commonly causes sagging due to fat redistribution and gravitational descent to be more prominent than, and appear before, other signs of facial aging.[1] These patients complain of lower face fullness and fat herniation, frequently with noticeable changes near the eyes, nasolabial fold, and jawline. This is in contrast to White patients, who often experience more worrisome wrinkles and folds.

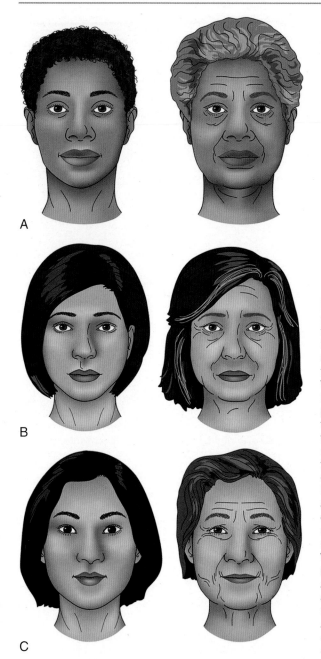

A

B

C

Fig. 1.4 (A) Typical African American faces, young and old. Compared to Whites, the young (left) African American face has relative malar hypoplasia. As the typical African American face ages (older face on right, younger on left), fat redistribution and descent, including in the submental area, is more notable than the fine lines, wrinkles, and skin laxity more often seen in aging Whites. (B) Typical Latino faces, young and old. Younger faces (left) tend to be wider and fuller, with thicker subcutaneous fat pads. Like Asians, Latinos have a wider intercanthal distance than Whites, with lateral canthi that are higher than medial canthi. Chins can be small and recessed, and noses slightly wide but not overall large in size. As Latinos age (right), thick folds but few fine wrinkles appear as the copious soft tissue sags. Eyelids and eyebrows become heavy and descend, suborbital fat accumulates, and nasolabial folds grow. (C) Typical Asian faces, young and old. Asians (left) tend to have the widest intercanthal distances and the most slant in the eyes, with lateral canthi markedly higher than medial canthi. Mouths are less wide and mandibles are more prominent and wider in Asians compared to Whites. Like Latinos, Asians have broader noses that are less protuberant at maximal elevation. Similar to Latinos and African Americans, Asians age (right) with fewer fine lines, wrinkles, and skin laxity than Whites. Sagging fat pads may also be less notable in aging Asians than those of other ethnicities. *(From Alam M, Tung R. Injection technique in neurotoxins and fillers: Planning and basic technique. J Am Acad Dermatol. 2018;79(3): 407-419.)*

Eyes and Midface

The area encompassing the infraorbital area and upper midface is often one of the first to show aging. There are notable differences in the periorbital region across ethnicities, and these variations determine the course of aging and treatment considerations (Fig. 1.5). In Black patients, there may be relative orbital proptosis and longer eye fissures.[13,26] With age, sagging of the malar fat pads in combination with relative ocular proptosis may contribute to appearance of midface concavity (Fig. 1.6).[21] Full-appearing upper eyelids may become a concern due to the relatively lower location of the upper

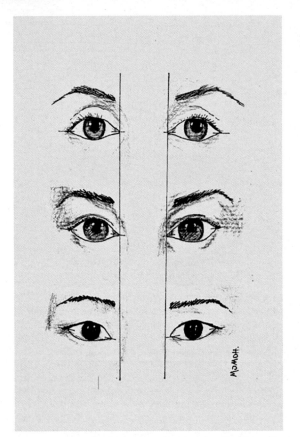

Fig. 1.5 Periorbital features of the White (top), African American (middle), and Asian (bottom) patient, with variations in intercanthal distance and the relationship of the medial canthus to the lateral canthus. *(From McKnight A, Momoh AO, Bullocks JM. Variations of structural components: Specific intercultural differences in facial morphology, skin type, and structures. Semin Plast Surg. 2009;23(3):163-167.)*

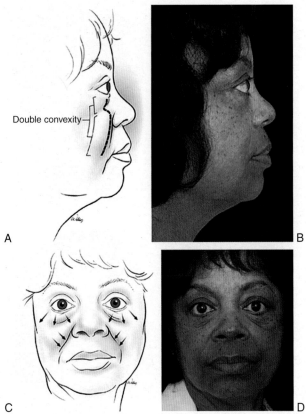

Fig. 1.6 Aging of the midface. (A) Lateral schematic showing the descent of the malar fat pad resulting in a double convexity of the midface. (B) Lateral view of a patient with a double convexity from midfacial aging. (C) Anterior schematic showing formation of tear troughs and nasojugal folds from descent of the malar fat pads. (D) Anterior view of a patient with tear troughs and prominent nasolabial folds. *(From Brissett AE, Naylor MC. The aging African-American face. Facial Plast Surg. 2010;26(02):154-163.)*

eyelid crease, medial orbital fat pad pseudoherniation, and lacrimal gland ptosis.[21,27]

In Asian, Latino, and Middle Eastern individuals, intercanthal and biocular widths tend to be wider compared to Whites, and eye fissure length smaller.[1,26,28] Individuals of East Asian descent tend to have high lateral canthi in relation to the medial canthi and full upper lids.[1,13] In Asians, including those from the Indian subcontinent, gravitational descent of flat but abundant malar fat tends to cause malar fat pad ptosis and formation of conspicuous tear troughs (Fig. 1.7).[13,29,30] Flat, broad noses (Fig. 1.8) may also cause patients to request soft tissue augmentation of this region.

Mestizo/Hispanic patients have been described as having broader, rounder faces with more prominent malar eminences, as well as smaller chins and flatter noses.[31] As these patients age, droopy eyebrows (often laterally), hooding of the upper eyelids, and prominent nasolabial folds may frequently develop (Fig. 1.9).

Due to descension of infraorbital fat pads, nearly all patients notice deepening of the nasolabial folds and formation of tear troughs.

Lower Face

In many ethnic groups, including Black, South Asian, and Hispanic/Latino, a primary concern in the appearance of

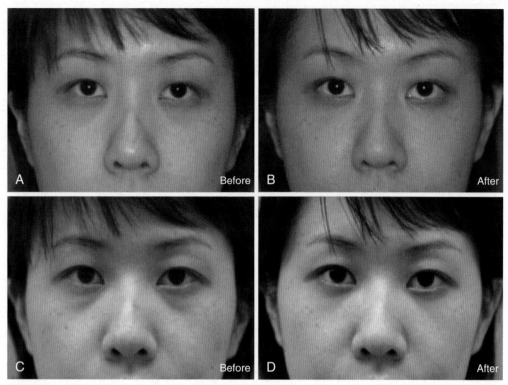

Fig. 1.7 (A, C) Preoperative views of a 28-year-old woman with tear trough deformity. (B, D) Postoperative views 1 year following transconjunctival orbital fat repositioning. *Note:* A and B were taken using the ring flashlight; C and D were taken under room ceiling light without the ring flashlight. *(From Momosawa A, Kurita M, Ozaki M, et al. Transconjunctival orbital fat repositioning for tear trough deformity in young Asians. Aesthet Surg J. 2008;28(3):265-271.)*

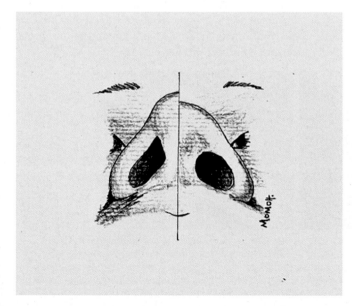

Fig. 1.8 Wider nasal base width and less tip projection in the Asian and the Black/African-American nose relative to the White nose. *(From McKnight A, Momoh AO, Bullocks JM. Variations of structural components: Specific intercultural differences in facial morphology, skin type, and structures. Semin Plast Surg. 2009;23(3):163-167.)*

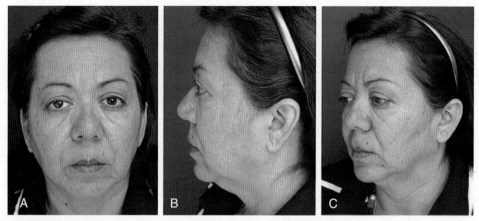

Fig. 1.9 (A–C) Aging Mestizo facial characteristics. With aging, Mestizo features become more prominent. Because of the thick S-STE, folds become more prominent without really having more wrinkles. Eyebrows tend to droop laterally, eyelid hooding becomes more prominent, nasolabial folds become pronounced, and lower eyelid fat herniation is more noticeable. *(From Cobo R, García CA. Aesthetic surgery for the Mestizo/ Hispanic patient: Special considerations. Facial Plast Surg. 2010;26(2):164-173.)*

lower face aging is blunting of the cervicomental angle. Fat pad atrophy permitting skin laxity, resorption of the mandible, and soft tissue accumulation contribute to excess subdermal tissue on a weakened framework and thus gradual loss of the jawline. Descent of thick, heavy skin and accumulation of fat also lead to jowl formation, a common sign of aging in patients with skin of color, especially Black and Latino patients.[24] Also in Black patients, descent of subplatysmal fat and accumulation of submental fat causing chin ptosis may further contribute to loss of the jawline (Fig. 1.10).[21]

In some East Asian populations, wide and prominent mandibles may be considered aesthetically undesirable,

and many patients request botulinum toxin injection into the masseter or other methods of facial slimming.[32] However, in older patients, reduction in lower face volume can exacerbate sagging and jowling. While thinning lips are a concern in patients of all ethnic groups, Asian patients in particular may request volume augmentation with a relatively larger upper lip compared to other ethnic groups, as this offers counterpoise to relative retrusion of the maxilla.

For Hispanic/Latino patients, retrusive chins combined with nearby sagging and jowl formation cause this area to be a primary concern.[33] Oral commissures and marionette lines also become more important treatment areas in this population.

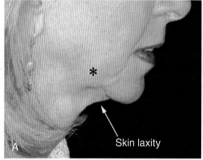
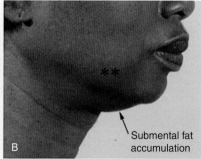

Fig. 1.10 Lower facial aging. The photographs illustrate the difference in lower facial aging between Black/ African-Americans and Whites. (A) White lower face. Asterisk denotes jowling from excess skin laxity, which is also responsible for the loss of the cervicomental angle. (B) African American lower face. Double asterisk denotes jowling from the descent of thick skin and subdermal tissues. Loss of the cervicomental angle occurs from accumulation of submental fat. *(From Brissett AE, Naylor MC. The aging African-American face. Facial Plast Surg. 2010;26(02):154-163.)*

TREATMENT CONSIDERATIONS

These differences in aging necessitate a tailored treatment approach. With regard to preservation of ethnic differentiation, volume correction and toxin injection should be targeted towards restoring a more youthful appearance based on the typical facial features of each patient's ethnicity, or multiple ethnicities, if they have mixed ethnicity. In patients with skin of color, stimulatory fillers (e.g., calcium hydroxylapatite and poly-L-lactic acid) that promote production of collagen and elastin and skin tightening may be appropriate in areas of the face requiring deeper volumization.[34–36] For patients with a wider mid-face region—a feature that may be seen more frequently in patients of East Asian descent—filler may be more preferentially injected into the medial, rather than lateral, cheek.[32] Injection of botulinum toxin requires targeting areas that may vary by ethnicity. Different dosing may be required, and toxin may be used more frequently for facial shaping in East Asian patients versus White patients. In patients of all ethnicities, combined treatment of facial aging with botulinum toxin and soft tissue filler may be more effective than either injection alone.[37]

Due to their safety in pigmented skin, and low risk of inducing pigmentary abnormalities, skin tightening procedures with energy-based devices such as radiofrequency and microfocused ultrasound may be considered to stimulate collagen and thus lessen the appearance of skin sagging.[36,38] Invasive procedures targeted at correcting excess skin and fat redistribution might also be discussed with patients with skin of color, but the risks of hypertrophic scar and incisional hyperpigmentation should be clearly conveyed and carefully considered.

In all patients with skin of color, the risk of scarring and postinflammatory hyperpigmentation should be discussed. With injectable fillers, linear threading versus serial puncture technique may help to reduce this risk.[39] When using energy-based treatments, conservative settings should be used.[11]

CONCLUSION

Aging is cross-cultural, and specific features of facial aging can vary according to self-identified racial/ethnic category or skin phototype, with certain features relatively more or less exaggerated. Successful treatment of aging requires awareness of potential racial/ethnic variations as well as understanding of the differences in youthful ideals across racial/ethnic groups, as these ideals are often the goal of treatment. Most importantly, regardless of racial/ethnic group or skin color, each individual's preferences and characteristics must be considered and used to develop a treatment plan.

REFERENCES

1. Alam M, Tung R. Injection technique in neurotoxins and fillers: Planning and basic technique. *J Am Acad Dermatol*. 2018;79(3):407-419. doi:10.1016/j.jaad.2018.01.034.
2. Sturm-O'Brien AK, Brissett AEA, Brissett AE. Ethnic trends in facial plastic surgery. *Facial Plast Surg*. 2010;26(2):69-74. doi:10.1055/s-0030-1253496.
3. Alexis AF, Alam M. Racial and ethnic differences in skin aging: Implications for treatment with soft tissue fillers. *J Drugs Dermatol JDD*. 2012;11(8):s30-s32; discussion s32.
4. Garn SM. *Human Races*. Thomas, Springfield, Illinois; 1961.
5. Rivara FP, Finberg L. Use of the terms race and ethnicity. *Arch Pediatr Adolesc Med*. 2001;155(2):119. doi:10.1001/archpedi.155.2.119.
6. Mays VM, Ponce NA, Washington DL, Cochran SD. Classification of race and ethnicity: Implications for public health. *Annu Rev Public Health*. 2003;24:83-110. doi:10.1146/annurev.publhealth.24.100901.140927.
7. Harding SG, ed. *The "Racial" Economy of Science: Toward a Democratic Future*. Indiana University Press, Bloomington, Indiana; 1993.
8. U.S. Census Bureau. Memorandum 2018.02: Using Two Separate Questions for Race and Ethnicity in 2018 End-to-End Census Test and 2020 Census. Published online January 26, 2018. Available at: https://www2.census.gov/programs-surveys/decennial/2020/program-management/memo-series/2020-memo-2018_02.pdf. Accessed August 1, 2021.
9. Sommers MS, Fargo JD, Regueira Y, et al. Are the Fitzpatrick skin phototypes valid for cancer risk assessment in a racially and ethnically diverse sample of women? *Ethn Dis*. 29(3):505-512. doi:10.18865/ed.29.3.505.
10. Ware OR, Dawson JE, Shinohara MM, Taylor SC. Racial limitations of Fitzpatrick skin type. *Cutis*. 2020;105(2):77-80.
11. Lancer HA. Lancer ethnicity scale (LES). *Lasers Surg Med*. 1998;22(1):9. Available at: https://doi.org/10.1002/(SICI)1096-9101(1998)22:1<9::AID-LSM4>3.0.CO;2-T.
12. Taylor SC, Cook-Bolden F. Defining skin of color. *Cutis*. 2002;69(6):435-437.
13. Talakoub L, Wesley NO. Differences in perceptions of beauty and cosmetic procedures performed in ethnic

patients. *Semin Cutan Med Surg.* 2009;28(2):115-129. doi:10.1016/j.sder.2009.05.001.

14. Muizzuddin N, Hellemans L, Van Overloop L, Corstjens H, Declercq L, Maes D. Structural and functional differences in barrier properties of African American, Caucasian and East Asian skin. *J Dermatol Sci.* 2010;59(2):123-128. doi:10.1016/j.jdermsci.2010.06.003.

15. Mekić S, Jacobs LC, Gunn DA, et al. Prevalence and determinants for xerosis cutis in the middle-aged and elderly population: A cross-sectional study. *J Am Acad Dermatol.* 2019;81(4):963-969.e2. doi:10.1016/j.jaad.2018.12.038.

16. Querleux B, Baldeweck T, Diridollou S, et al. Skin from various ethnic origins and aging: An in vivo cross-sectional multimodality imaging study. *Skin Res Technol.* 2009;15(3):306-313. Available at: https://doi.org/10.1111/j.1600-0846.2009.00365.x.

17. Taylor SC. Skin of color: Biology, structure, function, and implications for dermatologic disease. *J Am Acad Dermatol.* 2002;46(2 suppl 2):S41-S62. doi:10.1067/mjd.2002.120790.

18. Nouveau-Richard S, Yang Z, Mac-Mary S, et al. Skin ageing: A comparison between Chinese and European populations. A pilot study. *J Dermatol Sci.* 2005;40(3):187-193. doi:10.1016/j.jdermsci.2005.06.006.

19. Alexis AF, Obioha JO. Ethnicity and aging skin. *J Drugs Dermatol JDD.* 2017;16(6):s77-s80.

20. Alexis AF, Grimes P, Boyd C, et al. Racial and ethnic differences in self-assessed facial aging in women: Results from a multinational study. *Dermatol Surg.* 2019;45(12):1635-1648. doi:10.1097/DSS.0000000000002237.

21. Brissett AE, Naylor MC. The aging African-American face. *Facial Plast Surg.* 2010;26(02):154-163. doi:10.1055/s-0030-1253501.

22. Jothishankar B, Stein SL. Impact of skin color and ethnicity. *Clin Dermatol.* 2019;37(5):418-429. doi:10.1016/j.clindermatol.2019.07.009.

23. Kaidbey KH, Agin PP, Sayre RM, Kligman AM. Photoprotection by melanin—a comparison of black and Caucasian skin. *J Am Acad Dermatol.* 1979;1(3):249-260. doi:10.1016/S0190-9622(79)70018-1.

24. Alexis A, Boyd C, Callender V, Downie J, Sangha S. Understanding the female African American facial aesthetic patient. *J Drugs Dermatol.* 2019;18(9):858-866.

25. Fujimura T, Sugata K, Haketa K, Hotta M. Roughness analysis of the skin as a secondary evaluation criterion in addition to visual scoring is sufficient to evaluate ethnic differences in wrinkles. *Int J Cosmet Sci.* 2009;31(5):361-367. doi:10.1111/j.1468-2494.2009.00521.x.

26. McKnight A, Momoh AO, Bullocks JM. Variations of structural components: Specific intercultural differences in facial morphology, skin type, and structures. *Semin Plast Surg.* 2009;23(3):163-167. doi:10.1055/s-0029-1224794.

27. Harris MO. The aging face in patients of color: Minimally invasive surgical facial rejuvenation—a targeted approach. *Dermatol Ther.* 2004;17(2):206-211. Available at: https://doi.org/10.1111/j.1396-0296.2004.04021.x.

28. Farkas LG, Katic MJ, Forrest CR. International anthropometric study of facial morphology in various ethnic groups/races. *J Craniofac Surg.* 2005;16(4):615-646. doi:10.1097/01.scs.0000171847.58031.9e.

29. Momosawa A, Kurita M, Ozaki M, et al. Transconjunctival orbital fat repositioning for tear trough deformity in young Asians. *Aesthet Surg J.* 2008;28(3):265-271. doi:10.1016/j.asj.2008.02.002.

30. Shome D, Vadera S, Khare S, et al. Aging and the Indian face: An analytical study of aging in the Asian Indian face. *Plast Reconstr Surg Glob Open.* 2020;8(3):e2580. doi:10.1097/GOX.0000000000002580.

31. Cobo R, García CA. Aesthetic surgery for the Mestizo/Hispanic patient: Special considerations. *Facial Plast Surg.* 2010;26(2):164-173. doi:10.1055/s-0030-1253502.

32. Wu WTL, Liew S, Chan HH, et al. Consensus on current injectable treatment strategies in the Asian face. *Aesthetic Plast Surg.* 2016;40:202-214. doi:10.1007/s00266-016-0608-y.

33. Fabi S, Montes J, Aguilera S, Bucay V, Brown S, Ashourian N. Understanding the female Hispanic and Latino American facial aesthetic patient. *J Drugs Dermatol.* 2019;18(7):623-632.

34. Burgess C, Awosika O. Ethnic and gender considerations in the use of facial injectables: African-American patients. *Plast Reconstr Surg.* 2015;136(5S):28S. doi:10.1097/PRS.0000000000001813.

35. Grimes PE, Thomas JA, Murphy DK. Safety and effectiveness of hyaluronic acid fillers in skin of color. *J Cosmet Dermatol.* 2009;8(3):162-168. doi:10.1111/j.1473-2165.2009.00457.x.

36. Callender VD, Barbosa V, Burgess CM, et al. Approach to treatment of medical and cosmetic facial concerns in skin of color patients. *Cutis.* 2017;100(6):375-380.

37. Sundaram H, Liew S, Signorini M, et al. Global Aesthetics Consensus: Hyaluronic acid fillers and botulinum toxin type A-recommendations for combined treatment and optimizing outcomes in diverse patient populations. *Plast Reconstr Surg.* 2016;137(5):1410-1423. doi:10.1097/PRS.0000000000002119.

38. Alexis AF, Few J, Callender VD, et al. Myths and knowledge gaps in the aesthetic treatment of patients with skin of color. *J Drugs Dermatol.* 2019;18(7):616-622.

39. Taylor SC, Burgess CM, Callender VD. Safety of nonanimal stabilized hyaluronic acid dermal fillers in patients with skin of color: A randomized, evaluator-blinded comparative trial. *Dermatol Surg.* 2009;35:1653-1660. doi:10.1111/j.1524-4725.2009.01344.x.

2

Cultural Considerations in the Perception of Beauty

Melissa Laughter, Mayra B. C. Maymone, Omer Ibrahim, Neelam A. Vashi

SUMMARY AND KEY FEATURES

- Beauty perception is dynamic and involves individual subjective factors and personality traits as well as the sociocultural trends and influences.
- Asians tend to have a rounder face, when compared to White individuals, and delicate lower face in a "V" shape contour.
- Black/African-American faces may display increased facial convexity and broader nasal base with decreased nasal projection.
- White beauty typically includes round eyes, narrow faces, small noses, high cheekbones, and a thin figure.

- Larger eyes in Asians, lighter and more yellow skin tones in Black/African-American, and larger lips in Latinos has historically been deemed more attractive in these different ethnic groups.
- The perception of beauty is influenced by a person's environment and experiences. This concept is known as perceptual adaptation, which refers to the reshaping of ideals based on how we view our surroundings.
- Social media has amplified different forms of interaction and experiences that may impact perception of beauty.

INTRODUCTION

Beauty may be difficult to define, yet one knows when faced with a beautiful landscape or painting and even a beautiful face. The fascination with beauty dates back to ancient times. Plato described beauty as one of three gifts someone could wish for along with health and material wealth.[1] Although many centuries have passed, the influence of beauty remains undisputable. The theme of beauty influences many aspects of modern society, from the consistently perpetuated beautiful is good to ugly is evil seen in movies[2] to the effects of beauty on daily life. Studies have shown that beautiful people tend to marry equally beautiful partners,[3] influence the admission process in graduate education, are more frequently hired and promoted, and earn a higher income. Beauty may also have an influence in politics and legal sentencing, as studies have also shown that

unattractive people are more often found guilty and have longer sentences.[4–6]

Facial beauty is often associated with moral beauty and positive personality traits such as being sociable, sexually attractive, and trustworthy. This phenomenon is known as the "what is beautiful is good" effect.[7] As this controversial association between moral beauty and aesthetic beauty remains under debate, the focus on appearance and pursuit of physical beauty continues to grow. In 2019, Americans spent $8.2 billion on cosmetic procedures, and the beauty and cosmetic industry revenue was estimated to be approximately 49.2 billion United States (US) dollars in 2019.[8]

Although what is considered beautiful may vary, there appears to be universally accepted physical characteristics of beauty that span different cultures.[9] As the US population becomes more diverse, it is essential to recognize and understand the unique facial features and cultural influences of the perception of beauty in order to provide an individualized approach to cosmetic procedures between all races and ethnicities.

THE EYE OF THE BEHOLDER

Beauty perception is dynamic and involves individual subjective factors and personality traits as well as the sociocultural trends and influences.[10] The subjective component of beauty is influenced by the eye of the beholder and goes beyond scientific measurements and transcends cultural boundaries.[11] Whether the perception of beauty is innate or learned, there seems to be an agreement between beauty perception across cultures.[11,12] Studies evaluating facial attractiveness in different groups including South Africans and Scottish,[13] Americans, Brazilians, and Russians showed an overall agreement in attractiveness that was higher with familiar faces compared to unfamiliar.[14] First impressions are formed in approximately 100 milliseconds[15] and facial characteristics are the most common cue used to make this quick judgement. Research shows that having childlike facial features such as big eyes, a small chin and nose, race-related familiarity, and the objective components of beauty such as symmetry, averageness, and skin homogeneity, along with youthfulness and emotional resemblance, all impact perception of beauty.[16]

Interestingly, one study evaluating trustworthiness and attractiveness among Japanese and Israeli participants found similarities in the evaluation of attractiveness; however, more culturally typical faces were deemed more trustworthy.[17] One theory on the influence of culture in beauty perception is based on the "visual diet," which suggests that preferences are based on the faces that individuals are more commonly exposed to.

This can partially explain the variable perception of beauty and the facial features that are found to be attractive across different races and ethnicities.[18–20] Fig. 2.1 shows composite faces of different ethnicities.[21,22]

From the classic golden ratio to the modern anthropometric and photogrammetric measurements, many attempts have been made to soften the blurred lines between art and science. The golden ratio, also known as the Greek letter Phi, is a numerical value equal to approximately 1.618 and is frequently observed in nature, architectural structures, fashion, and even the human genome.[23] It is thought to represent perfect harmony and the perfect proportion.[24] Multiple studies have demonstrated that the Divine proportions may play a role in identifying the components of objective beauty that transcend different cultures and ethnicities.[24–27] However, one study comparing Miss Universe Thailand proportions with Neoclassic canons found that only oral and nasal width, nasal tip projection, and lower face proportions were similar to the golden ratio.[28] Moreover, anthropometric studies in African Americans,[29] Nigerians,[30] Saudi Arabians,[31] Southern Chinese,[32] and South Indians[33] did not conform to the neoclassical facial canons.

CULTURAL CONSIDERATIONS AND THE OBJECTIVE ASPECTS OF BEAUTY

Originally introduced by Sir Francis Galton, facial averageness refers to a mathematical mean and proposes that faces that are closer to the "norm" are easier and quicker to process compared to those that are far from this average.[34] Averageness is a major influencing factor in facial beauty and attractiveness and is thought to be associated with genetic heterozygosity, higher chance of successfully

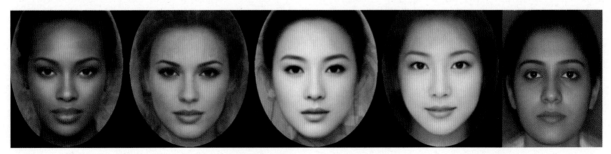

Fig. 2.1 Attractive composite faces of different ethnicities. *(From Rhee SC, Lee SH. Attractive composite faces of different races. Aesthetic Plast Surg. Published online 2010. doi:10.1007/s00266-010-9606-7.)*

passing genes to offspring, and overall health.[35] The preference for averageness appears to be a cross-cultural finding. One study evaluating attractiveness in Czechs, Czech Vietnamese, and Asian Vietnamese found a positive correlation between averageness and perceived attractiveness.[36] Another study used composite facial images of White and Japanese to show that both groups found the average composite more attractive.[9]

Symmetry is another universal component of facial attractiveness.[36] One study evaluated beauty ideals within cosmetic advertisements across 18 countries and found that symmetry was the top characteristic among models.[37] Fluctuating asymmetry is characterized by small variations in perfect symmetry due to genetics or stressors during development and is potentially associated with growth, good health, and survival.[38] A study assessing symmetry preferences among Hazda, a hunter population in Tanzania, and UK participants found that symmetry is attractive across both gender and cultures.[39]

Skin homogeneity refers to skin with even pigmentation and textures. Skin homogeneity has been commonly upheld as a desired human trait and an important component in perception of beauty.[34,40] Studies have corroborated this theory, showing that one's visible skin condition, coloration, skin surface, and texture all independently predict attractiveness.[40] Both texture and skin color homogeneity influence the positive perception of facial beauty. In one study, 10 females designated higher facial attractiveness in faces with foundation and more even

skin pigmentation.[40] Facial skin texture also plays an important role in the perception of the individual's health. One study conducted with Asian participants showed that homogenous skin texture positively predicted the apparent health of Malaysian and Chinese faces.

Having a youthful appearance is highly valued among society. A multicenter and ethnically diverse study found some variation on beauty perception and attractiveness within participants from China, Japan, France, South Africa, and India; however, a decline in attractiveness with aging was observed across all nationalities.[18] Another study evaluating perceived facial impressions among British and Chinese reported a cross-cultural agreement on youthfulness and attractiveness.[11]

Sexual dimorphism refers to sex-typical characteristics—men having masculine features and women feminine facial features; those traits are associated with increased perceived attractiveness.[41] A recent study using manipulated computer images of male and female faces found that sexual dimorphism and attractiveness were dissociable, and other variable clues possibly play a role in perceived attractiveness.[42] Interestingly, a large study including 28 countries reported an overall preference for feminine faces,[43] and another study further corroborated the findings that feminine features are preferred by males. However, no association between masculine faces and attractiveness was found across different populations.[44] A diagram illustrating the objective aspects of beauty can be found in Fig. 2.2.

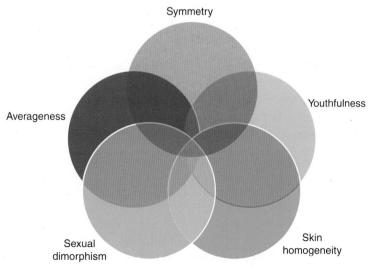

Fig. 2.2 Objective aspects of beauty diagram.

ASIAN BEAUTY

Unique Facial Features

Asians comprise over half of the world's population and represent a heterogenic group including East Asia, Southeast Asia, and Central Asia, each with facial characteristics that are unique to their respective ethnicity.[45] The facial shape is an important component of an attractive face. Asians tend to have a rounder face when compared to White individuals. Three dimensionally, Asians' maxilla, brow, nasal region, and chin are less projected, with more pronounced zygomatic arch and fuller lips.[45,46]

Cultural Influences

An oval face shape with a delicate lower face in a "V"-shape contour and larger eyes are considered attractive and are also a sign of good luck and happiness in certain countries. Understanding the facial features patients wish to be enhanced or minimized is key to harmonic aesthetic procedures. One nonvalidated recently published clinical assessment tool attempted to help individualize the different morphologic facial types that are considered desirable and beautiful among various Asian countries (Fig. 2.3).[47,48] Another study evaluating the ideals of facial beauty in Han Chinese population revealed a preference for an oval face with smooth jawlines.[49] The same study indicated that the desire for a defined chin is similar between both genders and most survey participants believed that being beautiful positively contributes to improved quality of life. Moreover, participants wanted to look beautiful but all while keeping with their ethnic features and not changing their appearance to be similar to White individuals.[47]

Although more than half of the Asian population has a small or absent supratarsal crease also known as "single eyelids," these groups perceive the presence of an upper eyelid crease as more attractive. Therefore, it is no surprise that blepharoplasty is one of the most common surgical cosmetic procedures in Asia.[50] Beyond facial features alone, having an unblemished and fair skin tone are perceived as beautiful among the Asian population.[37,51] Studies reported a high prevalence of skin-lightening products within these groups. The motivations behind this preference are to improve attractiveness, socioeconomic advantages, and marital prospects.[52]

The ideal body shape and size varies across cultures at any given time; however, the wait-to-hip ratio (WHR) is a universal measure of physical attractiveness. One study analyzing Miss Korea winners demonstrated a change overtime from a WHR of 0.645 in the 1970s to a ratio of 0.678 in the 2000s, indicating a move toward the universally accepted WHR of 0.7.[53] Studies on East Asians showed that women have a tendency to perceive themselves as being overweight despite normal or low BMI and are more influenced by thin social body ideals compared to men.[54]

BLACK BEAUTY

Unique Facial Features

Black/African-Americans represent decedents from multiple ethnicities. It is therefore extremely challenging to make generalizations concerning unique facial features within this group.[55] However, studies show that there are some key facial features more heavily represented within the Black/African-American population. Black/African-American faces may display increased facial convexity, broader nasal base with decreased nasal projection, bimaxillary protrusion, and orbital proptosis.[56,57] However, due to the aforementioned high level of interethnic variability, some features within Black/African-American groups can be very different, such as a high or low dorsum of the nasal structure.[58]

Cultural Influences

Studies have shown stark differences between what Black/African-American women perceive as beautiful versus what White women perceive as beautiful. The earliest studies suggest that Black/African-American women define attractiveness based on a myriad of factors that extend beyond having the "ideal body" or certain facial features.[59] Much of what comprises Black/African-American women's perception of beauty stems from their general presentation, including their dress attire and overall appearance.[60] There are mixed findings in terms of the effects of body weight on body image and perception of beauty. Some studies have shown that Black/African-American women are more focused on public image as well as having hips and femininity.[60] Within certain populations of Black/African-American women, being overweight or obese is not associated with body dissatisfaction.[61] However, another study showed that African populations from South Africa perceive thinner women with lower facial adiposity as

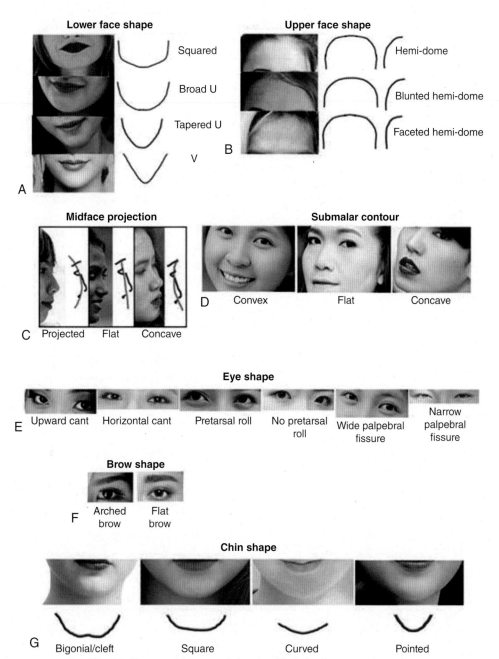

Fig. 2.3 Shape and features of the simplified visual assessment tool.

more attractive compared to their heavier peers. Within this study, over 20% of the images perceived as more attractive depicted underweight women, an interesting finding considering that within certain African countries low body weight is often associated with illness and disease.[62] Pale skin color is considered to be more attractive in many cultures, including within Black/African-American groups. More specifically, skin tones that have more yellow undertones have been shown to increase men's facial attractiveness within African populations.[63] Studies have shown that certain cultures perceive both lighter skin and more yellow skin as an indication of increased femininity and health.[64] This is dissimilar to the focus on tanned skin and darker skin tone within European and American societies.[65] Another, more comprehensive study showed that youthfulness, lighter and more yellow skin tones, and skin smoothness or homogeneity were all independent predictors of facial attractiveness in female African faces.[62]

WHITE BEAUTY

Unique Facial Features

White faces typically display a narrower nasal bridge paired with longer projection of the nasal tip when compared to Black/African-American, Latino, or Asian faces.[66] However, studies have shown that White faces have intercanthal widths identical to those of African descent and smaller when compared to Asian faces.[57] White individuals also generally have decreased lip volume when compared to other groups.[57]

Cultural Influences

There are significant variations across cultures as to what dictates feminine beauty and the "ideal" body image. In the time of globalization, Western European and American beauty ideals are becoming increasingly significant as cultures meld and share similar influences. In particular, fashion, media, and film within the United States represent a significant contribution to global culture and the construct of beauty ideals.[67] These Western ideals have integrated into many different countries even though women from these countries may look nothing like White women.[68] One study demonstrated that fashion magazines in Asia and Latin America preferred Western ideals of beauty and featured White models much more than models from their own respective

country. This exchange of beauty ideals did not ring true for Western countries, as the United Kingdom and the United States still mostly feature White models that fit their own standard of beauty.[69]

Western beauty ideals have typically included round eyes, narrow faces, small noses, high cheekbones, thin figure, small lips, and white skin amongst other characteristics.[70–73] Among these characteristics is the influence of body image and size on perception of beauty and Western beauty ideals. Our previous study showed that highly influential models that currently represent the popular brand, Victoria's Secret, have significantly smaller waist size, hip size, and bust size compared to Victoria's Secret models 20 years ago. The sizes of these models is dramatically smaller than the size of the average American woman.[74] Although the American beauty industry typically features lighter complexions, certain studies have shown that modern White women prefer more tanned skin, which may contribute to the increase in indoor tanning use.[60,65] The relationship between race and ideals of beauty are complex with limited studies being conducted on the topic. One study did show that Europeans have also been shown to prefer mixed-ethnicity face shapes compared to single-ethnicity face shapes as well as Black/African-American models compared to White models.[35,60] Of note, the use of cosmetics appear to play an important role in White beauty ideals. One study showed that White faces with full makeup were deemed more attractive than the same faces without makeup.[75] Other factors that have been shown to contribute to beauty ideals within Western society include bias against advancing age. Media has contributed to this perception that older women are less feminine or less employable.[67]

LATIN BEAUTY

Unique Facial Features

Beauty ideals have not been extensively studied within Latin populations. There also exist wide variations in terms of descent within the Hispanic ethnic group, as some people may be of African descent while others are from Central or South American descent. Common features within Hispanic populations regardless of descent include thick nasal skin, bimaxillary protrusion, prominent malar eminences, and noses with a broad base and wider tip.[76]

Cultural Influences

Importantly, studies have shown that Latin Americans distinguish attractiveness by decreased nasal prominence, less protrusive lips, and less bimaxillary protrusion.[77,78] These stark differences in beauty ideals and common characteristics of the Hispanic population are important considerations and have likely led to rhinoplasty being the most common plastic surgery request within this population.[79] One study comparing 3D-digitized images of contestants from the Miss Paraguay beauty pageant showed that Paraguayans favor rectangular faces, wide mouths, and lips. The proportion index of contestants also varied significant from the "golden ratio."[80] When considering lip measurements, laypersons in Latin America favored the largest lips when compared to Asian or European preferences. In addition, Latin American surgeons preferred larger lips.[72] In certain parts of Latin America, lighter skin is considered more aligned with beauty ideals and, importantly, women with darker complexions living in Brazil report higher likelihood of discrimination within society and the workplace.[81] In another study, researchers show that both American Hispanics and Chileans had a strong preference toward lighter complexions compared to darker complexions. Even more, participants in this study also showed a preference for White individuals over Hispanics with similar skin tones, lending to the influence of western beauty ideas within Latin America.[82] Among the Latin population, the ideal body is slightly larger than the White beauty ideal, with preference towards a bigger bust, smaller waist, and broader hips.[83] In Brazil, plastic surgery procedures have steadily increased along with the average size of implants for breast augmentation.[84]

MALLEABILITY OF BEAUTY AND COSMETIC TREATMENT

Previous studies have suggested that the perception of facial beauty is derived from objective measures such as symmetry, facial proportions, and various enhancement of certain features.[41,85] However, it is now thought that perception of beauty is malleable and subject to change. The perception of beauty and what we perceive to be beautiful is likely also influenced by a person's environment and experiences. This concept, also known of perceptual adaptation, refers to the reshaping of ideals based on how we view our surroundings.[86] It has even

been shown that small experiences and exposures to certain images can shift the perception of beauty toward that distortion.[87] The theory behind this observation is that people tend to prefer familiarity and thus shape what they perceive as beautiful by what they perceive as familiar. Perception of beauty can be thought of as an "average" image shaped by each person's individual experiences and environment to which they are exposed.

With the advent of social media, images are shared much more easily, and the consumption of these images continues to increase, influencing each person's perception of beauty. Social media also puts forth "ideal" images that have been filtered or photo-edited into sometimes unachievable outcomes. Unfortunately, this unrealistic beauty standard has led to the increase in cosmetic procedures and beauty products in an attempt to move closer to this frequently unattainable look. In fact, billions of dollars are spent annually on diet products, makeup, and hair and nail care, while millions of dollars are spent annually on cosmetic surgical procedures.[88] There are many motivations surrounding this increase in cosmetic surgery including fear of discrimination, coercion by others, shame, social anxiety, and career or societal development. All this said, the end goals of the patients are most likely going to focus on achieving their own perception or ideal of beauty that was shaped by their individual experiences and observations.[89]

BEAUTY INFLUENCE AND SOCIAL MEDIA

The use of social media has increased significantly over the past decade, with social media platforms infiltrating many aspects of our lives. This widespread use of social media has amplified different forms of interaction and experiences that may all impact perception of beauty. Our society can consume thousands of images through various social media platforms each day and each image that we view will be registered to shape what our society now perceives as beautiful. Users also look to social media to identify ideals or treads within ideals of beauty.[90] Taking selfies and sharing them with others on social media platforms has significantly increased in the recent years. In fact, studies have shown that people prefer the mirror image of themselves or their "selfie" compared to their true image, demonstrating the power of social media on perception.[91] Another study demonstrated that men and women prefer the most attractive modified image of themselves when compared to their actual appearance.[92]

Social media has had a significant impact on behavioral aspects of body image through the focus on specific body types as being more beautiful. Many social media platforms have a large portion of their posts dedicated specifically to fitness, body image, and body inspiration ("thinspiration").[93] Importantly, many images presented within social media are filtered, altered, or present an unattainable beauty ideal or body image. Many popular socialites and influencers have been criticized for posting heavily photoshopped and edited images that make themselves appear thinner or more toned, further propagating unrealistic beauty standards. For this reason, there are many concerns with body dissatisfaction and body image as social media use continues to rise. One study showed that girls consider the images shown in social media to be unrealistic and believe that society will evaluate them based on these images.[94] Another study demonstrated that increased exposure to idealized images and time spent on Facebook was linked to increased feelings of self-objectification, weight dissatisfaction, and body image dissatisfaction.[95]

CONCLUSION

Beauty is a combination of many characteristics; however, what one finds beautiful may be influenced by individual perception and cultural background. As the world population becomes more diverse, the traditional beauty stereotypes among the different races and ethnicities will tend to be less marked and a more individualized approach to cosmetic surgery and procedure will be essential in order to enhance each individual unique beauty.

REFERENCES

1. Alam M, Dover JS. On beauty: Evolution, psychosocial considerations, and surgical enhancement. *Arch Dermatol.* 2001;137(6):795-807.
2. Croley JA, Reese V, Wagner RF. Dermatologic features of classic movie villains: The face of evil. *JAMA Dermatol.* 2017;153(6)559-564. doi:10.1001/jamadermatol.2016.5979.
3. Elder GH. Appearance and education in marriage mobility. *Am Sociol Rev.* 1969;34(4):519-533. doi:10.2307/2091961.
4. Maxfield CM, Thorpe MP, Desser TS, et al. Bias in radiology resident selection: Do we discriminate against the obese and unattractive? *Acad Med.* 2019;94(11):1774-1780. doi:10.1097/ACM.0000000000002813.
5. Nahai F. The power of beauty. *Aesthetic Surg J.* 2018;38(9):1039-1041. doi:10.1093/asj/sjy038.
6. Karraker A, Sicinski K, Moynihan D. Your face is your fortune: Does adolescent attractiveness predict intimate relationships later in life? *J Gerontol B Psychol Sci Soc Sci.* 2017;72(1):187-199. doi:10.1093/geronb/gbv112.
7. Dion K, Berscheid E, Walster E. What is beautiful is good. *J Pers Soc Psychol.* 1972;24(3):285-290. doi:10.1037/h0033731.
8. Statista. Cosmetics industry worldwide. Statista. 2019.
9. Perrett DI, May KA, Yoshikawa S. Facial shape and judgements of female attractiveness. *Nature.* 1994;368(6468):239-242. doi:10.1038/368239a0.
10. Sutherland CAM, Rhodes G, Burton NS, Young AW. Do facial first impressions reflect a shared social reality? *Br J Psychol.* 2020;111(2):215-232. doi:10.1111/bjop.12390.
11. Sutherland CAM, Liu X, Zhang L, Chu Y, Oldmeadow JA, Young AW. Facial first impressions across culture: Data-driven modeling of Chinese and British perceivers' unconstrained facial impressions. *Pers Soc Psychol Bull.* 2018;44(4):521-537. doi:10.1177/0146167217744194.
12. Langlois JH, Kalakanis L, Rubenstein AJ, Larson A, Hallam M, Smoot M. Maxims or myths of beauty? A meta-analytic and theoretical review. *Psychol Bull.* 2000;126(3):390-423. doi:10.1037/0033-2909.126.3.390.
13. Coetzee V, Greeff JM, Stephen ID, Perrett DI. Cross-cultural agreement in facial attractiveness preferences: The role of ethnicity and gender. *PLoS One.* 2014;9(7):e99629. doi:10.1371/journal.pone.0099629.
14. Jones D, Hill K. Criteria of facial attractiveness in five populations. *Hum Nat.* 1993;4(3):271-296. doi:10.1007/BF02692202.
15. Willis J, Todorov A. First impressions: Making up your mind after a 100-ms exposure to a face. *Psychol Sci.* 2006;17(7):592-598. doi:10.1111/j.1467-9280.2006.01750.x.
16. Zebrowitz LA. First impressions from faces. *Curr Dir Psychol Sci.* 2017;26(3):237-242. doi:10.1177/0963721416683996.
17. Sofer C, Dotsch R, Oikawa M, Oikawa H, Wigboldus DHJ, Todorov A. For your local eyes only: Culture-specific face typicality influences perceptions of trustworthiness. *Perception.* 2017;46(8):914-928. doi:10.1177/0301006617691786.
18. Voegeli R, Schoop R, Prestat-Marquis E, Rawlings AV, Shackelford TK, Fink B. Cross-cultural perception of female facial appearance: A multi-ethnic and multi-centre study. *PLoS One.* 2021;16(1):e0245998. doi:10.1371/journal.pone.0245998.

19. Packiriswamy V, Kumar P, Bashour M. Photogrammetric analysis of eyebrow and upper eyelid dimensions in South Indians and Malaysian South Indians. *Aesthetic Surg J*. 2013;33(7):975-982. doi:10.1177/1090820X13503472.

20. Zhang L, Holzleitner IJ, Lee AJ, et al. A data-driven test for cross-cultural differences in face preferences. *Perception*. 2019;48(6):487-499. doi:10.1177/0301006619849382.

21. Rhee SC, Lee SH. Attractive composite faces of different races. *Aesthetic Plast Surg*. 2010;34(6):800-801. doi:10.1007/s00266-010-9606-7.

22. Duggal S, Kapoor DN, Verma S, et al. Photogrammetric analysis of attractiveness in Indian faces. *Arch Plast Surg*. 2016;43(2):160-171. doi:10.5999/aps.2016.43.2.160.

23. Perez JC. Codon populations in single-stranded whole human genome DNA are fractal and fine-tuned by the Golden Ratio 1.618. *Interdiscip Sci*. 2010;2(3):228-240. doi:10.1007/s12539-010-0022-0.

24. Hwang K, Park CY. The divine proportion: Origins and usage in plastic surgery. *Plast Reconstr Surg Glob Open*. 2021;22(9):e3419. doi:10.1097/GOX.0000000000003419.

25. Khan NA, Nagar A, Tandon P, Singh GK, Singh A. Evaluation of facial divine proportion in North Indian Population. *Contemp Clin Dent*. 2016;7(3):366-370. doi:10.4103/0976-237X.188566.

26. Pancherz H, Knapp V, Erbe C, Heiss AM. Divine proportions in attractive and nonattractive faces. *World J Orthod*. 2010;11(1):27-36.

27. Kaptein YE, Kaptein JS, Markarian A. Vertical localization of the malar prominence. *Plast Reconstr Surg Glob Open*. 2015;3(6):e411. doi:10.1097/GOX.0000000000000383.

28. Burusapat C, Lekdaeng P. What is the most beautiful facial proportion in the 21st century? Comparative study among Miss Universe, Miss Universe Thailand, neoclassical canons, and facial golden ratios. *Plast Reconstr Surg Glob Open*. 2019;7(2):e2044. doi:10.1097/GOX.0000000000002044.

29. Farkas LG, Forrest CR, Litsas L. Revision of neoclassical facial canons in young adult Afro-Americans. *Aesthetic Plast Surg*. 2000;24(3):179-184. doi:10.1007/s002660010029.

30. Olusanya AA, Aladelusi TO, Adedokun B. Anthropometric analysis of the Nigerian face: Any conformity to the neoclassical canons? *J Craniofac Surg*. 2018;29(7):1978-1982. doi:10.1097/SCS.0000000000004831.

31. Al-Sebaei MO. The validity of three neo-classical facial canons in young adults originating from the Arabian Peninsula. *Head Face Med*. 2015;11:4. doi:10.1186/s13005-015-0064-y.

32. Jayaratne YSN, Deutsch CK, McGrath CPJ, Zwahlen RA. Are neoclassical canons valid for southern Chinese faces? *PLoS One*. 2012;7(12):e52593. doi:10.1371/journal.pone.0052593.

33. Veerala G, Gandikota CS, Yadagiri PK, et al. Marquardt's facial golden decagon mask and its fitness with South Indian facial traits. *J Clin Diagnostic Res*. 2016;10(4):ZC49-ZC52. doi:10.7860/JCDR/2016/16791.7593.

34. Vashi NA. Objective aspects of beauty. In: Vashi NA, ed. *Beauty and body Dysmorphic Disorder: A Clinician's Guide*. Springer International Publishing/Springer Nature; 2015:17-43.

35. Little AC, Hockings KJ, Apicella CL, Sousa C. Mixed-ethnicity face shape and attractiveness in humans. *Perception*. 2012;41(12):1486-1496. doi:10.1068/p7278.

36. Rhodes G, Yoshikawa S, Clark A, Kieran L, McKay R, Akamatsu S. Attractiveness of facial averageness and symmetry in non-western cultures: In search of biologically based standards of beauty. *Perception*. 2001;30(5):611-625. doi:10.1068/p3123.

37. Spyropoulou GAC, Pavlidis L, Herrmann S, et al. Can cosmetics' advertisements be an indicator of different perceptions of beauty amongst countries? *Aesthetic Plast Surg*. 2020;44(5):1871-1878. doi:10.1007/s00266-020-01679-1.

38. Kočnar T, Adil Saribay S, Kleisner K. Perceived attractiveness of Czech faces across 10 cultures: Associations with sexual shape dimorphism, averageness, fluctuating asymmetry, and eye color. *PLoS One*. 2019;14(11):e0225549. doi:10.1371/journal.pone.0225549.

39. Little AC, Apicella CL, Marlowe FW. Preferences for symmetry in human faces in two cultures: Data from the UK and the Hadza, an isolated group of hunter-gatherers. *Proc Biol Sci*. 2007;274(1629):3113-3117. doi:10.1098/rspb.2007.0895.

40. Samson N, Fink B, Matts PJ. Visible skin condition and perception of human facial appearance. *Int J Cosmet Sci*. 2010;32(3):167-184. doi:10.1111/j.1468-2494.2009.00535.x.

41. Perrett DI, Lee KJ, Penton-Voak I, et al. Effects of sexual dimorphism on facial attractiveness. *Nature*. 1998;394(6696):884-887. doi:10.1038/29772.

42. Nakamura K, Watanabe K. A new data-driven mathematical model dissociates attractiveness from sexual dimorphism of human faces. *Sci Rep*. 2020;10(1):16588. doi:10.1038/s41598-020-73472-8.

43. Marcinkowska UM, Kozlov MV, Cai H, et al. Cross-cultural variation in men's preference for sexual dimorphism in women's faces. *Biol Lett*. 2014;10(4):20130850. doi:10.1098/rsbl.2013.0850.

44. Kleisner K, Tureček P, Roberts SC, et al. How and why patterns of sexual dimorphism in human faces vary across the world. *Sci Rep*. 2021;11:5978. doi:10.1038/s41598-021-85402-3.

45. Liew S, Wu WTL, Chan HH, et al. Consensus on changing trends, attitudes, and concepts of Asian beauty. *Aesthetic Plast Surg*. 2016;40(2):193-201. doi:10.1007/s00266-015-0562-0.

46. Venkatesh S, Maymone MBC, Vashi NA. Aging in skin of color. *Clin Dermatol*. 2019;37(4):351-357. doi:10.1016/j.clindermatol.2019.04.010.

47. Samizadeh S. The ideals of facial beauty among Chinese aesthetic practitioners: Results from a large national survey. *Aesthetic Plast Surg*. 2019;43(1):102-114. doi:10.1007/s00266-018-1241-8.

48. Corduff N, Chao YYY, Lam SCK, et al. A new simplified visual assessment tool describing facial morphotypes observed and desired in Asian populations. *J Clin Aesthet Dermatol*. 2020;13(4):23-34.

49. Samizadeh S, Wu W. Ideals of facial beauty amongst the Chinese population: Results from a large national survey. *Aesthetic Plast Surg*. 2018;42(6):1540-1550. doi:10.1007/s00266-018-1188-9.

50. Hwang HS, Spiegel JH. The effect of "single" vs "double" eyelids on the perceived attractiveness of Chinese women. *Aesthetic Surg J*. 2014;34(3):374-382. doi:10.1177/1090820X14523020.

51. Swami V, Henry A, Peacock N, Roberts-Dunn A, Porter A. Mirror, Mirror. A preliminary investigation of skin tone dissatisfaction and its impact among British adults. *Cultur Divers Ethnic Minor Psychol*. 2013;19(4):468-476. doi:10.1037/a0032904.

52. Shroff H, Diedrichs PC, Craddock N. Skin color, cultural capital, and beauty products: An investigation of the use of skin fairness products in Mumbai, India. *Front Public Health*. 2018;5:365. doi:10.3389/fpubh.2017.00365.

53. Hong YJ, Park HS, Lee ES, Suh YJ. Anthropometric analysis of waist-to-hip ratio in Asian women. *Aesthetic Plast Surg*. 2009;33(2):185-190. doi:10.1007/s00266-008-9200-4.

54. Noh JW, Kwon YD, Yang Y, Cheon J, Kim J. Relationship between body image and weight status in east Asian countries: Comparison between South Korea and Taiwan. *BMC Public Health*. 2018;18(1):814. doi:10.1186/s12889-018-5738-5.

55. Brissett AE, Naylor MC. The aging African-American face. *Facial Plast Surg*. 2010;26(2):154-163. doi:10.1055/s-0030-1253501.

56. Talakoub L, Wesley NO. Differences in perceptions of beauty and cosmetic procedures performed in ethnic patients. *Semin Cutan Med Surg*. 2009;28(2):115-129. doi:10.1016/j.sder.2009.05.001.

57. Vashi NA, De Castro Maymone MB, Kundu RV. Aging differences in ethnic skin. *J Clin Aesthet Dermatol*. 2016;9(1):31-38.

58. Porter JP, Olson KL. Anthropometric facial analysis of the African American woman. *Arch Facial Plast Surg*. 2001;3(3):191-197. doi:10.1001/archfaci.3.3.191.

59. Cash TF, Duncan NC. Physical attractiveness stereotyping among Black American college students. *J Soc Psychol*. 1984;122(1):71-77. doi:10.1080/00224545.1984.9713459.

60. Davis DS, Sbrocco T, Odoms-Young A, Smith DM. Attractiveness in African American and Caucasian women: Is beauty in the eyes of the observer? *Eat Behav*. 2010;11(1):25-32. doi:10.1016/j.eatbeh.2009.08.004.

61. Befort CA, Thomas JL, Daley CM, Rhode PC, Ahluwalia JS. Perceptions and beliefs about body size, weight, and weight loss among obese African American women: A qualitative inquiry. *Health Educ Behav*. 2008;35(3):410-426. doi:10.1177/1090198106290398.

62. Coetzee V, Faerber SJ, Greeff JM, Lefevre CE, Re DE, Perrett DI. African perceptions of female attractiveness. *PLoS One*. 2012;7(10):e48116. doi:10.1371/journal.pone.0048116.

63. Stephen ID, Scott IML, Coetzee V, Pound N, Perrett DI, Penton-Voak IS. Cross-cultural effects of color, but not morphological masculinity, on perceived attractiveness of men's faces. *Evol Hum Behav*. 2012;33(4):260-267. doi:10.1016/j.evolhumbehav.2011.10.003.

64. Stephen ID, Coetzee V, Perrett DI. Carotenoid and melanin pigment coloration affect perceived human health. *Evol Hum Behav*. 2011;32(3):216-227. doi:10.1016/j.evolhumbehav.2010.09.003.

65. Trekels J, Eggermont S, Koppen E, Vandenbosch L. Beauty ideals from reality television and young women's tanning behavior: An internalization and self-objectification perspective. *Commun Q*. 2018;66:325-343. doi:10.1080/01463373.2017.1381627.

66. Farkas LG, Katic MJ, Forrest CR, et al. International anthropometric study of facial morphology in various ethnic groups/races. *J Craniofac Surg*. 2005;16(4):615-646. doi:10.1097/01.scs.0000171847.58031.9e.

67. Rowe-Jones JM. Facial aesthetic surgical goals in patients of different cultures. *Facial Plast Surg Clin North Am*. 2014;22(3):343-348. doi:10.1016/j.fsc.2014.04.003.

68. de Zoysa DA, Appadurai A. Modernity at large: Cultural dimensions of globalization. *Int Migr Rev*. 1998;32(4):1073. doi:10.2307/2547675.

69. Yan Y, Bissell K. The globalization of beauty: How is ideal beauty influenced by globally published fashion and beauty magazines? *J Intercult Commun Res*. 2014;43(3):194-214. doi:10.1080/17475759.2014.917432.

70. Carneiro R, Zeytinoglu S, Hort F, Wilkins E. Culture, beauty, and therapeutic alliance. *J Fem Fam Ther*. 2013;25(2):80-92. doi:10.1080/08952833.2013.777873.

71. Bryant SL. The beauty ideal: The effects of European standards on black women. *Columbia Soc Work Rev.* 2013;11(1):80-91.

72. Heidekrueger PI, Szpalski C, Weichman K, et al. Lip attractiveness: A cross-cultural analysis. *Aesthetic Surg J.* 2017;37(7):828-836. doi:10.1093/asj/sjw168.

73. Erbay EF, Caniklio«ßlu CM. Soft tissue profile in Anatolian Turkish adults: Part II. Comparison of different soft tissue analyses in the evaluation of beauty. *Am J Orthod Dentofacial Orthop.* 2002;121(1):65-72. doi:10.1067/mod.2002.119573.

74. Maymone MBC, Laughter M, Anderson JB, Secemsky EA, Vashi NA. Unattainable standards of beauty: Temporal trends of Victoria's secret models from 1995 to 2018. *Aesthetic Surg J.* 2020;40(2):NP72-NP76. doi:10.1093/asj/sjz271.

75. Mulhern R, Fieldman G, Hussey T, Lévêque JL, Pineau P. Do cosmetics enhance female Caucasian facial attractiveness? *Int J Cosmet Sci.* 2003;25(4):199-205. doi:10.1046/j.1467-2494.2003.00188.x.

76. Daniel RK. Hispanic rhinoplasty in the United States, with emphasis on the Mexican American nose. *Plast Reconstr Surg.* 2003;112(1):244-256. doi:10.1097/01.PRS.0000066363.37479.EE.

77. Mejia-Maidl M, Evans CA, Viana G, Anderson NK, Giddon DB. Preferences for facial profiles between Mexican Americans and Caucasians. *Angle Orthod.* 2005;75(6):953-958. doi:10.1043/0003-3219(2005)75[953:PFFPBM]2.0.CO;2.

78. Scavone H, Zahn-Silva W, Do Valle-Corotti KM, Nahás ACR. Soft tissue profile in white Brazilian adults with normal occlusions and well-balanced faces. *Angle Orthod.* 2008;78(1):58-63. doi:10.2319/103006-447.1.

79. Cosmetic Surgery National Data Bank Statistics. *Aesthetic Surg J.* 2018;38(suppl_3):1-24. doi:10.1093/asj/sjy132.

80. Bayome M, Park JH, Shoaib AM, Lee N ki, Boettner V, Kook YA. Comparison of facial esthetic standards between Latin American and Asian populations using 3D stereophotogrammetric analysis. *J World Fed Orthod.* 2020;9(3):129-136. doi:10.1016/j.ejwf.2020.06.003.

81. Fattore GL, Amorim LD, Marques dos Santos L, dos Santos DN, Barreto ML. Experiences of discrimination and skin color among women in urban Brazil: A latent class analysis. *J Black Psychol.* 2020;46(2-3). doi:10.1177/0095798420928204.

82. Uhlmann E, Dasgupta N, Elguela A, Greenwald AG, Swanson J. Subgroup prejudice based on skin color among Hispanics in the United States and Latin America.

Soc Cogn. 2002;20(3):198-225. doi:10.1521/soco.20.3.198.21104.

83. Pompper D, Koenig J. Cross-cultural-generational perceptions of ideal body image: Hispanic women and magazine standards. *Journal Mass Commun Q.* 2004;81(1):89-107. doi:10.1177/107769900408100107.

84. Finger C. Brazilian beauty. *Lancet.* 2003;362(9395):1560. doi:10.1016/s0140-6736(03)14789-7.

85. Penton-Voak IS, Jones BC, Little AC, et al. Symmetry, sexual dimorphism in facial proportions and male facial attractiveness. *Proc R Soc B Biol Sci.* 2001;268(1476):1617-1623. doi:10.1098/rspb.2001.1703.

86. Rhodes G, Jeffery L, Watson TL, Clifford CWG, Nakayama K. Fitting the mind to the world: Face adaptation and attractiveness aftereffects. *Psychol Sci.* 2003;14(6):558-566. doi:10.1046/j.0956-7976.2003.psci_1465.x.

87. Cooper PA, Maurer D. The influence of recent experience on perceptions of attractiveness. *Perception.* 2008;37(8):1216-1226. doi:10.1068/p5865.

88. Jacobson N, Sullivan DA. Cosmetic surgery: The cutting edge of commercial medicine in America. *Contemp Sociol.* 2001;30(6):642. doi:10.2307/3089042.

89. Grossbart TA, Sarwer DB. Cosmetic surgery: Surgical tools - psychosocial goals. *Semin Cutan Med Surg.* 1999;18(2):101-111. doi:10.1016/S1085-5629(99)80034-0.

90. Henriques M, Patnaik D. Social media and its effects on beauty. 2020. doi:10.5772/intechopen.93322.

91. Mita TH, Dermer M, Knight J. Reversed facial images and the mere-exposure hypothesis. *J Pers Soc Psychol.* 1977;35(8):597-601. doi:10.1037/0022-3514.35.8.597.

92. Wen W, Kawabata H. Why am I not photogenic? Differences in face memory for the self and others. *Iperception.* 2014;5(3):176-187. doi:10.1068/i0634.

93. Lewallen J, Behm-Morawitz E. Pinterest or thinterest?: Social comparison and body image on social media. *Soc Media + Soc.* 2016;2(1). https://doi.org/10.1177/2056305116640559.

94. Milkie MA. Social comparisons, reflected appraisals, and mass media: The impact of pervasive beauty images on Black and White girls' self-concepts. *Soc Psychol Q.* 1999;62(2):190-210. doi:10.2307/2695857.

95. Meier EP, Gray J. Facebook photo activity associated with body image disturbance in adolescent girls. *Cyberpsychol Behav Soc Netw.* 2014;17(4):199-206. doi:10.1089/cyber.2013.0305.

3

Cosmetic Concerns and Special Considerations for Specific Populations: Populations of African Ancestry

Sara Hogan, Camille Robinson, Valerie D. Callender

SUMMARY AND KEY FEATURES

- There has been an increase in patients of African descent seeking cosmetic procedures, yet there are few studies and clinical trials discussing the aesthetic preferences and relevant treatment considerations for this patient population.
- Understanding the differences in cosmetic concerns and treatment approach when treating patients of African descent is vital to providing inclusive care.

- Patients of African descent commonly present with concerns regarding dyspigmentation, skin texture, hypertrophic scars/keloids, and skin aging. Knowing how to treat these concerns of patients of this patient population appropriately can minimize potential adverse effects.

INTRODUCTION

Populations of African descent include individuals with a mixture of African, White, and Indigenous American ancestries, Afro-Caribbeans, and individuals with only African ancestry, reflecting the diversity and complexity of the African diaspora and the kinetics of immigration. These populations encompass a myriad of lineages, multiple ethnicities, multicultural, and varying skin tones, also including an emergent group of individuals who are multiracial and multiethnic. Still, populations of African descent share commonalities with regard to skin biology, aging stigmata, and some anatomical features. Cultural themes also exist among this population regarding perceptions of beauty, skin and hair care practices, and openness to aesthetic treatments.[1,2]

The past two decades saw a marked increase in the number of individuals of African descent seeking cosmetic treatments. This is primarily due to the rise of minimally invasive cosmetic procedures that, with increased safety profiles and decreased downtime, allow for increased accessibility by and application among patients with deeper skin tones. The ever-expanding role of social media is also a likely contributor to this shift—increasing awareness of and destigmatizing aesthetic procedures among the general public. In 2018, Black/African-Americans received 1.6 million, or nine percent, of all cosmetic procedures performed in the United States.[3] This is a one-percent increase from 2017 and will likely continue to trend upward.

This growth in readiness and demand for aesthetic procedures, however, is met with a paucity of clinical data. The vast majority of cosmetic injectable and device clinical research trials, and cosmetic procedural literature, focuses on populations with lighter skin types. Little is published on the aging processes, aesthetic preferences, and treatment modifications for this patient population. Moreover, many physicians who perform cosmetic procedures are not confident in treating individuals of African descent given concerns for potential complications, such as postinflammatory hyperpigmentation and keloid formation. This chapter reviews the existing research on cosmetic considerations for populations of African descent, with the goal of providing a framework for tailoring treatment approaches and optimizing patient outcomes.

ANATOMICAL AND PHYSIOLOGICAL CONSIDERATIONS

Skin aging consists of two distinct processes that are driven by shared and unique molecular mechanisms. Photoaging is characterized by dyspigmentation, deep rhytids, and telangiectasias, while intrinsic aging is marked by xerosis, fine rhytids, and laxity. Photoaging is experienced by all populations and skin types, but to a lesser extent by patients of African descent. Darkly pigmented skin contains a greater number of melanosomes that are also larger, contain higher melanin content, are more broadly dispersed, and are slower to degrade than melanosomes in lighter skin. This results in a photoprotective effect among individuals of African descent.[1,4] Skin fibroblasts in studies of Black female facial skin are noted to be larger, bi- or multinucleated, and greater in number compared to fibroblasts in White female facial skin.[5] Additionally the fascial system enveloping soft tissue is thicker and heavier in individuals of African descent.[6] This translates into greater structural integrity of skin and, in the context of aging, the maintenance of youthful-appearing skin for a longer period of time than other populations similarly exposed to the sun.[7]

Facial aging among individuals of African descent is driven by reduced facial skeletal support, repositioning of the superficial musculoaponeurotic system, and gravity-induced displacement of fatty and muscular tissues.[4,6] These changes are focused in the midface. Upper and lower eyelid laxity is less likely to occur among this patient population, but if it does, is often more dramatic due to increased thickness of skin.[6–8] The upper eyelid crease in those of African descent is, on average, 6 to 8 mm from the lid margin compared to 8 to 10 mm in White individuals, causing soft tissue fullness with or without the presence of brow ptosis.[8] Pseudoherniation of the medial infraorbital fat pads is often observed and results in ocular proptosis with infraorbital shadowing.[9,10] Hypoplasia of the malar eminence combined with increased redundancy of soft tissue and descent of the malar fat pad results in formation of nasojugal and nasolabial folds and a so-called "double convexity" of the midface.[6] Given that this population has a decreased propensity to photodamage and lost lip volume, they are less likely to form perioral rhytids. Jowling, when it does occur, is more likely secondary to the thickness and heaviness of skin, rather than skin laxity.[6] The cervicomental angle, ideally between 90 and 120 degrees, is blunted with aging among populations of African descent. This, combined with bulky displacement of submental fat and retrogenia, results in the appearance of a "double chin."[6,9–10]

PATIENT EVALUATION

A detailed interview should be performed during the initial cosmetic consultation to elicit the chief concerns of the patient. Past medical and surgical history, current medications and supplements, and allergies should be reviewed. It is important to identify those patients having conditions with increased risk of koebnerization (i.e., lichen planus, vitiligo, or psoriasis) as this may affect treatment selection. Individual skin care routine practices should also be discussed as this can influence treatment outcomes. Evaluation of photographs taken when the patient was younger may also be helpful in setting patient expectations. The patient should be photographed from frontal, 45-degree, and 90-degree views to establish a baseline reference.

African ancestry, given its varied phenotypes, may not always be apparent to the physician based on patient appearance alone. It is therefore crucial to appreciate the cultural context of the patient and afford them the opportunity to self-identify their racial and ethnic background.[11] Skin phototype should be determined and documented. The Fitzpatrick skin type classification is the current standard for patient phototype assessment; with this system, however, there is risk of inaccurate conflation of race and ethnicity with phototype. Studies show that this occurs more frequently among physicians who do not identify as having skin of color.[12] Notably, the Fitzpatrick skin type classification is limited in its prediction of skin reactions, having particular implications for cosmetic procedures. The authors recommend utilization of the Roberts skin type classification, a four-part system that evaluates phototype, hyperpigmentation, photoaging, and scarring by review of ancestral and clinical history and visual examination.[13] During the patient evaluation, specific attention should be given to any prior history of hypertrophic scarring or keloids and hyperpigmentation. This is particularly helpful for treatment planning and minimization of potential cosmetic procedure complications.

COSMETIC CONCERNS

Dyschromia, Postinflammatory Hyperpigmentation, and Melasma

In the first large survey of women with skin of color regarding cosmetic concerns, 100 women (81 African Americans, 16 Hispanics, and 3 Asians) were compared with an age-matched population of 143 White women. The primary cosmetic concern among those surveyed was hyperpigmentation or dark spots (87%).[14] A 2019 survey of 401 female African American respondents on cosmetic concerns and treatments showed the biggest concern was also hyper-/hypopigmentation (64%), followed by looking tired (63%), uneven skin tone/color (57%), dark circles (48%), and bags under eyes (37%).[15] Dyschromia can occur in the form of both hyperpigmentation and hypopigmentation. Skin that is deeply melanated is the most vulnerable to pigmentary changes. This is in part due to labile responses by melanocytes. Postinflammatory hyperpigmentation (PIH) results from an overproduction and transfer of melanin by melanocytes to keratinocytes. PIH is mediated by prostaglandins D2 and E2, interleukin-1 and -6, and tumor necrosis factor-alpha.[16] This occurs in the setting of inflammatory processes (e.g., acne vulgaris, atopic dermatitis) and presents as dark macules or patches at the corresponding site of inflammation. Melasma is a complex, chronic condition mediated by genetic predisposition, hormonal influences, and exposure to heat, ultraviolet radiation, and visible light. It presents as tan to brown patches on the forehead, cheeks, nose, upper cutaneous lip, and, less frequently, chin. The treatment for both postinflammatory hyperpigmentation and melasma are similar and include a strict photoprotection, oral antioxidants, a wide range of topical medications (see Table 3.1), chemical peels, laser resurfacing, and oral tranexamic acid (Figs. 3.1 and 3.2).[15]

TABLE 3.1 Topical Agents Used in the Treatment of Melasma and Postinflammatory Hyperpigmentation
Antioxidants
Glutathione
Vitamin C (L-ascorbic acid)
Hesperidin
Tyrosinase inhibitors
Hydroquinone
Kojic acid
a-Arbutin and Arbutin
Aloesin
Azelaic acid
p-coumaric acid
Cysteamine
Mulberry extract
Glabridin
Melanosome transfer inhibitors
Niacinamide
Exfoliants
Willow bark extract
Glycolic acid
Lactic acid
Mandelic acid
Linoleic acid
Plasmin Inhibition
Tranexamic acid

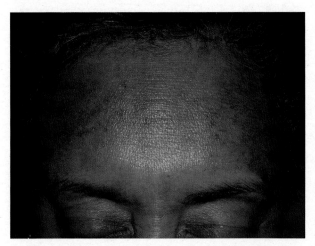

Fig. 3.1 Melasma of an Black/African-American woman.

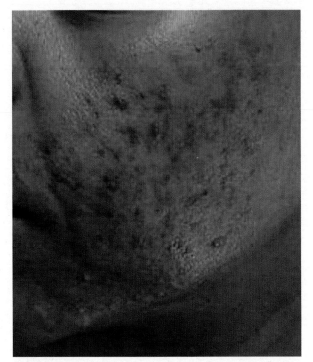

Fig. 3.2 Postinflammatory hyperpigmentation in Black/African-American woman.

SKIN TEXTURE

Skin texture and oiliness are also common concerns among individuals of African descent affecting 40% and 77% of women of color, respectively.[14] Studies show no difference between measurements of sebum between Black/African-American and White individuals.[16] There does exist a moderate amount of data to suggest that individuals of African descent have 2.5 times the corneocyte desquamation rate when compared to White individuals and Asians, contributing to higher rates of xerosis.[17] Black/African-American patients, when compared to other racial groups, have been found to have the lowest amount of ceramides in the stratum corneum.[18] Transepidermal water loss was also shown in older studies to occur at higher rates in Black patients, but a recent literature of review found no conclusive relationship between skin of color and transepidermal water loss.[19] Skin texture is best treated with tailored treatment regimen, including topical and oral retinoids, chemical peels, microneedling, and laser resurfacing.

DERMATOSIS PAPULOSA NIGRA

Dermatosis papulosa nigra (DPN) is a benign epithelial neoplasm of the head and neck found among individuals of African descent, occurring in 35% to 77% of this patient population.[20,21] There is a slight female predominance.[20] DPNs increase in number with age, although there is likely some role of sun exposure given anatomical distribution. Treatment for DPNs includes electrodessication, shave excision, curettage, cryosurgery, and laser removal (Fig. 3.3).[21]

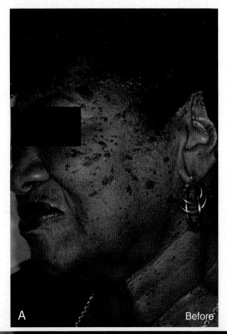

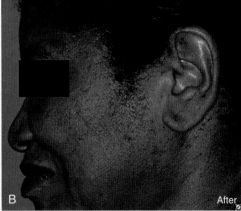

Fig. 3.3 Electrodessication dermatosis papulosa nigra. (A) Before (B) After.

UNWANTED HAIR

Unwanted facial and body hair is a cosmetic concern among many racial and ethnic groups, including individuals of African descent.[22] Curly and coily hair occurs in part due to hair follicle shape and predisposes patients of African descent to ingrown hairs. Among men of African descent, hair removal is frequently requested for medical conditions like pseudofolliculitis barbae, acne keloidalis nuchae, and dissecting cellulitis (Fig. 3.4).[22–24]

HYPERTROPHIC SCARS AND KELOIDS

Hypertrophic scars are characterized by an accumulation of extracellular matrix, resulting in varying degrees of thickening, induration, and elevation that do not extend beyond the borders of the original site of injury. These scars typically undergo a rapid period of growth followed by a period of regression. Keloids are characterized by abnormal proliferation of disorganized collagen that extends beyond the original margins of injury. Keloids do not undergo regression and may continue to grow for several years and can greatly affect patient quality of life. The risk of developing keloid scarring depends on genetic predisposition, abnormal cellular signaling (e.g., overproduction of TGF-beta), and anatomic location. The prevalence of keloids among individuals of African descent is unknown. Keloids was the eighth most common dermatologic diagnosis among Black/African-American the National Ambulatory Medical Care Survey whereas by comparison, it was not among the top 10 leading diagnoses in the other groups studied (including the White population, Asian/Pacific Islanders, Hispanic/Latinos).[25,26] Initial treatment of both hypertrophic scars and keloids includes intralesional steroids alone or combined with 5-fluorouracil and/or bleomycin, followed by vascular and fractional ablative or nonablative lasers in tandem or combined for laser-assisted drug delivery. Surgical resection of keloids is frequently unsuccessful, and recurrence is often observed (Fig. 3.5).

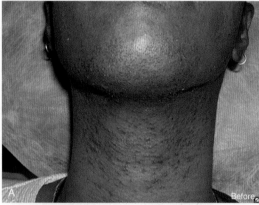

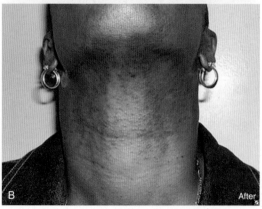

Fig. 3.4 Laser hair removal. (A) Before. (B) After.

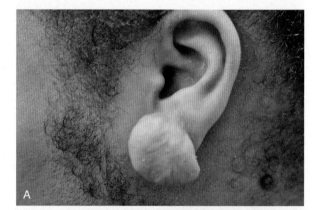

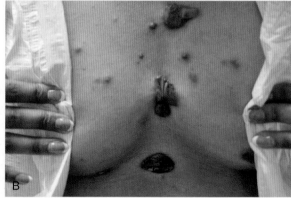

Fig. 3.5 Keloids. (A) Keloid scar in left earlobe. (B) Keloid scarring on upper chest and trunk.

ACNE VULGARIS

Epidemiological studies as early as 1908 have identified acne as one of the most common dermatoses affecting patients of African descent.[27–31] Even mild to moderate cases of acne commonly lead to the development of postinflammatory hyperpigmentation among black patients.[31,32] Postinflammatory lesions can last months to years longer than acne lesions and are a major reason for seeking dermatologic care.[32] One study of acne patients found that dyspigmentation, postinflammatory hyperpigmentation, and atrophic scars were more common among Black and Hispanic females when compared to other ethnicities.[33] In addition, studies have shown that PIH is often associated with overall greater acne severity, specifically targeting the jawline and trunk. The management of acne among patients of African descent must concurrently address postinflammatory hyperpigmentation. Daily photoprotection is essential. Topical retinoids, topical hydroquinone, and compounded lightening formulations with a variety of components including ascorbic acid, kojic acid, and corticosteroids are mainstay treatments for this patient population. When creating a treatment regimen for patients of African descent it is especially important to utilize a plan that is effective in reducing PIH, while being mindful to avoid causing irritation or dermatitis-induced PIH. Including gentle cleansers and moisturizers are necessary adjunctive agents to achieve and maintain tolerability of treatment (Fig. 3.6).[34]

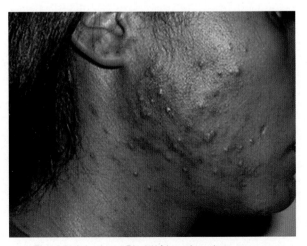

Fig. 3.6 Acne in an Black/African-American woman.

FACIAL REJUVENATION AND CONTOURING

A 2019 survey of 401 African American respondents identified the most bothersome facial areas among younger respondents (aged 30–44) as the under eye (28%) and crow's feet (21%), while older respondents (aged 45–65) were most concerned about a sagging/double chin (35%).[15] This is consistent with the midfacial aging that is characteristic of patients of African descent. Soft tissue augmentation with dermal fillers is the initial treatment of choice. The same survey explored attitudes towards cosmetic treatments. Among those who would consider injectables (64%), the majority were motivated by wanting their face to look good for their age (67%) and to look more youthful (51%). The top three barriers for not having tried injectable treatments were cost (50%), concerns about potential side effects (43%), and concerns about starting treatments they would have to repeat (31%).[15] These findings underscore the importance of clear communication of procedure technique, costs, and potential adverse effects during the cosmetic consult (Fig. 3.7).

TREATMENT APPROACHES IN PATIENTS OF AFRICAN DESCENT

Chemical Peels

Chemical peels are characterized as superficial, medium, or deep. Superficial peels target the stratum corneum to papillary dermis and include salicylic acid, glycolic acid 20% to 70%, trichloroacetic acid (TCA) 10% to 30%, resorcinol 30% to 50%, Jessner's solution, pyruvic acid, and solid carbon dioxide. Medium-depth peels target the papillary dermis to upper reticular dermis and include TCA 30% to 50%, combination glycolic acid 70% with TCA 25%, Jessner's solution with TCA 35%, solid carbon dioxide with TCA 35%, and phenol 88%. Deep chemical peels target the mid-reticular dermis and include the Baker-Gordon formula (e.g., croton oil 1.2%, phenol 35%).

Chemical peel selection in patients of African descent is paramount to achieve optimal outcomes while minimizing risk. A histologic study in patients with Fitzpatrick skin types IV to VI was performed 24 hours after application of salicylic acid 30%, glycolic acid 70%, TCA 25% and 30%, and Jessner's solution.[33] The most

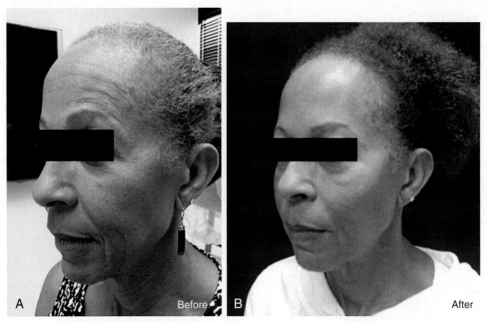

A   Before   B   After

Fig. 3.7 Facial rejuvenation with neuromodulators, radiofrequency, and fillers. (A) Before. (B) After.

significant stratum corneum necrosis was observed with the glycolic acid peel. TCA 25% and 30% caused deep epidermal necrosis and dense papillary dermal lymphohistiocytic infiltrates, resulting in postinflammatory hyperpigmentation.[35] Although postinflammatory hyperpigmentation can occur with any chemical peel—depending on individual susceptibility and procedural technique—it can be concluded that salicylic acid, glycolic acid, and Jenner's solution carry decreased risk compared to TCA 25% and 30%.[36]

Test spots on the preauricular skin with 1-week follow up may be required. Pretreatment with hydroquinone for 2 to 4 weeks—or kojic acid or azelaic acid in patients who develop irritation to hydroquinone—is thought by some dermatologists to help decrease risk of postinflammatory hyperpigmentation. Topical retinoids (e.g., retinol, tretinoin, tazarotene) should be held for 1 to 2 weeks prior to chemical peels. Retinoids increase epidermal turnover and the depth of chemical peels, which may be desired in Fitzpatrick types I–III, but increases the risk of post-peel complications (i.e., excessive erythema, desquamation, postinflammatory hyperpigmentation) in Fitzpatrick types IV–VI.[36]

Chemical peels in patients of African descent should be administered using a titration method.[36–38] The lowest concentration of salicylic acid (20%–30%), glycolic acid (20%–30%), and TCA (10%–15%) should initially be used. Peels should be performed at 3- to 4-week intervals, with slow increase in peel concentration after two to three treatments (e.g., increase from glycolic acid 30% to 70%, TCA 15% to TCA 20%). Medium-depth peels (e.g., Jessner's solution with TCA 20%) can be employed safely in some patients of African descent after a significant titration period. Deep-depth chemical peels carry significantly higher risk of hypopigmentation and scarring in this patient population. A series of five to six peels is routinely performed before appreciable improvement in dyschromia, acne, or skin texture may be observed.[37]

Post-peel care consists of bland cleanser and emollients for five to seven days. If excessive irritation, erythema, or desquamation occurs, topical corticosteroids may be employed. Strict photoprotection with broad-spectrum sunscreen is imperative (Fig. 3.8).

NEUROMODULATORS

Botulinum toxin type A (BoNT-A) injection is the most commonly performed minimally invasive cosmetic procedure, with 7.8 million procedures performed in 2018.[3]

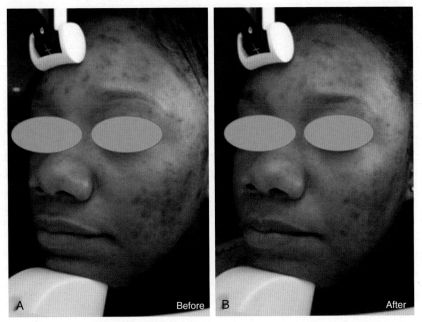

Fig. 3.8 Chemical peels. (A) Before. (B) After.

From its inception as a cosmetic procedure, BoNT-A has been primarily studied and performed on White women.[39-41] One large, randomized, double-blind, placebo-controlled trial of abobotulinumtoxin-A found no difference in in glabellar muscle mass distribution between White and Black patients.[42] Notably, the same study found Black/African-American study participants had a higher response and marginally longer duration of action—117 days versus 109 days—compared to other study participants.[42] A randomized double-blind study of onabotulinumtoxin-A in glabellar folds of women with Fitzpatrick V and VI found no difference in cosmetic outcome between 20 or 30 U and no increased incidence of adverse events.[43] Additionally, a post-hoc analysis of six abobotulinumtoxin-A clinical trials found a similar onset of cosmetic effect with no difference in rates of adverse events among White patients and patients with skin of color. The analysis also found that patients with skin of color had a greater response rate 30 days after treatment.[44] The existing data on BoNT-A among patients of African descent are limited, with clinical trials listing patient demographic data having 10% or less of Black/African-American participants.[45-47] The existing evidence suggests that no treatment modifications with regard to administration or dosing are needed, and that possibly these patients may experience cosmetic improvement for a longer period of time compared to their White counterparts (Fig. 3.7).

SOFT TISSUE AUGMENTATION

For patients of African descent, soft tissue augmentation is of particular importance given the central role of midfacial aging. Studies of soft tissue fillers among this patient population are few in number. It was previously postulated that patients of African descent are at higher risk of adverse events such as postinflammatory hyperpigmentation and hypertrophic scarring, but this has since been disproven.

Two prospective studies of 160 subjects with Fitzpatrick skin types IV, V, and VI treated with hyaluronic acid and/or collagen fillers in the nasolabial folds found no incidence of keloid or hypertrophic scar formation, and only three cases of mild hyperpigmentation up to 24 weeks post-treatment.[48] Another study of 100 subjects with Fitzpatrick skin types IV to VI injected subdermally with calcium hydroxylapatite into the nasolabial folds found no reports of hypertrophic scarring, keloid formation, or dyspigmentation.[49] A randomized split-face trial of 150 subjects with Fitzpatrick skin types IV, V, and VI treated with nonanimal stabilized hyaluronic acid dermal fillers into the nasolabial folds demonstrated no difference or tolerability in adverse events (e.g., bruising, edema) when compared with White patients.[50] And a study of cohesive polydensified matrix hyaluronic acid in treatment of nasolabial folds among 93 subjects with Fitzpatrick skin types IV, V, and VI found no association with dyspigmentation or scarring.[51] Additionally, pooled data from subjects with Fitzpatrick skin types IV, V, and VI treated with hyaluronic acid fillers for lip and perioral enhancement found 85% of subjects were positive responders and injection site adverse events (e.g., site mass, bruising) were mild to moderate in severity and resolved within 2 weeks.[52] It can therefore be concluded that soft tissue fillers of varying types (e.g., hyaluronic acid, calcium hydroxylapatite, and collagen) can all be used safely in patients of African descent.

LASER AND LIGHT-BASED DEVICES

There are several factors that can influence laser treatment outcomes in patients of African descent (see Table 3.2). The increased size and number of melanosomes present in skin of color places these patients at increased risk of

---

TABLE 3.2 Factors Influencing Laser Complications Among Patients of African Descent

Practical Factors
- Access to laser and light-based devices
- Cost of procedure

Patient Factors
- Skin phototype
- Predisposition to development of dyspigmentation and/or scarring
- Type of cosmetic concern (e.g. laxity, skin lesion, skin discoloration, skin texture)
- Anatomical area treated
- Inadequate peri-procedural skin care

Operator Factors
- Training in laser technology and safety
- Experience in laser treatment of patients with darker skin
- Incorrect parameter selection (e.g., wavelength, fluence, pulse duration, cooling)
- Poor technique
- Knowledge of the management of adverse effects

---

hypo- and hyperpigmentation after laser procedures, particularly those laser devices with wavelengths targeting melanin as a chromophore. The authors propose that the bulk heating of tissue during laser treatment also leads to increased activation of melanocytes and the development of postinflammatory hyperpigmentation, though this is debated by other laser experts. Eliciting a complete medical history, performing test spots, and counseling patients of potential adverse events is imperative.

The proper selection of laser devices and treatment parameters is extremely important. In general, longer wavelengths, longer pulse durations, and cooling mechanisms are safer in darker skin types as they allow for decreased heating of the epidermis and epidermal-dermal junction and increased depth of penetration.[53] Nonablative fractional laser resurfacing has been demonstrated in several studies to be safe and effective in Black patients, resulting in improvement of skin texture (i.e., in cases of acne scarring) and even skin laxity.[53–55] When performing laser procedures, it is key to utilize lower fluences administered over multiple treatments, as well as proper technique (e.g., holding handpieces perpendicular skin at the proper distance from skin).

Pre- and post-laser procedural skin care is essential to minimization of risk for adverse treatment outcomes. The use of pre-procedure hydroquinone is promoted by many dermatologists, but studies demonstrating the efficacy of hydroquinone in preventing laser-induced postinflammatory hyperpigmentation are lacking.[56] Post-procedural topical corticosteroid application may also be beneficial in mitigating erythema and the development of dyspigmentation and is used by the authors. Strict photoprotection with broad-spectrum sunscreen remains key for patients and should be strongly encouraged.

SURGICAL APPROACH

The skin of patients of African descent maintains its elasticity longer than that of other populations, including White populations. For some patients, however, with advanced skin laxity and midfacial aging, a surgical approach may be required. The double convexity described earlier in this chapter may be addressed by a lower eyelid blepharoplasty or sculpting of retro-orbital ocular fat.[56] Submental fullness may be addressed with submental liposuction. It is likely that the increased skin integrity among patients of African descent may even allow for satisfactory outcomes after minimally invasive surgical procedures.[57]

CONCLUSION

Individuals of African descent represent a range of ancestries with a diversity of phenotypes but share some commonalities with regard to anatomic features, predisposition to certain skin and hair conditions, tissue response to dermatologic procedures, as well as cosmetic concerns. There is a dearth of clinical studies on cosmetic procedures in this patient population, which has led to a paucity in evidence regarding cosmetic treatments in patients of African descent. It is incumbent upon those in the industry who are involved in the development of injectable and laser and light devices to increase the representation of patients of African descent in clinical trials so that this knowledge gap may be addressed. Special consideration of cosmetic treatment selection and administration can result in optimal results while minimizing adverse events.

REFERENCES

1. Alexis AF, Few J, Callender V, et al. Myths and knowledge gaps in the aesthetic treatment of patients with skin of color. *J Drugs Dermatol.* 2019;18(7):616-622.
2. Davis EC, Callender VD. Aesthetic dermatology for aging ethnic skin. *Dermatol Surg.* 2011;37(7):901-917.
3. American Society of Plastic Surgeons. 2018 Plastic Surgery Statistics Report. ASPS National Clearinghouse of Plastic Surgery Procedural Statistics. 2018.
4. Alexis AF, Grimes P, Boyd C, et al. Racial and ethnic differences in self-assessed facial aging in women: Results from a multinational study. *Dermatol Surg.* 2019;45(12):1635-1648.
5. Montagna W, Carlisle K. The architecture of Black and White facial skin. *J Am Acad Dermatol.* 1991;24:929-937.
6. Brissett AE, Naylor MC. The aging African-American face. *Facial Plast Surg.* 2010;26(2):154-163.
7. Taylor SC. Skin of color: Biology, structure, function, and implications for dermatologic disease. *J Am Acad Dermatol.* 2002;46(2, Suppl Understanding):S41-S62.
8. Mattory WE. *Ethnic Considerations in Facial Aesthetic Surgery.* Philadelphia, PA: Lippincott-Raven; 1998.
9. Alexis AF, Obioha JO. Ethnicity and aging skin. *J Drugs Dermatol.* 2017;16(6):s77-s80.
10. Brissett AE, Zevallos JP. Rejuvenation of the aging African face. In: Trustwell WH, ed. *Surgical Facial Rejuvenation;*

11. Barbosa VH. Impact of traditional African American cultures on healthcare practices. In: Kelly AP, Taylor S, eds. *Taylor and Kelly's Dermatology for Skin Color, 2e.* New York, NY: McGraw Hill; 2016.
12. Ware OR, Dawson JE, Shinohara MM, et al. Racial limitation of Fitzpatrick skin type. *Cutis.* 2020;105(02):77-80.
13. Roberts WE. The Roberts skin type classification system. *J Drugs Dermatol.* 2008;7(5):452-456.
14. Grimes PE. Skin and hair cosmetic issues in women of color. *Dermatol Clin.* 2000;18:659-665.
15. Alexis A, Boyd C, Callender V, Downie J, Sangha S. Understanding the female African American facial aesthetic patient. *J Drugs Dermatol.* 2019;18(9):858-866.
16. Grimes P, Edison BL, Green BA, et al. Evaluation of inherent differences between African American and White skin surface properties using subjective and objective measures. *Cutis.* 2004;73:392-396.
17. Wesley NO, Maibach HI. Racial (ethnic) differences in skin properties: The objective data. *Am J Clin Dermatol.* 2003;4(12):843-860.
18. Jungersted JM, Hiøgh JK, Hellgren LI, Jemec GBE, Agner T. Ethnicity and stratum corneum ceramides. *Br J Dermatol.* 2010;163(6):1169-1173.
19. Peer RA, Burli A, Maibach H. Did human evolution in skin of color enhance the TEWL barrier? *Arch Dermatol Res.* 2021;314:121-132.
20. Grimes PE, Arora S, Minus HR, et al. Dermatosis papulosa nigra. *Cutis.* 1983;32:385-386.
21. Kauh YC, McDonald JW, Rapaport JA, et al. A surgical approach for dermatosis papulosa nigra. *Int J Dermatol.* 1983;22:590-592.
22. Awosika O, Burgess CM, Grimes PE. Considerations when treating cosmetic concerns in men of color. *Dermatol Surg.* 2017;43 suppl 2:S140-S150.
23. Callender VD. Commentary on considerations when treating cosmetic concerns in men of color. *Dermatol Surg.* 2017;43 suppl 2:S151-S152.
24. Callender VD, Barbosa V, Burgess CM, et al. Approach to treatment of medical and cosmetic facial concerns in skin of color patients. *Cutis.* 2017;100(6):375-380.
25. Brissett AE, Sherris DA. Scar contractures, hypertrophic scars, and keloids. *Facial Plast Surg.* 2001;17:263-272.
26. Davis SA, Narahari S, Feldman SR, et al. Top dermatologic conditions in patients of color: An analysis of nationally representative data. *J Drugs Dermatol.* 2012;11:466-473.
27. Fox H. Observations on skin diseases in the Negro. *J Cutan Dis.* 1908;26:67-79.
28. Hazen HH. Personal observations upon skin diseases in the American Negro. *J Cutan Dis.* 1914;32:705-712.

29. Hazen HH. Syphilis and skin disease in the American Negro: Personal observations. *AMA Arch Derm Syphilol.* 1935;31:316-323.

30. Kennedy JA. Management of dermatoses peculiar to Negroes. *Arch Dermatol.* 1965;91:126-129.

31. Halder RM, Grimes PE, McLaurin CI, et al. Incidence of common dermatoses in a predominately Black dermatologic practice. *Cutis.* 1983;32:388-390.

32. Davis EC, Callender VD. A review of acne in ethnic skin: Pathogenesis, clinical manifestations, and management strategies. *J Clin Aesthet Dermatol.* 2010;3:24-38.

33. Perkins AC, Cheng CE, Hillebrand GG, et al. Comparison of the epidemiology of acne vulgaris among Caucasians, Asian, Continental Indian and African American women. *J Eur Acad Dermatol Venereol.* 2011;25:1054-1060.

34. Alexis AF, Woolery-Lloyd H, Williams K, et al. Racial/ethnic variations in acne: Implications for treatment and skin care recommendations for acne patients with skin of color. *J Drugs Dermatol.* 2021;20(7):716-725.

35. Grimes PE. Agents for ethnic skin peeling. *Dermatol Ther.* 2000;13:159-164.

36. Grimes PE. The safety and efficacy of salicylic acid chemical peels in darker racial-ethnic groups. *Dermatol Surg.* 1999;25(1):18-22.

37. Quarles FN, Brody H, Johnson BA, Badreshia S. Chemical peels in richly pigmented patients. *Dermatol Ther.* 2007;20(3):147-148.

38. Vemula S, Maymone MBC, Secemsky EA, et al. Assessing the safety of superficial chemical peels in darker skin: A retrospective study. *J Am Acad Dermatol.* 2018;79(3):508-513.e2.

39. Carruthers JA, Lowe NJ, Menter MA, Gibson J. A multicenter, double-blind, randomized, placebo-controlled study of the efficacy and safety of botulinum toxin type A in the treatment of glabellar lines. *J Am Acad Dermatol.* 2002;46:840-849.

40. Carruthers JD, Lowe NJ, Menter MA, Gibson J. Double-blind, placebo-controlled study of the safety and efficacy of botulinum toxin type A for patients with glabellar lines. *Plast Reconstr Surg.* 2003;112:1089-1098.

41. Carruthers A, Carruthers J, Cohen J. A prospective, double-blind, randomized, parallel-group, dose-ranging study of botulinum toxin type A in female subjects with horizontal forehead rhytides. *Dermatol Surg.* 2003;29:461-467.

42. Kane MA, Brandt F, Rohrich RJ, et al. Evaluation of variable-dose treatment with a new U.S. Botulinum Toxin Type A (Dysport) for correction of moderate to severe glabellar lines: results from a phase III, randomized, double-blind, placebo-controlled study. *Plast Reconstr Surg.* 2009;124:1619-1629.

43. Grimes PE, Shabazz D. A four-month randomized, double-blind evaluation of the efficacy of botulinum toxin type A for the treatment of glabellar lines in women with skin types V and VI. *Dermatol Surg.* 2009;35:429-435; discussion 435-436.

44. Taylor SC, Callender VD, Albright CD, Coleman J, Axford-Gatley RA, Lin X. AbobotulinumtoxinA for reduction of glabellar lines in patients with skin of color: post hoc analysis of pooled clinical trial data. *Dermatol Surg.* 2012;38(11):1804-1811.

45. Schlessinger J, Dover JS, Joseph J, et al. Long-term safety of abobotulinumtoxinA for the treatment of glabellar lines: Results from a 36-month, multicenter, open-label extension study. *Dermatol Surg.* 2014;40(2):176-183.

46. Kane MC, Gold M, Coleman WP III, et al. A randomized, double-blind trial to investigate the equivalence of incobotulinumtoxinA and onabotulinumtoxinA for glabellar frown lines. *Dermatol Surg.* 2015;41(11):1310-1319.

47. Carruthers JD, Fagien S, Joseph JH, et al. DaxibotulinumtoxinA for injection for the treatment of glabellar lines: Results from each of two multicenter, randomized, double-blind, placebo-controlled, phase 3 studies (SAKURA 1 and SAKURA 2). *Plast Reconstr Surg.* 2020;145(1):45-58.

48. Grimes PE, Thomas JA, Murphy DK. Safety and effectiveness of hyaluronic acid fillers in skin of color. *J Cosmet Dermatol.* 2009;8:162-168.

49. Marmur ES, Taylor SC, Grimes PE, Boyd CM, Porter JP, Yoo JY. Six-month safety results of calcium hydroxylapatite for treatment of nasolabial folds in Fitzpatrick skin types IV to VI. *Dermatol Surg.* 2009;35(suppl 2):1641-1645.

50. Taylor SC, Burgess CM, Callender VD. Safety of nonanimal stabilized hyaluronic acid dermal fillers in patients with skin of color: A randomized, evaluator-blinded comparative trial. *Dermatol Surg.* 2009;35 suppl 2:1653-1660.

51. Downie JB, Grimes PE, Callender VD. A multicenter study of the safety and effectiveness of hyaluronic acid with a cohesive polydensified matrix for treatment of nasolabial folds in subjects with Fitzpatrick skin types IV, V, and VI. *Plast Reconstr Surg.* 2013;132(4 suppl 2):41S-47S.

52. Taylor SC, Downie JB, Shamban A, et al. Lip and perioral enhancement with hyaluronic acid dermal fillers in individuals with skin of color. *Dermatol Surg.* 2019;45(7):959-967.

53. Munavalli GS, Weiss RA, Halder RM. Photoaging and nonablative photorejuvenation in ethnic skin. *Dermatol Surg.* 2005;31(9 Pt 2):1250-1260; discussion 1261.

54. Alexis AF, Coley MK, Nijhawan RI, et al. Nonablative fractional laser resurfacing for acne scarring in patients with Fitzpatrick skin phototypes IV-VI. *Dermatol Surg.* 2016;42(3):392-402.

55. Alexis AF. Laser resurfacing for treatment of acne scarring in Fitzpatrick skin types V to VI: Practical approaches to maximizing safety. *Cutis.* 2013;92(6):272-273.

56. Wong ITY, Richer V. Prophylaxis of post-inflammatory hyperpigmentation from energy-based device treatments: A review. *J Cutan Med Surg.* 2021;25(1): 77-86.

57. Harris MO. The aging face in patients of color: Minimally invasive surgical facial rejuvenation-a targeted approach. *Dermatol Ther.* 2004;17:206-211.

4

Populations of East Asian Ancestry

Henry H. L. Chan, Nicole Y. Lee

SUMMARY AND KEY FEATURES

- Beauty in the age of globalization requires an understanding of the distinctive ethnic features that are inherently alluring within each race. This Chapter first introduces the ethnic features of Asians, and photoaging of East Asians. Popular

Cosmetic treatments for East Asians were introduced, including injectables, laser and energy-based device treatment, and body contouring. The skills and approaches of these cosmetic treatments, and the tips to avoid complications will be discussed.

INTRODUCTION

The concept of a universal standard of beauty has been extensively debated over the centuries. Renaissance neoclassical canons and Marquardt's phi mask are examples of attempts to objectively define the ideal facial archetype. However, it is now widely accepted that while they provide an aesthetic guideline for which to analyze the face, they are not universally applicable. It is understood that the perception of beauty and attractiveness can vary based on cultural norms, but recent studies have shown that a general appreciation for the overarching ideals of beauty does exist independent of societal and racial influences.[1,2] Possessing an oval facial shape with symmetry and balance are key to being universally regarded as beautiful. Beauty in the age of globalization also requires an understanding of the distinctive ethnic features that are inherently alluring within each race so that they can be optimized. All aesthetically attractive people exhibit both the broader ideals of beauty while also maintaining their distinct ethnic features.[3] In terms of photoaging, East Asians differ from populations of European descent (commonly referred to as Caucasians) and tend to present with more pigmentary changes and less wrinkling. Furthermore, postinflammatory hyperpigmentation (PIH) is a common issue after laser procedures. Therefore, a less aggressive

approach to treatment will result in a better cosmetic outcome. In this chapter, we will review the ethnic considerations as well as the cultural nuances that should guide the evaluation and cosmetic treatments in those of East Asian ancestry.

STRUCTURAL AND CULTURAL CONSIDERATIONS

Historically, Asian culture has always placed an emphasis on beauty since certain facial features have traditionally been regarded as a reflection of one's character and determining one's future prospects in life.[4] Although variability exists among East Asian populations (defined as Chinese, Korean, and Japanese), the facial anatomy is predominantly characterized by an increased bizygomatic, bitemporal, and bigonial width, a regressed central face (forehead, cheeks, chin), increased intercanthal distance, a shorter palpebral fissure, and fuller lips with a prominent upper lip.[2,5,6] White facial structure, on the other hand, is narrow in comparison with a pronounced anterior three-dimensional projection, increased vertical height, larger eyes, and thinner lips.[6] Although the overarching concept of beauty has not changed throughout history and across cultures, specific ideals of beauty and perceived attractiveness are very much influenced by the nuances of sociocultural ideologies.

In Asia, there has been an increase in demand for nonsurgical aesthetic treatments sought out by younger patients in their 20s and 30s with the goal of improving upon ethnically distinct anatomic proportions, such as slimming of the lower face and improving the anterior projection of the midface.[7] Older patients seek out traditional cosmetic treatments focused on correcting the classic signs of aging. Furthermore, Asian ideals of beauty are centered on having clear and flawless skin as is reflected in the rapidly growing Korean and Japanese skincare industry that has now taken a hold in North American and European countries. The current ideals of beauty for an Asian female in Asia consist of having clear and unblemished skin, an oval facial shape, a small but prominent nose and chin, proportionately full lips with a defined cupid's bow, a "v-shaped" jawline, and large eyes.[6] Asians that have been raised in Western society, on the other hand, have different attitudes about their ideals of beauty. Attractiveness is associated with facial contouring and sharper angles, such as the jawline and lateral cheek, that is similar to their non-Asian peers. In contrast, softer features and obtuse jawlines are favored in Asia. Also, while Western society regards tanned skin as attractive, Asian society has traditionally preferred untanned and unblemished fair skin. However, with globalization, these distinctions have started to blur as Western societies have embraced Asian food, pop culture, and beauty standards while Asian societies, in turn, have been influenced by Western culture.

Due to the unique pathophysiologic properties of Asian skin and the distinct features of their facial anatomy, aging in Asian patients presents in a different manner and is often perceived as occurring at a slower rate when compared to their White counterparts of similar age. Among East Asian populations, the skin tends to be thicker, containing more collagen, and possesses more melanin, which is protective against the textural changes from cumulative UV exposure.[8] As a result of the increase in melanin, Asians develop pigmented lesions, such as macular seborrheic keratoses and solar lentigines, at an earlier age; thus, pigmented lesions are often seen as a marker of aging among Asians. While Asian skin during the second and third decades may appear to be less wrinkled and, thereby, more visually youthful, the aging process ultimately "catches up" by the sixth decade.[9] Aging in Asian faces is slowed down due to ligamentous support and the dense fibrous attachments of the fascial layers, which delays midface soft tissue

descent, while the thicker dermis and increased superficial fat reduces the appearance of superficial rhytides.[10] Ultimately, aging occurs in a similar fashion as in all ethnicities from soft tissue volume loss, increase in skin laxity and atrophy, and loss of structural support with bone remodeling. Aging in Asian faces predominantly occurs by gravitational descent of the soft tissue in the absence of midface structural skeletal support.[11,12] These changes eventually result in early tear-trough hollowing and sagging of the face over time. Furthermore, cultural nuances that dictate how an individual articulates and the use of facial expressions as part of day-to-day social interaction may also play a part in the formation of wrinkles. Asians tend to be less dynamic in their facial expression and do not use as many muscles with speech, which may minimize the development of dynamic rhytides[6,13]; however, Asians raised in Western cultures do tend to develop more dynamic lines in comparison, similarly to their non-Asian peers.

An understanding of the unique anatomic facial features and properties of the skin as well as an awareness of the nuances of cultural and social norms are vital to the evaluation and aesthetic treatment of Asian patients. The goal of treatment is to not appear "Westernized" as had been previously thought, but to improve overall facial attractiveness by optimizing intrinsic ethnic features consistent within an individual's own racial/ethnic norms.

INJECTABLES

Neuromodulators

Treatment with botulinum toxin has rapidly become one of the most popular noninvasive aesthetic treatments worldwide. While it is typically used to address dynamic facial rhytides, botulinum toxin is often used by Asian patients as a method to reshape and recontour the face as well as areas of the body, such as the calf and deltoids. Ethnic, anatomic, and cultural considerations must be made since there is variability even among Asians on their perception of how beauty is defined. Asian patients do not develop as many dynamic lines as their non-Asian peers. Therefore, when creases do start to appear, Asian patients tend to want them addressed at an earlier age. Furthermore, Asian patients often require less botulinum toxin to achieve the desired results in the classically treated areas due to having smaller facial muscles as well as a preference for a more natural and unfrozen look.

While the glabella is usually the most treated area in White, it is second after the periorbital area in Asian patients.[7,14] When treating the glabella, it must be noted that Asian corrugators tend to be shorter and narrower in comparison to White corrugators. As a result, smaller doses of botulinum toxin are often used, and it is typically administered as three point injections rather than the traditional five, although the latter can be used as well if appropriate for a given individual.[15] This will prevent unintentional widening of the eyebrows, ptosis, and medial brow heaviness. At times, a half unit of product may also be needed at the lateral forehead to address arching of the eyebrows, which is generally considered aesthetically unattractive by Asian patients. Brow position must be considered since Asians typically do not want to enhance the lateral brow in the same manner that is popularized in non-Asian populations. Enhanced arching of the lateral brow unattractively widens the appearance of Asian faces and creates an angry "Samurai" look. Asians often prefer a flatter arch to their brow; treating the lateral forehead in addition to the glabella will address this aesthetic preference. The frontalis muscle is frequently smaller and less dynamic, thus warranting lower doses of botulinum toxin. There is some variability in proposed injection techniques where the placement can be standard as in White patients, or as two rows of a series of injections, or as microdroplets with a higher saline-to-product ratio where each injection point is around half a unit.[15]

The development of crow's feet in Asian populations tends to begin at least a decade later than in European populations with lighter phototypes and more extensive sun exposure. Similar to the other areas, smaller doses of botulinum toxin are typically used to achieve the desired response in the periorbital region. Neuromodulators can also be used to address lower eyelid rhytides. However, one must be aware that in certain cultures, such as in Korea, the pretarsal roll is considered a sign of youthfulness and is often enhanced with the use of filler.[14] Therefore, when treating lower eyelid rhytides, it is advised to place the injection points at the junction of the preseptal and orbicularis muscle to prevent flattening of the pretarsal roll. If the intent is to increase the eye opening, placement of the injection point closer to the inferior ciliary margin would create this result but

with the loss of the "charming roll." It is advised to avoid injecting the lower eyelid if the skin elasticity is poor and to use lower doses to prevent lower eyelid edema.

In addition to the standard dynamic areas of treatment, neuromodulators are also widely used in Asia to modify areas of the body in order to achieve perceived notions of beauty. Numerous papers have discussed the utilization of botulinum toxin to intentionally reduce the size of the masseters and to relax the hyperactive mentalis muscle in order to narrow and lengthen the face. Asian faces typically have a wider mandible, hypertrophic masseters, and increased subcutaneous adipose tissue resulting in a square-shaped and wide lower face.[16] This can be exacerbated by certain medical conditions such as bruxism or temporomandibular joint disorders or even certain ethnic diets that require increased chewing. An overlying enlarged parotid gland can also add to the width of the lower face; reports have shown successful reduction in size with botulinum treatment.[15] Proper evaluation and setting of expectations are important in selecting the correct patient since botulinum treatment will not address prominent mandibular prominence or the overlying subcutaneous adipose tissue. Of note, older patients with increased cutaneous laxity may not be appropriate candidates for botulinum toxin treatment of the masseter in that reduction of the masseters will lead to the increased appearance of excess skin along the jawline.[17]

Multiple injection techniques have been described in the literature, but the most common reported technique involves three injection points to the lower third of the masseter. The area for treatment is located within the borders of an imaginary line connecting the tragus to the oral commissure, the mandible, and the anterior and posterior edges of the masseter.[18] Keeping the injection points at least 1 cm within these margins minimizes potential complications of unintended diffusion of the product. The amount of product used varies depending on the size of the muscle and can range between 20 to 60 units of botulinum toxin A per side. Clinical results begin to be apparent at 2 weeks but progresses to reach peak atrophy at 3 months before returning to baseline after 6 to 9 months from injection.[16] Consistent and repeated treatments lead to chronic atrophy and volume reduction of the masseter, thereby requiring less product with each session.[18] Side effects are uncommon and include weakness with chewing, facial asymmetry with expression from unintended diffusion to the risorius muscle, prominence of the zygomatic arch from infra-zygomatic hollowing, and paradoxical masseter bulging.[19] Muscle weakness with mastication becomes apparent at 2 weeks while the strength starts to return after 3 to 4 months.[16] The other reported side effects can typically be prevented with keeping the injection points within the borders previously mentioned. Paradoxical bulging is uncommon but is thought to occur from uneven diffusion of product from inadequate dosing, concentration of product, or inconsistent injection point depth.[17] This results in persistent activity of the superficial belly of the masseter while the deep belly of the masseter has been paralyzed. Anatomic analysis of the muscle has shown a deep inferior tendon within the superficial masseter that can prevent this diffusion.[20] Bulging typically appears within 2 weeks after injection and, if not improved by week 4, can be corrected with additional units to the areas of residual activity.[19,21] There is also some concern of mandibular osteopenia from chronic treatment; however, further research is needed to determine long-term functional consequences from these bony changes.[17]

The use of neuromodulators for contouring has also been utilized beyond the face to areas such as the calves, shoulders,[22] and deltoids.[15] Asians tend to have increased leg circumference and shorter legs relative to their torso. By thinning the calves, the legs appear visually longer.[23] Although botulinum treatment of calves is widely accepted in East Asian countries, the available literature is limited and the approach for treatment varies widely. Even though there is variability in the placement of injection points, the overarching approach to treatment focuses on treating the medial and lateral bellies of the gastrocnemius muscle. In certain situations, treatment of the soleus and peroneus longus muscle may also be needed for optimal results.[24] Dosing is dependent based on the size of the muscle and shape of the leg as determined by having the patient stand on their toes.[25] Pinching the skin while the patient is in tiptoe position allows the physician to differentiate between muscle and subcutaneous fat and dermis.[26] Doses are typically between 100 to 200 units of botulinum toxin per leg. Reduction in calf size starts to become apparent by 1 month with 50% of the muscle volume returning after 6 months.[15,25] Muscle strength will start to return by the second to third month.[24] Side effects associated with treatment typically include bruising or cramping with walking that resolves by 1 to 2 months

after injection.[27] However, there are no reports of difficulty with gait or exercise that would affect quality of life.[24] Patients are advised to minimize physical exertion in order to prevent regeneration of the calf muscle and to maintain results.

Filler

As previously described, distinctions of East Asian facial anatomy include broad width, flat to concave T-zone, and short vertical height. Younger Asian patients tend to seek out filler treatments to reshape and recontour the face in order to improve upon these unique ethnic anatomic features while older Asian patients are more likely to be interested in overall volume restoration. The overarching goal with filler augmentation in Asian faces is to enhance the anterior mid projection while lengthening the vertical height of the face, which creates the visual illusion of a narrow and slimmer face.[7] This is achieved by treating the forehead, temples, nose, medial cheeks, and chin.

The flat, hypoplastic skeletal framework of the anterior maxillary wall and inferior orbital rim results in midface soft tissue ptosis that lends to early tear-trough hollowing,[12] which is often a concern at an earlier age in Asian patients. It is recommended to first augment the medial cheek as this will often improve the appearance of the tear-trough area without overfilling.[28] Also, treating the medial and apex of the cheek as well as the submalar hollow will enhance the anterior projection of the face and address the nasolabial folds and lower face.[28] As a result, it is advised to first address the midface when planning treatment followed by the nasolabial folds if needed. However, it must be noted that since Asian faces tend to be anatomically broad, filling the lateral zygoma is often not advised as this will undesirably widen the face.

Treating the nose and forehead are two other areas that will also improve the 3D projection of the face. Nonsurgical rhinoplasties are one of the most popular treatments in Asia. Asian noses tend to be broad with a low-set nasal bridge, short in length with a flattened nasal tip, and with overlying thicker skin.[29] Correcting the nasal bridge and tip improves the overall appearance and projection of the nose. However, it should only be attempted by advanced injectors with an awareness of the vascular anatomy of the nose in order to avoid accidental intravascular occlusion, which can lead to soft tissue necrosis and, in rare cases, blindness (Fig. 4.1A and B).

Augmentation of the forehead is rarely performed in Western communities where neurotoxins are much

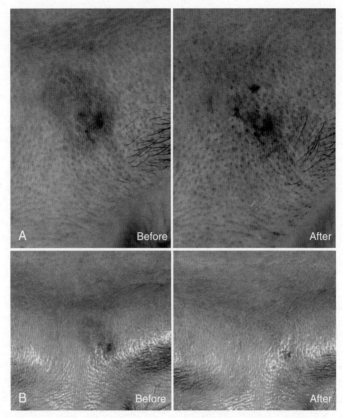

Fig. 4.1 (A) Arterial occlusion after filler injection. Left: Before hyaluronidase; Right: Immediately after hyaluronidase. (B) Arterial occlusion after filler injection. Left: Immediately; Right: 1 month after hyaluronidase.

more commonly requested. Age-related bony changes of the forehead exacerbate the receded appearance of the upper face in Asians. Therefore, volumizing the forehead, lateral brow, and temple is important in improving the anterior projection of the upper face and thereby creating the appearance of a more youthful convex forehead. It is recommended to combine filler with neuromodulators when treating the forehead and to be careful with placement to reduce the risk for nodules and textural irregularities from filler migration.[7] From an anatomic standpoint, caution must also be taken to avoid the supraorbital, supratrochlear, and frontal branch of the superficial temporal arteries when injecting the forehead and glabella while staying along the supraperiosteal level when injecting temples.[28]

Asian women tend to prefer a narrow lower face, pointed narrow chin, and a delicate, obtuse mandibular angle. This can be achieved by the combination of neuromodulators to the masseters and mentalis muscle as well, along with filler augmentation of the chin, pre-jowl and post-jowl sulcus, marionettes, and jawline. The hypoplastic chin in Asian faces results in the appearance of increased submental fullness which can be improved by increasing the prominence of the chin.[11,30] Asian lips tend to be fuller than White lips where the upper lip is often more prominent than the lower lip. Lip augmentation is not as commonly requested by Asian patients when compared to their White counterparts. However, when requested, the goal is to enhance the shape rather than to increase volumization. The larger upper lip also diminishes the appearance of the hypoplastic maxillary bone in Asian faces.[7] Treatment is generally focused on enhancing the central portion of the upper lip and enhancing the borders for a natural appearance.

Laser- and Energy-Based Devices

Laser and light sources have long been established to be effective for the treatment of acquired pigmentary conditions including freckles and solar lentigines among Asians. While both nanosecond and picosecond lasers can achieve significant improvement within one to two treatment sessions, the risk of PIH remains to be an issue and occurs among about 5% of treated patients[31] (Fig. 4.2). The appropriate clinical endpoint is important to ensure success and minimize complications. For nanosecond and picosecond lasers, the smallest spot size together with the lowest fluence to achieve immediate whitening should be used (for example, picosecond 532 Nd:YAG laser, 4-mm spot size 0.3–0.4 J/cm^2). Long-pulsed lasers with less photomechanical impact have been found to be associated with a lower incidence of PIH but will require more treatment sessions in comparison.[32] The clinical endpoint is a grey ashen appearance that can be rather subtle (for example, 532-nm KTP laser with contact cooling at 10°C, fluence range of 8.6–9.6 J/cm^2, 3-mm spot size, 2-ms pulse duration).[33] An advantage of using a long-pulsed laser is the ability to combine the treatment with other modalities during the same office visit. This allows a patient to address other aspects of photoaging in one appointment, such as diffuse erythema and telangiectasia with vascular lasers; pore size and skin texture with low-energy, low-density, nonablative fractional laser resurfacing or with fractionated picosecond focus lens lasers (Fig. 4.3).[34] Previous studies have shown greater patient satisfaction when patients experience minimal downtime, multiple modalities are used in a given office visit, and the treatments are spaced as multiple monthly sessions. It is

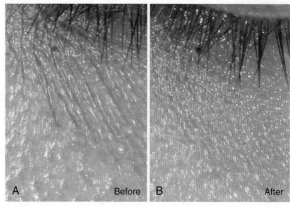

Fig. 4.3 Before and after treatment with picosecond laser. (A) Left: Baseline; (B) Right: 1 month after fifth treatment of nonablative skin rejuvenation with pulsed dye laser, fractionated picosecond 755 nm focus lens, and low-density, low-energy 1440 nm nonablative fractional laser.

important that a small spot size be used when treating lentigines in Asians with a long-pulsed laser in order to minimize unintended lightening of adjacent skin since there is less contrast in color between pigmented lesions and background skin in Asian patients.

High-energy nonablative fractional resurfacing can be associated with PIH among Asians and previous studies indicated that while both energy and density are important factors, density is of particular importance (Fig. 4.4).[35] Using low-density settings with an increase in the number of treatment sessions can reduce the risk of PIH.

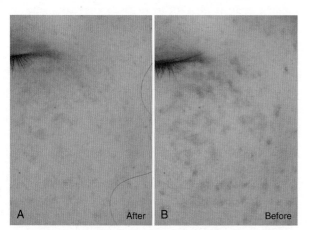

Fig. 4.2 PIH after picosecond laser. (A) Left: Baseline; (B) Right: PIH, 1 month after picosecond laser (532 nm Nd:YAG, 0.40 J/cm^2, 4 mm, 5 Hz).

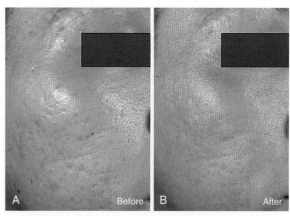

Fig. 4.4 Before and after treatment with nonablative fractional resurfacing. (A) Left: Baseline; (B) Right: after eighth NA-FR.

Although previous studies looking at the long-term effects of ablative fractional carbon dioxide (CO_2) laser resurfacing for the treatment of photoaging among Chinese patients indicated sustained efficacy for up to 5 years, the downtime and adverse effects, specifically the high prevalence of PIH (up to 58%), has limited its application in Asian skin.[36,37] Fractionated Erbium-YAG tends to have a lower degree of PIH than carbon dioxide but is also associated with reduced efficacy. Other means to reduce the risk of PIH include the use of a bleaching cream pre- and posttreatment, a topical steroid after treatment, and the use of oral tranexamic acid.

Another important means to ensure the patient's satisfaction for nonablative and ablative fractional resurfacing is patient selection. The treatment of surgical and acne scars tends to result in better patient satisfaction compared to the treatment of photoaging among Asian patients. In the authors' experience, the risk for PIH is generally more acceptable to Asian patients with scarring than in those who are interested in the antiaging benefit of laser resurfacing.

Monopolar radiofrequency has gained increased popularity as a noninvasive mean to improve skin laxity and has shown histologically to have a significant degree of improvement among Koreans 6 months after treatment.[38] It is advocated to treat at a lower fluence, with multiple passes, and with the endpoint of immediate tightening. Newer-generation models have improved the vibration in the handpieces, which has reduced the pain and provided a more accurate assessment of impedance to improve outcomes.[39] Adverse effects with newer devices are generally mild with rare crust formation and subsequent PIH. This can be due to cryoinjury when the tip is inappropriately placed or when there is a defect of the tip.

In more recent years, radiofrequency microneedling (RFMN) has gained increased popularity for skin rejuvenation, skin laxity, and acne-scar treatment among Asians due to the lower risk of PIH. Many RFMN devices are now on the market offering different levels of depth, with or without insulation. Noninsulated needle devices are associated with a greater risk for PIH.[40]

High-intensity focused ultrasound (HIFU) has been used for skin tightening in the last decade. A study looking at 22 Korean patients indicated both clinical and histological improvement with 77% improvement of the nasolabial fold and 73% improvement along the jaw line.[41] Some have since advocated the use of moderate parameters (lower energy) with an increase in the number of lines delivered per treatment or to increase the number of treatment sessions to reduce the discomfort associated. Complications are unusual but blister and scar formation can occur due to poor contact.[42] More recently, a device utilizing synchronous ultrasound parallel beam that delivers ultrasound energy to 1.5 mm has obtained FDA approval for skin tightening. Limited peer-reviewed data are currently available to compare it with existing technologies.

Body Contouring

Noninvasive body contouring using cryolipolysis, radiofrequency, focused ultrasound, and neuromuscular electrical stimulation have been advocated as alternative options to traditional surgical procedure. Asians tend to have a smaller physique and, therefore, device modification is sometimes necessary to achieve the desirable outcome.

Cryolipolysis involves controlled cold exposure to subcutaneous fat tissue by the means of heat withdrawal and, in doing so, results in cold-induced panniculitis leading to fat reduction in the region of 20% over a 2- to 6-month period. Studies among Asians indicated it is a safe procedure without any pigmentary changes.[43] Paradoxical adipose hyperplasia is a rare but significant complication that can be seen among Asians and the appropriate informed consent is important. Recent applicators have been modified to allow even smaller areas to be treated and can be specifically beneficial to Asians.

High-intensity focused ultrasound has also been used for body contouring by inducing thermal injury at a focal depth of 1.3 cm to destroy subcutaneous fat. For Asians, such depth can be an issue given the smaller physique in many instances. Furthermore, the pain and bruising associated with its use has limited its application.[44] Ultrasound-induced mechanical disruption of the fat, with or without radiofrequency, has also been used with some success. Other noninvasive devices used to reduce subcutaneous fat include low-level laser therapy and noncontact radiofrequency. Limited data are available in their application among Asians.

Neuromuscular electrical stimulation has been used to further improve body contouring and recent data indicate that its effect among Asians is similar to the White population with a significant reduction in abdominal circumference after 3 months with six, twice-weekly treatments.[45]

Laser-assisted lipolysis has been used with the proposed advantages of combining liposuction with skin tightening; different wavelength lasers have been used

(980-nm diode laser, 1064-nm Nd:YAG, 1064/1320-nm Nd:YAG). Side effects such as skin infection and burns have been reported. However, multiple factors have led to its lack of popularity, which include the cost of the device and the lack of data demonstrating its effectiveness when compared to traditional liposuction.

Deoxycholic acid injection for submental fullness has been shown to produce better results when compared to cryolipolysis and is also less invasive than neck liposuction. Although common side effects such as swelling, numbness, and nodules are usually transient and manageable, recent reports of rare but significant complication including vascular injury, nerve injury, and scarring must be taken into consideration as part of the informed consent process.[46]

CONCLUSION

For cosmetic procedures among Asians, ethnic consideration is important to achieve optimal outcomes. During the consultation, cultural expectations and personal upbringing are important factors to be taken into account before planning treatment. Asians tend to age less in the second and third decade, but by the sixth decade, aging tends to be similar to their White counterparts. Anatomic features unique to Asians, such as facial shape and body physique, coupled with population-specific cultural norms, lend to different approaches with injectables as well as with body contouring. Neuromodulators are used to widen eyes and treat masseter hypertrophy—creating the V-shape appearance that is popular among young Asians. The use of neuromodulators on nonfacial sites are commonly used for body contouring in East Asian populations and include treatment areas such as the calves, shoulders, and deltoids. For facial augmentation, the use of fillers to improve forehead, chin, and nose contour or shape are common requests among Asian patients. Filler injection for nose augmentation requires advance anatomical knowledge and skill, given the potential greater risk of vascular complication. PIH is an important factor to consider in the dermatological application of lasers and energy-based devices in Asians. Less is often more and therefore, more gentle treatment parameters but increased number of treatment sessions should be considered. Noninvasive devices that carry low risk regardless of skin type such as mono-polar radiofrequency, high-intensity focused ultrasound, or cryolipolysis can be of particular advantage among Asians.

REFERENCES

1. Fink B, Neave N. The biology of facial beauty. *Int J Cosmet Sci.* 2005;27(6):317-325.
2. Samizadeh S, Wu W. Ideals of facial beauty amongst the Chinese population: Results from a large national survey. *Aesthetic Plast Surg.* 2020;44(4):1173-1183.
3. Chan IL, Cohen S, da Cunha MG, Maluf LC. Characteristics and management of Asian skin. *Int J Dermatol.* 2019;58(2):131-143.
4. McGrath C, Liu KS, Lam CW. Physiognomy and teeth: An ethnographic study among young and middle-aged Hong Kong adults. *Br Dent J.* 2002;192(9):522-525.
5. Le TT, Farkas LG, Ngim RC, Levin LS, Forrest CR. Proportionality in Asian and North American Caucasian faces using neoclassical facial canons as criteria. *Aesthetic Plast Surg.* 2002;26(1):64-69.
6. Liew S, Wu WTL, Chan HH, et al. Consensus on changing trends, attitudes, and concepts of Asian beauty. *Aesthetic Plast Surg.* 202;44(4):1186-1194.
7. Wu WTL, Liew S, Chan HH, et al. Consensus on current injectable treatment strategies in the Asian face. *Aesthetic Plast Surg.* 2020;44(4):1195-1207.
8. Tsukahara K, Fujimura T, Yoshida Y, et al. Comparison of age-related changes in wrinkling and sagging of the skin in Caucasian females and in Japanese females. *J Cosmet Sci.* 2004;55(4):351-371.
9. Nouveau-Richard S, Yang Z, Mac-Mary S, et al. Skin ageing: A comparison between Chinese and European populations. A pilot study. *J Dermatol Sci.* 2005;40(3):187-193.
10. Sykes JM. Management of the aging face in the Asian patient. *Facial Plast Surg Clin North Am.* 2007;15(3):353-360, vi-vii.
11. Shirakabe Y, Suzuki Y, Lam SM. A new paradigm for the aging Asian face. *Aesthetic Plast Surg.* 2003;27(5):397-402.
12. Talakoub L, Wesley NO. Differences in perceptions of beauty and cosmetic procedures performed in ethnic patients. *Semin Cutan Med Surg.* 2009;28(2):115-129.
13. Tzou CH, Giovanoli P, Ploner M, Frey M. Are there ethnic differences of facial movements between Europeans and Asians? *Br J Plast Surg.* 2005;58(2):183-195.
14. Kane MA. Commentary: Asian consensus recommendations on the aesthetic usage of botulinum toxin type A. *Dermatol Surg.* 2013;39(12):1861-1867.
15. Sundaram H, Huang PH, Hsu NJ, et al. Aesthetic applications of botulinum toxin A in Asians: An international, multidisciplinary, pan-Asian consensus. *Plast Reconstr Surg Glob Open.* 2016;4(12):e872.
16. Kim NH, Chung JH, Park RH, Park JB. The use of botulinum toxin type A in aesthetic mandibular contouring. *Plast Reconstr Surg.* 2005;115(3):919-930.

17. Cheng J, Hsu SH, McGee JS. Botulinum toxin injections for masseter reduction in East Asians. *Dermatol Surg.* 2019;45(4):566-572.

18. Kim NH, Park RH, Park JB. Botulinum toxin type A for the treatment of hypertrophy of the masseter muscle. *Plast Reconstr Surg.* 2010;125(6):1693-1705.

19. Yeh YT, Peng JH, Peng HP. Literature review of the adverse events associated with botulinum toxin injection for the masseter muscle hypertrophy. *J Cosmet Dermatol.* 2018;17(5):675-687.

20. Lee HJ, Kang IW, Seo KK, et al. The anatomical basis of paradoxical masseteric bulging after botulinum neurotoxin type A injection. *Toxins (Basel).* 2016;9(1):14.

21. Lee SJ, Kang JM, Kim YK, Park J, Kim DY. Paradoxical bulging of muscle after injection of botulinum neurotoxin type A into hypertrophied masseter muscle. *J Dermatol.* 2012;39(9):804-805.

22. Jeong SY, Park KY, Seok J, Ko EJ, Kim TY, Kim BJ. Botulinum toxin injection for contouring shoulder. *J Eur Acad Dermatol Venereol.* 2017;31(1):e46-e47.

23. Ahn BK, Kim YS, Kim HJ, Rho NK, Kim HS. Consensus recommendations on the aesthetic usage of botulinum toxin type A in Asians. *Dermatol Surg.* 2013;39(12):1843-1860.

24. Cheng J, Chung HJ, Friedland M, Hsu SH. Botulinum toxin injections for leg contouring in East Asians. *Dermatol Surg.* 2020;46(suppl 1):S62-S70.

25. Lee HJ, Lee DW, Park YH, Cha MK, Kim HS, Ha SJ. Botulinum toxin a for aesthetic contouring of enlarged medial gastrocnemius muscle. *Dermatol Surg.* 2004;30(6):867-871; discussion 871.

26. Han KH, Joo YH, Moon SE, Kim KH. Botulinum toxin A treatment for contouring of the lower leg. *J Dermatolog Treat.* 2006;17(4):250-254.

27. Bogari M, Tan A, Xin Y, et al. Treatment of gastrocnemius muscle hypertrophy with botulinum toxin injection followed by magnetic resonance imaging assessment and 3-dimensional evaluation. *Aesthet Surg J.* 2017;37(10):1146-1156.

28. Rho NK, Chang YY, Chao YY, et al. Consensus recommendations for optimal augmentation of the Asian face with hyaluronic acid and calcium hydroxylapatite fillers. *Plast Reconstr Surg.* 2015;136(5):940-956.

29. Seo KK. Nose. In: Carruthers J, Carruthers A, eds. *Soft Tissue Augmentation.* New York: Elsevier; 2012:112-122.

30. Moon HJ, Gao ZW, Hu ZQ, Wang H, Wang XJ. Expert consensus on hyaluronic acid filler facial injection for Chinese patients. *Plast Reconstr Surg Glob Open.* 2020;8(10):e3219.

31. Kung KY, Shek SY, Yeung CK, Chan HH. Evaluation of the safety and efficacy of the dual wavelength picosecond laser for the treatment of benign pigmented lesions in Asians. *Lasers Surg Med.* 2019;51(1):14-22.

32. Ho SG, Chan NPY, Yeung CK, Shek SY, Kono T, Chan HHL. A retrospective analysis of the management of freckles and lentigines using four different pigment lasers on Asian skin. *J Cosmet Laser Ther.* 2012;14(2):74-80.

33. Wanner M, Sakamoto FH, Avram MM, et al. Immediate skin responses to laser and light treatments: therapeutic endpoints: How to obtain efficacy. *J Am Acad Dermatol.* 2016;74(5):821-833; quiz 834, 833.

34. Wat H, Yee-Nam Shek S, Yeung CK, Chan HH. Efficacy and safety of picosecond 755-nm alexandrite laser with diffractive lens array for non-ablative rejuvenation in Chinese skin. *Lasers Surg Med.* 2019;51(1):8-13.

35. Chan HH, Manstein D, Yu CS, Shek S, Kono T, Wei WI. The prevalence and risk factors of post-inflammatory hyperpigmentation after fractional resurfacing in Asians. *Lasers Surg Med.* 2007;39(5):381-385.

36. Tan J, Lei Y, Ouyang HW, Gold MH. The use of the fractional CO2 laser resurfacing in the treatment of photoaging in Asians: Five years long-term results. *Lasers Surg Med.* 2014;46(10):750-756.

37. Chan NP, Ho SG, Yeung CK, Shek SY, Chan HH. The use of non-ablative fractional resurfacing in Asian acne scar patients. *Lasers Surg Med.* 2010;42(10):710-715.

38. Suh DH, Ahn HJ, Seo JK, Lee SJ, Shin MK, Song KY. Monopolar radiofrequency treatment for facial laxity: Histometric analysis. *J Cosmet Dermatol.* 2020;19(9):2317-2324.

39. Consensus recommendations for 4th generation nonmicroneedling monopolar radiofrequency for skin tightening: a Delphi consensus panel. *J Drugs Dermatol.* 2020;19(1):20-26.

40. Tan MG, Jo CE, Chapas A, Khetarpal S, Dover JS. Radiofrequency microneedling: A comprehensive and critical review. *Dermatol Surg.* 2021;47(6):755-761.

41. Suh DH, Shin MK, Lee SJ, Rho JH, et al. Intense focused ultrasound tightening in Asian skin: clinical and pathologic results. *Dermatol Surg.* 2011;37(11):1595-1602.

42. Friedmann DP, Bourgeois GP, Chan HHL, Zedlitz AC, Butterwick KJ. Complications from microfocused transcutaneous ultrasound: Case series and review of the literature. *Lasers Surg Med.* 2018;50(1):13-19.

43. Oh CH, Shim JS, Bae KII, Chang JH. Clinical application of cryolipolysis in Asian patients for subcutaneous fat reduction and body contouring. *Arch Plast Surg.* 2020;47(2):200.

44. Shek SY, Yeung CK, Chan JCY, Chan HHL. Efficacy of high-intensity focused ultrasonography for noninvasive body sculpting in Chinese patients. *Lasers Surg Med.* 2014;46(4):263-269.

45. Manuskiatti W, Nanchaipruek Y, Gervasio MK, Lektrakul N. Efficacy and safety of electrical multidirectional stimulation for abdominal contouring in Thai subjects with normal body mass index. *Dermatol Surg.* 2022;48(5):591-593.

46. Metzger KC, Crowley EL, Kadlubowska D, Gooderham MJ. Uncommon adverse effects of deoxycholic acid injection for submental fullness: Beyond the clinical trials. *J Cutan Med Surg.* 2020;24(6):619-624.

5

Populations of Hispanic/Latino Ancestry

Autumn L. Saizan, Mara Weinstein Velez, Maritza Perez

SUMMARY AND KEY FEATURES

- This chapter will discuss various skin conditions, cosmetic concerns, and appropriate treatments for Hispanic and Latino patients.
- As the United States becomes more diverse, understanding the unique dermatologic concerns of patients with skin of color, particularly those of Hispanic and Latino descent, is imperative.
- Education on the unique concerns and skin conditions amongst various racial and ethnic groups is important for avoiding adverse outcomes, increasing patient satisfaction, and optimizing aesthetic results in individuals of color.

- With respect to skin disorders, this chapter mainly focuses on disorders of hyperpigmentation, specifically postinflammatory hyperpigmentation, melasma, lichen planus pigmentosum, and erythema dyschromicum perstans.
- This chapter also discusses the properties of intrinsic and extrinsic aging, with specific emphasis on Hispanic and Latino populations as well as cosmetic treatments and procedures, including neuromodulators, topical depigmenting therapies, chemical peels, microdermabrasion, radio frequency, ultrasound, infrared devices, laser therapy, and fillers.

INTRODUCTION

As the United States becomes more diverse, understanding the unique dermatologic concerns of patients with skin of color is imperative. The United States Hispanic population is suspected to double over the next 40 years.[1] The term "Hispanic" refers to individuals whose place of birth, ancestry, heritage, nationality, and/or culture originate from Spanish-speaking countries, including Mexico, Cuba, Puerto Rico, Dominican Republic, and South and Central America.[2–4] It is important to recognize the various races and ethnicities, and thus skin types, that the Hispanic population encompasses. While the incidence of skin disease is equivalent between the Hispanic and general population,[5,6] there are several cutaneous disorders with increased prevalence amongst Hispanic and Latino patient populations, particularly those relating to pigmentary disorders.[5]

Dermatologists should recognize the unique psychosocial impact of certain disorders in relation to a patient's cultural, racial, and ethnic background. A degree of cultural competency is required when forming treatment plans. Additionally, dermatologists should be aware of the appropriate treatments with respect to patient skin type, as racial and ethnic differences may greatly influence clinical presentation as well as treatment options and outcomes. This chapter will discuss various skin conditions, cosmetic concerns, and appropriate treatments for Hispanic and Latino patients.

DISORDERS OF HYPERPIGMENTATION

Postinflammatory Hyperpigmentation
Introduction

Postinflammatory hyperpigmentation (PIH) is an acquired pigmentary disorder that may occur in all skin types but is most prevalent in patients of color.[7] PIH has a multitude of etiologies, all of which trigger an inflammatory response that subsequently results in hyperpigmentation of the affected skin. Common triggers include acne, infection, trauma, and procedures. The psychosocial impact of PIH seems to be greater in patients of color, particularly those of Hispanic and Latin descent.

Clinical Features

Patients present with dark brown to blue-gray macules and patches in areas of previous inflammation. The severity of hyperpigmentation depends on the inciting factor as well as the patient's skin type, in which those with darker skin types may present with a greater degree of hyperpigmentation.[7] PIH may be categorized into epidermal and dermal PIH. Epidermal PIH is characterized by dark brown macules and typically has a better prognosis and treatment response than dermal PIH. Dermal PIH, however, presents as blue to gray macules that are often more resistant to treatment, and in some

patients, may be permanent. Occasionally, patients present with a mixture of the two.

Pathogenesis and Etiology

The pathogenesis of postinflammatory hyperpigmentation is unclear. However, inflammation causing increased prostaglandins, leukotrienes, and thromboxanes likely results in local melanocyte stimulation with subsequent dispersion of melanocytes and increased melanin production.[7]

Treatment

PIH requires treatment of both the underlying cause and the associated hyperpigmentation. First-line treatments are limited to topical depigmenting products (see Table 5.1). Second- and third-line treatments include chemical peels (see Table 5.2) and laser therapy (see Table 5.3), respectively.[7] Chemical peels may be considered as monotherapy or as adjuvant therapy to topical depigmenting agents for patients who are refractory to topical products or who wish to achieve significant

TABLE 5.1	Topical Depigmenting Therapies
Treatment	**Mechanism of Action (MOA)**
Hydroquinone	• Inhibits tyrosinase enzyme • Melanocyte cytotoxicity
Retinoids	• Decrease tyrosinase activity • Melanosome transfer inhibition • Increased epidermal turnover
Azelaic Acid	• Dicarboxylic acid • Direct and indirect inhibitor of tyrosinase enzyme • Acts only on overactive melanocytes
Kojic Acid	• Inhibits tyrosinase enzyme by chelating copper at the active site
Mequinol	• Substrate for tyrosinase resulting in competitive inhibition
Arbutin	• Inhibits tyrosinase enzyme • Prevents melanosome maturation
Niacinamide	• Melanosome transfer inhibition
N-acetylglucosamine	• Prevents glycosylation of tyrosinase enzyme
Ascorbic acid (Vitamin C)	• Interferes with L-dopa to L-dopa-quinone conversion by interacting with copper • Reduces melanogenesis
Licorice	• Inhibits tyrosinase enzyme • Increases melanin dispersion
Soy	• Inhibits protease-activated 2 receptor and blocks keratinocyte uptake of melanosomes
Cysteamine	• Unclear MOA, known to facilitate intracellular production of glutathione, which is known to suppress melanogenesis through a variety of mechanisms

TABLE 5.2 Superficial Chemical Peels

Treatment	Mechanism of Action (MOA)
Salicylic Acid[40]	• Lipophilic properties • Desquamation/Increased exfoliation of superficial layers of epidermis • Keratolytic • Comedolytic • Reduction of sebum production • Antiinflammatory • Antibacterial • Neocollagenesis
Alpha Hydroxy Acids (Glycolic Acid, Lactic Acid)[40]	• Desquamation • Epidermolysis • Antiinflammatory • Antibacterial • Neocollagenesis • Increased dispersion of melanin in basal layer
Jessner's Solutions (salicylic acid + lactic acid + resorcinol)	• Refer to MOA of each ingredient
Retinol[32]	• Increased exfoliation of superficial layers of epidermis • Decreased tyrosinase activity resulting in decreased hyperpigmentation • Decreased matrix metalloproteinase (MMP) activity (collagenase) • Neocollagenesis

clinical improvement in a shorter period, as peels help to increase penetration and absorption, and thus efficacy, of topical depigmenting agents (see Fig. 5.1). For skin of color, particularly those with skin types III-VI, superficial chemical peels, which are limited to the papillary dermis, are preferred.[7,8] Medium or deep chemical peels should be avoided in patients with skin of color. (See "Chemical Peels" under "Cosmetic Treatments and Procedures") Laser therapy for PIH should generally be reserved for recalcitrant cases due to risk of dyschromia.[5] (See "Laser Therapy" under "Cosmetic Treatments and Procedures") Regardless of the treatment modality, however, adequate sunscreen with SPF 30 or higher and additional sun protective measures are essential to preventing new or worsening hyperpigmentation.[7]

Melasma

Introduction

Melasma is one of the most common acquired pigmentary disorders in patients of color. It has an increased prevalence amongst women of child-bearing age, particularly those that are Fitzpatrick skin types III-VI.[9,10] The exact prevalence of melasma within the Hispanic population is unknown.[11,12] Based on previous reports, prevalence may range from 8.2%[6,11] to 8.8%.[13] Another study found a prevalence as high as 66% amongst Mexican women during pregnancy.[12] There are several contributing factors to the development of melasma including both ultraviolet and visible light exposure, hormones, particularly the hyperestrogenic state of pregnancy, and genetics.[10,14] Depending on geographic location, there are several names for melasma in the Spanish language. In Mexico, the word for melasma is "paño," while in Central or South America the word is "manchas" or "mascara del embarzo," which translate to "stains" and "mask of pregnancy," respectively.[12]

Clinical Features

Patients present with asymptomatic, ill-defined, often symmetric, light to dark brown patches on sun-exposed areas of the face.[4,9] Hyperpigmented, reticulated patches commonly affect the centrofacial region, including the cheeks, nose, forehead, upper lip, and chin. The malar region followed by the mandibular region is less common.[11] Extra-facial melasma is another rare presentation.[11] Time of onset may be influenced by underlying skin type, in which those with lighter skin have an earlier onset than those with darker skin.[9] Melasma is often characterized as epidermal, dermal, or mixed hyperpigmentation.[11]

Quality of Life. Many patients presenting with melasma will report a reduced quality of life. There are a few health-related quality of life indices designed to assess the psychosocial impact of skin disease, including Skindex-16 and Melasma Quality of Life (MELAS-QOL). MELASQOL is a validated scale that is useful for identifying the areas of life most affected by melasma and quantifying the severity of its negative psychosocial impact. In 2006, Dominguez et al., translated the MELASQOL to Spanish (Sp-MELASQOL) and modified it so that it would integrate well with any version of

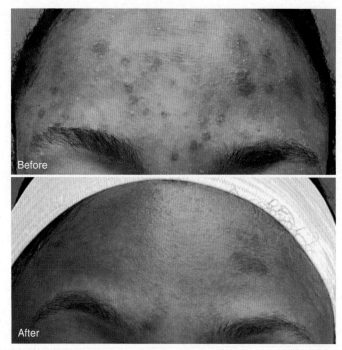

Fig. 5.1 Postinflammatory hyperpigmentation secondary to acne in a young Fitzpatrick skin type V female, demonstrating notable improvement with topical lightening agents and six chemical peels.

the Spanish language. Dominguez et al., reported significantly higher Sp-MELASQOL scores, and thus a reduced quality of life, amongst those with lower education, a longer duration of disease, and those who previously sought treatment.[12] Previous reports in the literature document increased anxiety and depression, decreased social engagement, and low self-esteem amongst patients with melasma.[15] It is important to understand the psychosocial stressors of melasma amongst patients with skin of color, given its increased prevalence in more darkly pigmented skin.[15] Clinicians, particularly those with large Spanish-speaking patient populations, should consider using the Sp-MELASQOL to monitor the psychosocial impact of disease in their melasma patients.

Pathogenesis and Etiology

The exact pathogenesis of melasma is unknown. Ultraviolet (UV) light, visible light, near-infrared regions, and hormones such as estrogen and progesterone are proposed to trigger the development of melasma in genetically predisposed individuals. While all spectral regions of the solar radiation cause upregulation of melanogenesis via the activation of reactive oxygen species as well as keratinocytes and fibroblasts,[11] certain components of the spectrum have been shown to have a greater effect on skin types IV-V.[16] A previous study found that a majority of free radicals produced in Fitzpatrick skin types IV–V were induced by visible light plus near-infrared regions, while a majority of free radicals in skin type II were produced by UV radiation.[16] Given the higher content of eumelanin in skin of color, the decreased production of UV-induced free radicals is expected.[16] Such differences in sensitivity to solar radiation, however, may suggest that individuals with skin types IV–VI require an additional form of sun protection compared to their skin type I-III counterparts. Sebocytes and increased vascularity may also play a role in pathophysiology.[9] With respect to hormones, recent literature suggest they may play less of a role in pathogenesis than previously thought. Recent observations note that melasma occurs in up to 10% of postmenopausal women and can progress even after the cessation of oral contraceptives.[9] With respect to genetic predisposition, a family history of melasma may be present in 55% to 64% of affected individuals. It is likely certain genes influence the pigmentary, hormonal, inflammatory, and vascular responses associated with melasma development. Additionally, those with Fitzpatrick skin types IV or higher are more likely to have a positive family history compared to those with lighter skin types.[11]

Prognosis and Treatment

Melasma is a benign, asymptomatic pigmentary disorder. Without treatment, melasma may persist throughout life. Treatment for melasma is similar to that of PIH, with first-line treatments limited to strict sun protection and topical depigmenting agents followed by chemical peels and laser therapy as second and third line, respectively (See "Cosmetic Treatments and Procedures"). It is important to note that there has been reported benefit of combined therapy with topical depigmented agents, specifically hydroquinone (HQ) and oral tranexamic acid (TA).[17] Arreola et al., reports a 49% decrease in Sp-MELASQOL score amongst patients on combined therapy with 4% HQ compared to 29%

decrease with oral TA alone.[17] Patients should avoid potential triggers, such as UV exposure (see Figs. 5.2, 5.3, 5.4(A), and 5.4(B)).

Lichen Planus Pigmentosus
Introduction

Lichen planus pigmentosus (LPP), a variant of lichen planus, is a pigmentary disorder commonly affecting middle-aged individuals, particularly those Fitzpatrick skin type III and above.[18] It is more prevalent in females.[18] Associations with hepatitis C, autoimmune diseases, and endocrinopathies have been reported. LPP may also occur after contact with various topical products, including mustard oil, henna, alma oil, nickel, and hair dye.[18] While typically asymptomatic, LPP can greatly affect quality of life.

Clinical Features

LPP presents as dark brown to gray, irregularly defined, round or oval macules and patches in sun-exposed areas

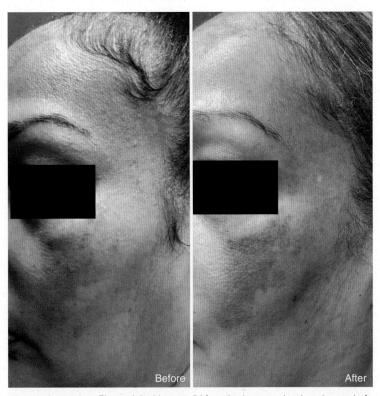

Fig. 5.2 Refractory melasma in a Fitzpatrick skin type IV female that remained unchanged after 6 months of topical lightening agents and a series of picosecond laser therapy.

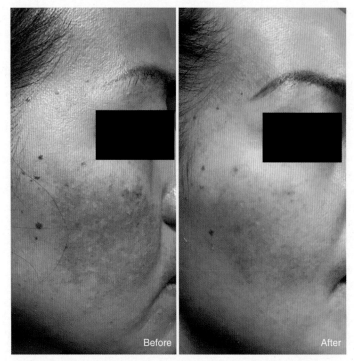

Before   After

Fig. 5.3 Melasma in a Fitzpatrick skin type IV female demonstrating notable improvement with topical lightening agents, oral tranexamic acid, and resurfacing therapy using the 1927-nm nonablative fractional diode laser.

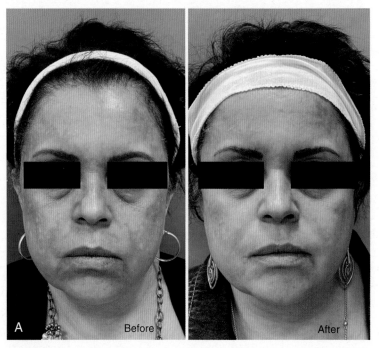

A   Before   After

Fig. 5.4 (A) and (B) Melasma in Fitzpatrick skin type III female demonstrating notable improvement after two months of topical lightening agents and sunscreen alone.

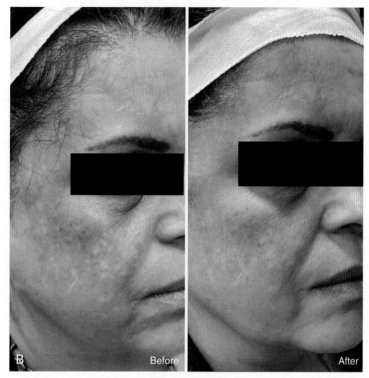

Fig. 5.4, cont'd

of the face and neck, particularly the temporal and peri-auricular regions. The arms are more commonly affected than the legs or trunk. Individuals with lighter skin types present with violaceous or maroon macules and patches. Lesions may increase in size and coalesce over time.[18]

Pathogenesis and Etiology

LPP is likely caused by an altered cellular immune response involving CD8+ T cells that recognize and destroy epidermal keratinocytes. Eventually, the inflammatory infiltrate resolves, resulting in dermal pigment incontinence that may persist for several months to years. CD4+ T cells and Langerhans cells may also be involved in the inflammatory response. Sun exposure, hormones, particularly in women undergoing menopause, hepatitis C, topical use and consumption of various products, and environmental pollution can all trigger LPP.[18]

Prognosis and Treatment

LPP can persists for months to years and may have an unpredictable course, sometimes spontaneously resolving without treatment. Other patients may experience relapses after treatment. Currently, there is no gold standard therapy and response to treatment is often gradual.[18] Treatment options should include avoidance of triggers and sun protection. Topical therapies include medium to high potency corticosteroids, tacrolimus, and various topical depigmenting agents (see Table 5.1). Of the topical therapies, tacrolimus remains the most used. Some patients benefit from systemic treatments, including steroids, dapsone, or isotretinoin as well as laser therapy.[18]

Erythema Dyschromicum Perstans
Introduction

Erythema dyschromicum perstans (EDP), sometimes referred to as ashy dermatosis, is an asymptomatic pigmentary disorder with increased prevalence in Central and South America. It was first described by Oswaldo Ramirez in El Salvador as "Los Cenicientos," which translates to the "ashen ones" and describes the ash-colored, gray macules commonly seen.[19] Later in Venezuela, Convit officially referred to this clinical presentation as "erythema dyschromicum perstans."[20]

Some clinicians debate whether EDP and ashy dermatosis are the same clinical entity, although most agree they are identical. EDP is common in individuals Fitzpatrick skin type III–V, particularly women in their second decade of life. EDP can cause significant psychosocial distress.[19]

Clinical Features

EDP presents as symmetric, ashy to blue-gray macules and patches involving the neck, face, upper extremities, and trunk. Lesions gradually progress, with many starting at roughly three millimeters, later increasing in size and coalescing. Some lesions have a peripheral, occasionally palpable, erythematous border, usually in the early stages of the disease as well as associated pruritus and scaling.[19] The erythematous border may be difficult to appreciate depending on the patient's phototype.

Pathogenesis and Etiology

The pathogenesis is unknown. A multitude of etiologies and predisposing factors have been proposed. This includes various infections, such as human immunodeficiency virus, hepatitis C, or enterovirus; various drugs, such as ethambutol, fluoxetine, or omeprazole; environmental insults, such as oral intake of ammonium nitrate or X-ray contrast medium; and finally, genetic factors, with one study reporting HLA-DR4 allele as a risk factor in Mexican mestizos.[19]

Prognosis and Treatment

EDP has a gradual, persistent, but asymptomatic course.[19] The clinical course often persists throughout life in adults, although some experience spontaneous remission. While there are no defined first-line treatments, a variety of topical and/or systemic treatments have proven beneficial. Topical therapies include steroids, hydroquinone, tretinoin, and calcineurin inhibitors. Systemic treatments include dapsone, minocycline, tranexamic acid, macrolides, and vitamin A.[21] Light therapy, picosecond laser treatments, and nonablative fractional laser therapy used in conjunction with topical 0.1% tacrolimus have also proven beneficial (see Fig. 5.5).

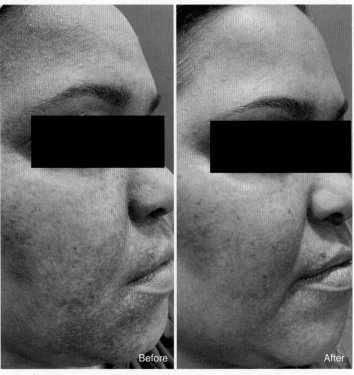

Fig. 5.5 Erythema dyschromicum perstans in Fitzpatrick V female demonstrating improvement with oral hydroxychloroquine, two topical nonsteroidal antiinflammatory agents, two treatment sessions with the picosecond laser, and two treatments with the pulse-dye laser.

COSMETIC CONCERNS

INTRODUCTION

Anatomic features, aging, and aesthetic preferences vary with patient race, ethnicity, and skin type.[4] Such variation exists just within the Hispanic population alone, in which individuals may share features with those of Asian, Northern European, and/or African descent.[2] For example, Hispanic patients with Central or South American ancestry may have facial features that are more similar to White individuals. This is in contrast to those of Caribbean ancestry who are more likely to have features observed in Black or African American individuals.[2,22,23] Previous reports, however, state that common Hispanic facial features include a broad, round face with a prominent midface as well as heavy eyelids, a shortened nasal length with a broad nasal bridge, increased width between the zygomatic processes, prominent maxillary regions, and slightly recessive chins.[2,4,22] There are few reports discussing the lip measurements of Hispanic/Latino populations, although they appear to be larger and more protrusive when compared to their White counterparts.[24] While this is preferred amongst most Hispanic/Latino populations, physicians should always account for ethnic variation.[24]

With respect to facial aging, Hispanic/Latino individuals tend to exhibit signs of aging before their Black counterparts, but after their White counterparts. Such differences, however, are greatly attributed to variation in skin phototype. Overall, Hispanic women do not demonstrate advanced signs of aging, including rhytides and facial sagging, until the fifth and sixth decades of life, respectively.[25] Earlier signs of aging in the fourth decade of life in the Hispanic/Latino population, particularly those skin phototypes V/VI, is typically limited to the nasolabial folds.[25] Dermatologists should acknowledge and be well versed in the racial and ethnic variances of cosmetic preferences and aging.

AGING

Aging occurs through several mechanisms, both intrinsic and extrinsic. Intrinsic, or chronologic aging, refers to those processes that are determined by genetics, anatomic structure, hormones, and race/ethnicity, while extrinsic aging refers to maturation secondary to environmental processes including gravity, ultraviolet exposure, and lifestyle.[2] Visible signs of aging include increased fine lines, deep furrowing and wrinkling, and dyspigmentation.[26]

Intrinsic Aging

Sun-protected, intrinsically aged skin tends to be thinner, finely wrinkled with less elasticity, fat atrophy, increased soft tissue distribution, and more even pigmentation compared to those with photoaged skin.[22,27] There are several changes that occur on a microscopic level during the aging process. This includes thinning of the epidermis, along with a decrease in lipid and water content as well as blood vessels, sweat glands, collagen, and elastic fibers.[2] Intrinsic aging is characterized by decreased cellular metabolism, particularly decreased cell replication and increased cellular senescence.[26]

Genetics

A study conducted by Kimball et al., demonstrated the relationship between gene expression and visible aging.[26] Genes involved in epidermal structure and barrier function as well as various molecular processes, such as cellular metabolism, DNA repair, cell replication, chromatin remodeling, and response to oxidative stress, all influence intrinsic aging.[26] In this study, White women ages 20 to 74 were found to have various levels of gene expression.[26] $CDH1$, $DSC3$, and $LAMA5$ are three examples of genes related to epidermal structure and barrier function. $CDH1$ and $DSC3$ are critical for cell–cell junctions in the epidermis, while $LAMA5$ ensures attachment of keratinocytes to the basement membrane. The level of expression varies with age, with older women or older-appearing skin more likely to have decreased expression of these genes.[26] Genes associated with cellular metabolism include but are not limited to $COX7A2L$, required for mitochondrial respirasome assembly and estrogen-stimulated energy production; $GLUD1$, required for energy homeostasis and glutamate and nitrogen metabolism; and $NKRK1$ and $PANK4$, required for the synthesis of energy cofactor. Any decrease in these genes involving cellular metabolism ultimately results in visible signs of aging.[26] Finally, genes involved in cell senescence, specifically $CDKN2A$, are expected to have increased expression in photoexposed skin. $CDK2NA$ codes for several proteins, including $p16^{INK4A}$, which decreases cell replication and induces cell senescence.[26] To further emphasize the influence of genes on age-related changes, Kimball et al., notes the presence of 2100 epidermal genes involved in skin appearance and age-related changes.[26]

It is important to note that visible appearance is not always concordant with chronological age.[26] Similar to their younger counterparts, older women with a more youthful appearance had higher expression of certain genes associated with appearance and aging, specifically those involved cellular metabolism and mitochondrial function, despite being chronologically older.[26] The generalizability of this study is limited and further investigation of intrinsic aging within the skin of color population is needed.[26] Previous reports in the literature, however, note that individuals of color experience the sequalae of intrinsic aging to a lesser degree and often a decade later than their White counterparts.[22,25]

Hormones

Hormones play a role in skin aging, particularly amongst women, in which estrogen is suspected to influence collagen synthesis as well as keratinocyte and fibroblast activity. Postmenopausal women are at increased risk for rhytides and skin laxity. There are several other hormones that contribute to intrinsic aging including, but not limited to, melatonin, cortisol, and insulin-like growth factor.[2]

Structural Aging

Rhytides. Rhytides, or wrinkles, occur secondary to reduction and degradation of collagen and elastic fibers. Rhytides occur primarily in areas with repetitive muscle activation, such as the periorbital and perioral regions. Reduced elasticity promotes sagging of excess skin, especially along the bilateral cheeks, specifically the jowl, as well as the nasolabial folds and submental region.[2] Dermal atrophy further contributes to the development of rhytides. Skin thickness, however, is directly proportional to skin pigmentation, with individuals of color more likely to have greater lipid content and cornified layers of the epidermis.[22] These additional layers of the stratum corneum are often more tightly compact with increased cellular adhesion.[25] Additionally, darker-skinned individuals typically have a greater number of fibroblasts that are larger and more active.[25] Finally, the collagen bundles are usually arranged parallel to the overlying epidermis.[25] Cobo and Garcia refer to the heavier, thicker, and often more oily skin seen in Hispanic individuals as the "soft-tissue envelope."[23] As the skin-soft tissue envelope loses elasticity, the skin begins to sag and look heavier. The appearance of wrinkles in those with robust soft-tissue envelopes remains minimal.[23]

Loss of Volume. Volume loss is the result of fat atrophy and redistribution within the hypodermis. It commonly occurs along the lateral portions of the face, including the chin, cheeks, and temples. Sagging of these areas exaggerates the nasolabial folds (See Video 5.1).[2] Bone resorption and atrophy, especially along the maxilla and mandible, further accentuates these findings. There may also eyebrow and eyelid sagging, hooding of the eyelids, herniation of the lower eyelid fat pads, and hollowing and darkening of the infraorbital region.[22] Older individuals present with a narrow forehead, decreased facial length, and increased facial width.[2]

Extrinsic Aging
Photoaging/Photodamage

Ultraviolet exposure leads to the production of reactive oxygen species and subsequent cellular damage.[26,27] Ultraviolet radiation degrades elastic fibers and collagen, promoting rhytides and skin laxity. Nonfunctional elastin and unorganized collagen fibril structures is commonly referred to as solar elastosis and is more common in photodamaged skin versus non-photoexposed, intrinsically aged skin.[26] Hyperpigmentation, xerosis, telangiectasias, and keratosis also occur secondary to sun exposure. Photodamage to cutaneous blood vessels can also damage nutritional supply to the skin and cause thinning.[2]

Photoaging and Skin of Color. Skin color and melanin content influence the degree of photodamage and subsequent photoaging, with darker individuals less susceptible to the effects of ultraviolet radiation.[2] Melanocyte-stimulating hormone and associated DNA repair is increased in darker skin types, leading to increased protection from UV exposure. In a multinational survey study, Black women reported the less severe and later onset in signs of photoaging compared to White women. Hispanic and Asian individuals demonstrated intermediate severity.[25] Skin phototype, however, is the best predictor for onset and severity of photomaturation. Photomaturation may occur as early as the fourth decade of life amongst White individuals but not until the fifth and sixth decades of life amongst skin of color.[4,25]

Amongst Hispanic women, the first signs of aging are limited to the nasolabial folds and occur in the

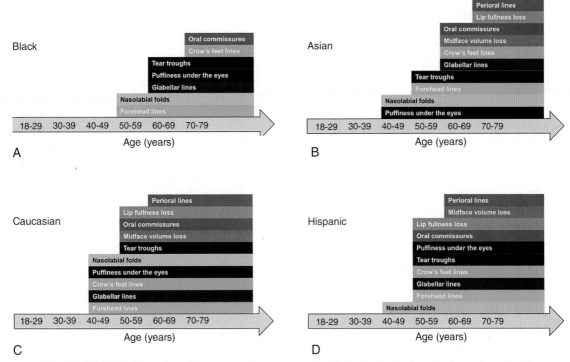

Fig. 5.6 (A)–(D) In this series of bar graphs from a study by Alexis et al., the decade of age (organized by 10-year age cohorts) by which certain signs of aging appeared in 30% or more women is categorized by race/ethnicity, specifically (A) Black, (B) Asian, (C) Caucasian, and (D) Hispanic. In (A), it is noted that less than 30% of Black women reported perioral lines, loss of lip fullness, or midface volume loss even by the seventh decade of life. *(From Alexis AF, Grimes P, Boyd C, et al. Racial and ethnic differences in self-assessed facial aging in women: Results from a multinational study. Dermatologic Surgery. 2019;45(12):1635-1648.)*

fourth decade of life.[25] It is not until they reach the fifth decade of life that more advanced signs of aging, including forehead lines, glabellar lines, and crow's feet along with formation of tear troughs, undereye puffiness, oral commissures, and loss of lip fullness, begin to appear.[25] Finally, in the sixth decade of life, Hispanic women tend to exhibit mid-facial volume loss and perioral line formation.[25] Each of these signs of aging occur a decade later in Black women, while some occur a decade earlier in White women (see Figure 5.6).[25]

COSMETIC TREATMENTS AND PROCEDURES

INTRODUCTION

Understanding and addressing the cosmetic concerns of various racial and ethnic groups is important for avoiding adverse outcomes, increasing patient satisfaction, and optimizing aesthetic results in individuals of color. The cosmetic industry has developed significantly over the recent years and racial and ethnic minorities are seeking cosmetic treatments at an increasing rate. In the last decade, there has been a 52% increase in the number of Hispanic/Latino individuals receiving cosmetic treatment. This population has also remained the largest racial and ethnic minority patient population to receive neuromodulator and dermal filler treatments over the last five years.[28] A survey study looking to identify the unique cosmetic concerns of the Hispanic/Latino population found that the areas of most concern were periorbital rhytides and the undereye region, forehead rhytides, and the submental region. Concerns regarding the submental region may be related to the increased prevalence of recessive chins in the Hispanic population. The survey also found decreased interest in injectable therapy, possibly highlighting a need for patient education on treatment options within this population.[28] Various reports in the literature highlight the importance of catering to the patient's predominant phenotype, unique anatomy and facial structure, skin phototype, and personal goals to develop the most appropriate, patient-centered treatment plan.[28]

Neuromodulators

Neuromodulators treat and prevent rhytides. Commonly involved areas include the forehead and glabellar lines, the periorbital region or crow's feet, and the perioral region.[29,30] Hispanic/Latino women receiving neurotoxin injections are in their fifties and are more likely to treat the entire face, while men typically limit treatment to the upper face.[30] Currently, onabotulinumtoxinA and abobotulinumtoxinA remain the only two FDA-approved neuromodulators for cosmetic use. The injection sites, injection techniques, dosing, and potential adverse outcomes remain the same across all ethnic groups.[29]

Topical Depigmenting Therapies

See Table 5.1.

Chemical Peels

Chemical peels, while effective for evening pigmentation and texture, should be used with caution in darker skin types. Superficial peels are safe for patients of color. Superficial peels include salicylic acid, alpha hydroxy acids, and Jessner's[31,32] (see Table 5.2). Medium, trichloroacetic acid, and deep phenol peels should be avoided in skin of color due to increased risk of dyspigmentation and scarring. Clinicians can start patients on hydroquinone and tretinoin 2 to 4 weeks prior to the peel to reduce the risk of hyperpigmentation. Additionally, adequate sun protection in the weeks leading up to the procedure is crucial to reducing risk of dyspigmentation, especially amongst those with darker skin types who have the misconception they do not require sunscreen.[32] Some patients may consider mineral sunscreens, although the white residue makes them a less desirable option for many patients of color.[4]

Microdermabrasion

Microdermabrasion is a minimally invasive negative pressure system used for epidermal resurfacing and to treat postinflammatory hyperpigmentation, melasma, uneven skin texture, and scarring. Microdermabrasion involves abrasive, usually aluminum hydroxide, crystals to resurface and exfoliate the skin. This results in a new epidermal layer and is reportedly safe in all Fitzpatrick skin types, although decreasing the power settings for patients with darker skin types is recommended.[29]

Radio Frequency, Ultrasound, Infrared Devices

Radiofrequency, microfocused ultrasound, and infrared therapies spare the epidermis and have proven to be safe and effective for increasing elasticity in ethnic skin.[29,32] These "skin-tightening devices" penetrate the deep dermis, promoting collagen breakdown, contraction, and remodeling. Some devices have additional features that include cooling effects, vacuum, or ultrasound. Side effects include temporary pain, swelling, and/or erythema.[32]

Laser Therapy

Specific laser and light therapies are useful for evening texture and pigmentation in skin of color. Laser therapy previously had limited use in ethnic skin, particularly those Fitzpatrick skin type IV or higher, due to an increased risk of hyperpigmentation, hypopigmentation, or scarring (see Fig. 5.7).[32] With the appropriate laser device and the correct wavelengths and parameters, however, laser therapy may be used in any Fitzpatrick skin type.[33,34] A previous study conducted by Leal-Silva et al., revealed that palmar and digital creases may help predict the risk of postinflammatory hyperpigmentation, specifically amongst those of Hispanic descent, who possess a wide range of skin phototypes.[35] Palmar and digital creases were categorized into levels zero to three, with the higher number representing a darker tissue response.[33,35,36] Clinical trials in darker skin types report optimal patient outcomes with longer wavelengths, low pulse duration, low fluence with increased time for cooling, and decreased treatment density.[32-34] There are several lasers that are useful amongst Latino individuals with skin of color (see Table 5.3).

Fillers

Dermal fillers restore facial balance after fat atrophy, collagen loss, and bone remodeling (see Videos 5.1 and 5.2). Midfacial aging involving the malar fat pads, infraorbital rim, tear troughs, and nasolabial folds tend to be the areas of most concern amongst Hispanic patients.

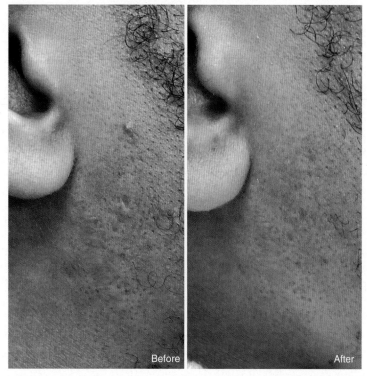

Before   After

Fig. 5.7 Scar along the right cheek of a Fitzpatrick skin type IV male demonstrating notable improvement in pigmentation and texture one month after four treatments of picosecond fractionated laser therapy.

TABLE 5.3 Laser Therapies for Skin of Color

Laser Therapies	Additional Comments
Radiofrequency Microneedling	Safe in skin of color, particularly for those with acne scarring
Picosecond	Can be useful for hyperpigmentation, safe in mixed skin as there is no emission of heat
Potassium Titanyl Phosphate (KTP)	
Intense Pulsed Light (IPL)	Extreme caution should be exercised with IPL in darker skin, starting with very low energies and possibly a test spot
Pulse-dye	Useful at low fluences for rosacea and vascular change
Diode	Can treat individuals up to Fitzpatrick skin type (FST) IV
Nd:YAG	Can treat individuals up to FST VI
Ablative	Limited use in FST V or VI due to increased risk for dyschromia and scarring
Ablative Fractional Lasers	Few reports documenting their safety and efficacy in darker skin types
Nonablative Fractional Lasers	Lower treatment densities recommended to reduce risk of PIH in FST IV-VI
Nonablative	Safer in darker skin types, as it does not remove epidermal layer

Additionally, increased subcutaneous tissue with decreased skeletal support amongst those with darker skin may further contribute to increased facial drooping.[29] Consequently, structural aging seems to be of greater concern to individuals of color compared to fine lines and wrinkling, thus emphasizing the utility of dermal fillers in skin of color.[37] Clinical studies have reported positive results with hyaluronic acid (temporary), calcium hydroxyapatite (semi-temporary), poly-L-lactic acid (semi-temporary), and polymethyl-methacrylate (permanent) fillers amongst patients of color.[37] One author notes a preference for poly-L-lactic acid for skeletal and soft-tissue loss and hyaluronic acid products to refine or augment facial contuor.[30] Additional therapies include autologous fat transfers and human collagen.[29] Of particular concern in the SOC population is dyspigmentation, hypertrophic scarring, and/or keloid formation.[32,37] Few studies report temporary dyspigmentation. There have been no reports of hypertrophic scarring or keloid formation secondary to filler injections.[32,37] Nevertheless, providers can reduce the number of injections using a linear or fanning technique to reduce postinjection erythema and postinflammatory hyperpigmentation.[32,34,37] A study conducted by Taylor et al., found that 2% of patients experience postinjection hyperpigmentation after using a linear threading technique compared to 13% of patients who underwent serial punctures.[32,38] Additional consideration is the use of a cannula versus a needle, as the cannula is less likely to cause bruising.[32] Persistent postinjection erythema is treated with topical corticosteroids, which also help prevent postinflammatory hyperpigmentation.[37] Other complications of filler include soft tissue necrosis, blindness, and stroke.[39]

Cheek Augmentation

Dermal fillers injected into subcutaneous and supraperiosteal sites help augment the zygomaticomalar region, anterior malar fat pads, and the submalar region. They also reduce the appearance of the nasolabial folds and tear troughs. Some patients experience therapeutic effects up to 2 years post-treatment. Clinicians should be careful not to inject the filler superficially to avoid bluish tinting of the skin, a result of the Tyndall effect. Hyaluronidase may be used to address the blue discoloration if the patient was treated with hyaluronic acid fillers.[39]

Chin Augmentation

Coralline calcium hydroxyapatite is commonly used to augment the maxilla and mandibular region.[39]

Facial Fat Transplantation

Autologous fat, usually from the thighs or anterior abdomen, injected subcutaneously or supraperiostally can augment and add volume to the nasolabial, malar, and submalar regions.[39]

CONCLUSION

As the Hispanic/Latino population continues to increase, understanding the unique clinical manifestations, cosmetic concerns, and treatment options for this demographic is crucial to achieving positive health outcomes and excellence in patient care.

REFERENCES

1. Vespa J, Medina L, Armstrong DM. *Demographic Turning Points for the United States: Population Projections for 2020 to 2060.* The United States Census Bureau; 2018. Available at: https://www.census.gov/library/publications/2020/demo/p25-1144.html. Accessed November 29, 2020.
2. Venkatesh S, Maymone MBC, Vashi NA. Aging in skin of color. *Clin Dermatol.* 2019;37(4):351-357. doi:10.1016/j.clindermatol.2019.04.010.
3. *Hispanic Origin.* The United States Census Bureau. Available at: https://www.census.gov/topics/population/hispanic-origin.html. Accessed January 31, 2021.
4. Talakoub L, Wesley NO. Differences in perceptions of beauty and cosmetic procedures performed in ethnic patients. *Semin Cutan Med Surg.* 2009;28(2):115-129. doi:10.1016/j.sder.2009.05.001.
5. Hexsel D, Arellano I, Rendon M. Ethnic considerations in the treatment of Hispanic and Latin-American patients with hyperpigmentation. *Br J Dermatol.* 2006;156(suppl 1):7-12. Available at: https://doi.org/10.1111/j.1365-2133.2006.07589.x.
6. Sanchez MR. Cutaneous diseases in Latinos. *Dermatol Clin.* 2003;21(4):689-697. doi:10.1016/S0733-8635(03)00087-1.
7. Davis EC, Callender VD. Postinflammatory hyperpigmentation. *J Clin Aesthetic Dermatol.* 2010;3(7):20-31. PMID: 20725554; PMCID: PMC2921758.
8. Castillo DE, Keri JE. Chemical peels in the treatment of acne: patient selection and perspectives. *Clin Cosmet Investig Dermatol.* 2018;11:365-372. doi:10.2147/CCID.S137788.

9. Passeron T, Picardo M. Melasma, a photoaging disorder. *Pigment Cell Melanoma Res.* 2018;31(4):461-465. doi:10.1111/pcmr.12684.

10. Hexsel D, Lacerda DA, Cavalcante AS, et al. Epidemiology of melasma in Brazilian patients: a multicenter study. *Int J Dermatol.* 2014;53(4):440-444. doi:10.1111/j.1365-4632.2012.05748.x.

11. Ogbechie-Godec OA, Elbuluk N. Melasma: An up-to-date comprehensive review. *Dermatol Ther.* 2017;7(3): 305-318. doi:10.1007/s13555-017-0194-1.

12. Dominguez AR, Balkrishnan R, Ellzey AR, Pandya AG. Melasma in Latina patients: Cross-cultural adaptation and validation of a quality-of-life questionnaire in Spanish language. *J Am Acad Dermatol.* 2006;55(1):59-66. doi:10.1016/j.jaad.2006.01.049.

13. Werlinger KD. Prevalence of self-diagnosed melasma among premenopausal Latino women in Dallas and Fort Worth, Texas. *Arch Dermatol.* 2007;143(3):423. doi:10.1001/archderm.143.3.424.

14. Pérez M, Sánchez JL, Aguiló F. Endocrinologic profile of patients with idiopathic melasma. *J Invest Dermatol.* 1983;81(6):543-545. doi:10.1111/1523-1747. ep12522896.

15. Pawaskar MD, Parikh P, Markowski T, Mcmichael AJ, Feldman SR, Balkrishnan R. Melasma and its impact on health-related quality of life in Hispanic women. *J Dermatol Treat.* 2007;18(1):5-9. doi:10.1080/ 09546630601028778.

16. Albrecht S, Jung S, Müller R, et al. Skin type differences in solar-simulated radiation-induced oxidative stress. *Br J Dermatol.* 2019;180(3):597-603. doi:10.1111/ bjd.17129.

17. Arreola Jauregui IE, Huerta Rivera G, Soria Orozco M, et al. A cross-sectional report on melasma among Hispanic patients: Evaluating the role of oral tranexamic acid versus oral tranexamic acid plus hydroquinone. *J Am Acad Dermatol.* 2020;83(5):1457-1458. doi:10.1016/ j.jaad.2020.02.072.

18. Robles-Méndez JC, Rizo-Frías P, Herz-Ruelas ME, Pandya AG. Lichen planus pigmentosus and its variants: Review and update. *Int J Dermatol.* 2018;57(5):505-514. doi:10.1111/ijd.13806.

19. Correa MC, Memije EV, Vargas-Alarcón G, et al. HLA-DR association with the genetic susceptibility to develop ashy dermatosis in Mexican Mestizo patients. *J Am Acad Dermatol.* 2007;56(4):617-620. doi:10.1016/j. jaad.2006.08.062.

20. Numata T, Harada K, Tsuboi R, Mitsuhashi Y. Erythema dyschromicum perstans: Identical to ashy dermatosis or not? *Case Rep Dermatol.* 2015;7(2):146-150. doi:10.1159/000437414.

21. Amatya B. Ashy dermatosis: A comprehensive review. *Our Dermatol Online.* 2017;8(2):143-148. doi:10.7241/ ourd.20172.39.

22. Vashi NA, Buainain De Castro Maymone M, Kundu RV. Aging differences in ethnic skin. *J Clin Aesthetic Dermatol.* 2016;9(1):31-38. PMID: 26962390; PMCID: PMC4756870.

23. Cobo R, García CA. Aesthetic surgery for the Mestizo/ Hispanic patient: Special considerations. *Facial Plast Surg.* 2010;26(02):164-173. doi: 10.1055/s-0030-1253502

24. Kollipara R, Walker B, Sturgeon A. Lip measurements and preferences in Asians and Hispanics: A brief review. *J Clin Aesthet Dermatol.* 2017;10(11):19-21. PMID: 29399256; PMCID: PMC5774906.

25. Alexis AF, Grimes P, Boyd C, et al. Racial and ethnic differences in self-assessed facial aging in women: Results from a multinational study. *Dermatol Surg.* 2019;45(12):1635-1648. doi:10.1097/DSS. 0000000000002237.

26. Kimball AB, Alora-Palli MB, Tamura M, et al. Age-induced and photoinduced changes in gene expression profiles in facial skin of Caucasian females across 6 decades of age. *J Am Acad Dermatol.* 2018;78(1):29-39.e7. doi:10.1016/j.jaad.2017.09.012.

27. Fisher GJ, Kang S, Varani J, et al. Mechanisms of photoaging and chronological skin aging. *Arch Dermatol.* 2002;138(11):1462-1470. doi:10.1001/archderm. 138.11.1462.

28. Fabi S, Faad VB. Understanding the female Hispanic and Latino American facial aesthetic patient. *J Drugs Dermatol.* 2019;18(7):623-632. PMID: 31329400.

29. Davis EC, Callender VD. Aesthetic dermatology for aging ethnic skin. *Dermatol Surg.* 2011;37(7):901-917. doi:10.1111/j.1524-4725.2011.02007.x.

30. Montes JR. Ethnic and gender considerations in the use of facial injectables: Latino patients. *Plast Reconstr Surg.* 2015;136:32S-39S. doi:10.1097/PRS.0000000000001789.

31. Rendon MI. Hyperpigmentation disorders in Hispanic population in the United States. *J Drugs Dermatol.* 2019;18(3):s112-s114. PMID: 30909363.

32. Henry M, Sadick N. Aesthetic considerations in female skin of color: What you need to know. *Semin Cutan Med Surg.* 2018;37(4):210-216. doi:10.12788/j. sder.2018.053.

33. Rossi AM, Perez MI. Laser therapy in Latino skin. *Facial Plast Surg Clin North Am.* 2011;19(2):389-403. doi:10.1016/j.fsc.2011.05.002.

34. Rossi A, Alexis AF. Cosmetic procedures in skin of color. *G Ital Dermatol Venereol.* 2011;146(4):265-272. PMID: 21785392.

35. Leal-Silva H. Predicting the risk of postinflammatory hyperpigmentation: The palmar creases pigmentation scale.

J Cosmet Dermatol. 2021;20(4):1263-1270. doi:10.1111/jocd.13968.

36. Jalalat S, Weiss E. Cosmetic laser procedures in Latin skin. *J Drugs Dermatol.* 2019;18(3):s127–s131. PMID: 30909360.

37. Heath CR, Taylor SC. Fillers in the skin of color population. *J Drugs Dermatol.* 2011;10(5):494-498. PMID: 21533295.

38. Taylor SC. Skin of color: Biology, structure, function, and implications for dermatologic disease. *J Am Acad Dermatol.* 2002;46(2 Supplement 2):S41-S62. doi:10.1067/mjd.2002.120790.

39. Whitehead DM, Schechter LS. Cheek augmentation techniques. *Facial Plast Surg Clin North Am.* 2019;27(2):199-206. doi:10.1016/j.fsc.2018.12.003.

40. Kontochristopoulos G, Platsidaki E. Chemical peels in active acne and acne scars. *Clin Dermatol.* 2017; 35(2):179-182. doi:10.1016/j.clindermatol.2016.10.011.

6

Populations of Middle Eastern Ancestry

Hassan Galadari, Farah Moustafa, Cindy Wassef

SUMMARY AND KEY FEATURES

- The Middle Eastern population is a heterogenous group represented by various Fitzpatrick skin types.
- Cosmetic skin discoloration concerns unique for Middle Eastern populations include skin discoloration such as melasma and hyperpigmentation.
- In addition to addressing concerns regarding volume loss and rhytides, enhancement of the nasal dorsum and chin are also a leading reason for cosmetic consultation in Middle Eastern populations.
- Excess hair, such as hirsutism, and alopecia such as female pattern hair loss are common concerns in the Middle Eastern population.

INTRODUCTION

The Middle East is defined as a region along the southern and eastern portions of the Mediterranean Sea. While its exact boundaries have changed over the years, it currently encompasses Bahrain, Cyprus, Egypt, Iran, Iraq, Israel, Jordan, Kuwait, Lebanon, Libya, Oman, Palestine, Qatar, Saudi Arabia, United Arab Emirates, and Yemen. Due to proximity and culture, Tunisia, Algeria, and Morocco are often included in this definition as well.[1] Even within these areas and the wide representation of all Fitzpatrick skin types, there are varied racial differences and beauty standards. This diversity adds to the uniqueness of this region and has led to less consensus information regarding aesthetic concerns in comparison to Asian and other cultures where there is a level of homogeneity. Historically, aesthetic standards of beauty extend as far back as Queen Nefertiti, whose name now is cosmetically synonymous with a sharply defined jawline. The modern-day Middle East draws much of its aesthetic inspiration from royal families, actresses, and others in the performing arts.[2]

The proximity and cultural similarities to other regions have also led to shared beliefs in beauty standards. However, the Middle East beauty standard is generally regarded as an oval, full symmetric face with arched thick eyebrows surrounding almond eyes. Other favorable features include a thin straight nose, full lips, and a well-defined jawline with a pointed chin.[2] Changes in overall aesthetic standards have started to change due to globalization and media influence. A 2017 study amongst university students in the United Arab Emirates found that 16.4% of those surveyed reported tanning at least once in their lifetime—a larger than expected number given the traditional emphasis on lighter skin and beauty.[3] A shift in hair styling from the Westernized straightening to embracing natural curly and wavy hair was noted to coincide with the Arab Spring and reembraced ideas of freedom and cultural heritage.[4]

Both extrinsic and intrinsic factors contribute to the aesthetic outcome in Middle Eastern skin. Ultraviolet radiation is the most cited cause of premature aging and a factor to consider in the equatorial-located Middle East. Depending on Fitzpatrick skin type, the effects on the Middle Eastern skin can vary with those with naturally darker skin tones possessing an intrinsic difference in epidermal melanin. These increased amounts lead to less photodamage albeit a stronger propensity for dyschromia. Smoking is also more socially acceptable compared to Western societies with one study reporting usage rates as high as 53.9% in Lebanon.[5] This can contribute to significant premature aging. Lentigines, seborrheic keratoses, and dermatoses papulosa nigra are also noted in increased frequency within this population. Preserved elasticity is aided by an intrinsically thicker dermis and numerous fibroblasts. These same fibroblasts also contribute to increasing keloids and hypertrophic scarring, which is an important consideration when considering surgical or cosmetic procedures in this ethnic group.[6]

Continued evolution in aesthetic standards has branched into cosmetic procedures. The demand for cosmetic procedures in the Middle East is rising with Dubai reporting the highest ratio of plastic surgeons per capita in the world.[7] The influence of social media and friends is the most cited reason for seeking cosmetic procedures amongst young Middle Eastern women. Those over 40 cite their preference, friends, and their husbands as driving factors. Desired results are also different for each age group. While those over 40 may desire a more natural appearance, younger females influenced by social media often desire more exaggerated results.[2] With this growing desire and demand in a burgeoning cultural center of the world, the aesthetic clinician needs to be knowledgeable of the needs of the Middle Eastern community. In this chapter, we will explore the major aesthetic concerns and goals of the Middle Eastern population as well as treatments available and those unique to this area.

SKIN DISCOLORATION

Melasma

Melasma is characterized by hyperpigmented jagged patches of the forehead, cheeks, and upper cutaneous lips that are believed to be due to an interplay of ultraviolet radiation, inflammation, and hormones. Factors that play a role in the development of the condition include multiple pregnancies and the use of oral contraceptive pills. The majority of those affected are women and this is often a distressing cosmetic concern. A Saudi Arabian study found that melasma made up 2.88% of

dermatology visits in one national hospital between 1995 and 1997.[8] Interestingly, amongst Middle Eastern Americans surveyed in Dearborn, Michigan, in 2007, 14.5% noted melasma as a significant cosmetic concern.[9] Due to hormonal influence and a higher pregnancy rate amongst Middle Eastern women, melasma continues to be an ongoing concern that drives patients into a dermatologist's office.

While there are many treatment options available for melasma, care should be taken when choosing the right one in this population. Postinflammatory dyspigmentation is a significant concern when using treatments such as energy-based devices such as Q-switched lasers, chemical peels, and topical lightening agents. Specifically, it is our expert opinion that if a peel is to be chosen as a treatment option, the depth should not exceed a light to medium depth given the risk of dyspigmentation from deep chemical peels is great. Topical steroids in the Middle East are often mixed with retinoids and hydroquinone to aid in the treatment of melasma in addition to achieving a lighter skin tone. The accessibility to these medications is high due to a prescription not being required to procure them. Patients, thus, often self-medicate or combine dermatologist-prescribed treatments with those suggested by or requested from the pharmacy. Often, it is not realized that these are duplicate treatments, leading to cumulative effects and possible atrophy, cataracts, irritation, and exogenous ochronosis.[10]

HYPERPIGMENTATION

Hyperpigmentation or darkening of the skin is an area of specific concern in the Middle Eastern population. This represents a broad category but specific areas of concern in this population include perioral and periorbital hyperpigmentation, flexural areas, in addition to elbows and knees.

Periorbital pigmentation is defined as circular or semicircular hyperpigmented patches around the upper and lower eyelids. Various factors can contribute to their presence, including superficial vasculature, tear trough depression, periorbital edema, genetic factors, and other medical dermatologic conditions.[11] While in practice this is often cited as an area of concern, our review did not find any specific literature pertaining to this topic and the Middle Eastern community. Care should be taken not to mistake these patches with acanthosis nigricans of the periorbital skin, a condition that is also quite common in the Middle East, given the high incidence of insulin resistance in the region.[12] It is also important to distinguish various facial hyperpigmentation from pigmentary demarcation lines. These are abrupt physiologic transitions between hyperpigmented skin and lighter areas. A Saudi Arabian study screening 1033 patients found 144 patients to have at least one of the described facial pigmentary demarcation lines.[13]

General treatment recommendations are similar to those for other populations and target the underlying cause. Increased vasculature leading to a bluish or purple discoloration of the skin may be treated with a long-pulsed Nd Yag 1064 nm laser, pulsed dye laser, or topical caffeine preparations. It is important to keep in mind the potential adverse effects that come with the use of these vascular lasers. With a pulsed dye laser, the high absorption coefficient melanin makes permanent eyebrow hair loss a possibility. The horizontally oriented hairs of the eyebrow are not as deep and thus susceptible to this effect. Pulsed dye lasers also come with the potential of developing vitreous floaters, for both the patient and the physician operating the laser. This is attributed to a lack of eye protection that allows the shock wave of a pulsed dye layer to disrupt the vitreous gel and cause the release of floaters.[14] Eye protection (including intraocular shields where indicated) is paramount when performing the aforementioned laser procedures. Constitutional pigmentation, often brown in color, can be treated with both q-switched lasers and light chemical peels.[15] Periorbital hyperpigmentation due to volume loss is best treated with expertly placed filler in the deep medial cheek subcutaneous fat and posterior to the orbicularis oculi muscle with care to avoid the Tyndall effect and related bluish discoloration that can further exacerbate the patient's concerns.

Postinflammatory hyperpigmentation relating to both medical conditions and cosmetic procedures is a common complication. In one study, 87.2% of acne patients reported postinflammatory hyperpigmentation with 69% attributing it to excoriation of acne lesions and 52.6% indicating that their hyperpigmentation had been present for more than 1 year.[16] The time required for hyperpigmentation to resolve can often be longer than that required for the resolution of the underlying condition. In another study examining body dysmorphic disorder amongst Saudi Arabian dermatologic patients, hyperpigmentation was noted by 29% and was the top concern of those with the condition.[17] In a survey of 318 Jordanian women, 50% of those with fair skin reported using skin-lightening cream to treat hyperpigmentation as opposed to those with a darker skin tone who used it mainly for lightening of their baseline skin tone.[18] This highlights the prevalence of hyperpigmentation concerns amongst various ranges of Fitzpatrick skin types in the Middle Eastern community. Treatment commonly used for this condition is similar to those used for other conditions of hyperpigmentation including topical lightening agents, superficial chemical peels, and lasers.

VOLUME LOSS

Injection of fillers for soft tissue augmentation aids to maintain and enhance the preferred oval full face. This baseline facial preference is important to keep in mind when performing volume-enhancing treatments in this population. Consensus recommendations for treating Middle Eastern faces include filling the temples to preserve the "triangle of youth." Temporal filling can lift the lateral cheek and lift corners of the lateral eye and maintain the desired almond shape. In addition, sagging of the skin and appearance of jowls are more prominent in the Middle Eastern face and the goal of fillers should be lateral placement to lift the mid-cheek and to enhance jawline contour.[2] For lips, both patients and medical professionals favor a slightly protruded lip. In one study comparing acceptable profile and jaw patterns, the bimaxillary protrusion with lip protrusion was found to be the least acceptable for men but slightly more acceptable for women. The authors concluded that when treating an orthodontic patient in particular, lip protrusion may be more acceptable in women than in men.[19] This is an important concept to keep in mind when treating lips as treatment of the cheeks and jawline may result in accentuated protrusion of the lips. Volume enhancement via filler improved facial contour, and lip vermillion contour is a common request among Middle Eastern women.[2]

FACIAL LINES

The main areas targeted for facial line improvement include forehead lines and crow's feet. Consensus opinion indicates that contrary to their Western counterparts, women in the Middle East prefer to be more expressive and have a less frozen appearance. Crow's feet are a less common occurrence in Middle Eastern population and are a result more of muscular rather than skin quality related; the use of neurotoxin with a discussion about the degree of muscle relaxation should be performed with each patient seeking treatment.[2]

FACIAL AUGMENTATION

Two common areas of desired facial augmentation and correction in this population include the nasal dorsum and chin.

NASAL DORSUM

The nasal dorsum is a common area of injection of fillers in the Middle Eastern population. In a study of facial profiles, Emirati laypeople surveyed ranked the nose as the most important factor in determining facial attractiveness. Both lay and medical personnel agreed that a straight profile was the most desirable.[19] Common issues that are addressed in this population include widened nasal structure, poorly defined nasal tip, alar flaring, bulk in the infratip area, a high dorsum, and a narrowed columellar labial angle.[20] The severity of defects often requires surgical correction although a small minority may benefit from nonsurgical correction including downward/rotated nose, hump, widened tip, or flatness.[2] Nonsurgical correction is achieved with the use of hyaluronic acid-based dermal fillers. Middle Eastern patients account for a large and growing percentage of rhinoplasty cases worldwide, particularly females. Important considerations when counseling patients include avoidance of overcorrection and seeking Western nasal styles as this can lead to incongruity in the face given the other more classic Middle Eastern facial features present on the face.[20]

CHIN

The chin represents another major structural area of concern. In a survey of Emirati laypeople as well oral physicians, laypersons found a female with a retruded chin to be the most unattractive whereas orthodontic specialists felt the protruded chin to be the least attractive in women. These differences were attributed to education and knowledge base.[19] However, this brings up the relevant point that what may be considered the most beautiful or correct in a medical sense may not harmonize with what is considered most desirable amongst those seeking cosmetic consultation. It is important to gather from the patient not only what they believe to be the most acceptable outcome but overall, the least acceptable when planning any intervention. (Figs. 6.1 and 6.2).

Other examples of facial soft tissue augmentation performed by the senior author in Middle Eastern patients can be seen in Figs. 6.3 to 6.6.

HAIR

Hair grooming in the Middle East has a storied history. Historical records indicate that as far back as 762 to 1258 AD, Arabs took advantage of their central location in the perfume trade to acquire products for hair and beard scent. Camel's urine was used to give hair its shine while ghee was a favorite conditioner.[21]

In contrast to previous pressures to conform to more Westernized hairstyles, the Middle East is seeing a resurgence of curly hairstyles. Men who often kept hair short are now allowing for longer growth while women are embracing more natural hairstyles.[4] Racial/ethnic differences in hair characteristics have been described; African hair is the curliest, with a more elliptical shape and less force required for breakage. Areas of kinking and twisting of the hair shafts are believed to be crucial weak points where hair breakage may occur.[22] It is important to note that our knowledge of Middle Eastern hair is often extrapolated from African hair studies given similarities in texture; however, specific studies are needed to identify properties about Middle Eastern hair that may or may not be present in African counterparts.

Both hair excess and paucity are often raised concerns in the Middle East as well as changes and loss of hair color. These topics will be addressed below.

EXCESS HAIR

Excess hair growth in areas such as the face, axilla, trunk, pubic areas, and extremities is a common cosmetic concern amongst Middle Eastern women. The Middle Eastern population is generally accepted as having a greater amount of excess body hair growth as compared with White and Asian counterparts. When assessing for hyperandrogenism in premenopausal women, the Ferriman-Gallwey (FG) score is used. This scoring system assigns a 0–4 rating scale for hair growth

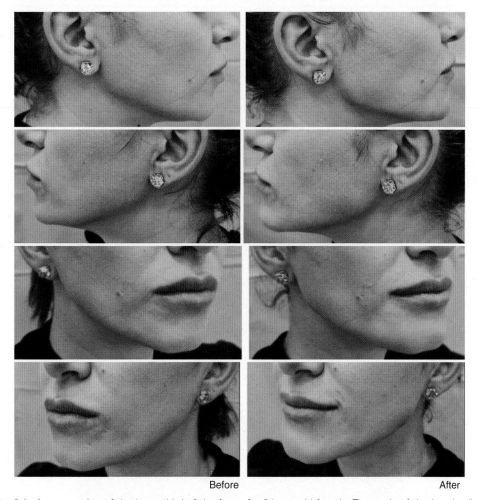

Before   After

Fig. 6.1. Augmentation of the lower-third of the face of a 34-year-old female. The angle of the jaw, jawline, as well as chin were injected with 3 ml of calcium hydroxylapatite.

in nine body areas. Scoring criteria are given to indicate when hyperandrogenism should be a concern when assessing a patient. Among the Middle Eastern population, a higher score is needed to raise concern for hyperandrogenism compared to their White, Black, and Asian counterparts. Updated guidelines now define an FG score greater than 8 in White and Black women, 2–7 in Asian women, and 9–10 or greater in Hispanic and Middle Eastern women as necessitating a workup for increased androgens.[23] Removal of body hair in Middle Eastern culture is considered an issue of hygiene and tradition. It has been promoted in Islamic teachings for many centuries, which has contributed to its popularity.[24]

Pubic hair removal is an area unique to the Middle East with ancient texts as far back as the 16th century detailing Egyptian female pubic hair epilation traditions and ceremonies. In a 2014 survey of 61 Turkish women, over 90% endorsed regular pubic hair removal with 95% having done so in the last month. Hair removal methods in order of decreasing frequency were waxing, shaving, depilatory cream, laser, and electronic depilatory devices. The most common sources of knowledge regarding pubic hair removal were mothers, cited by 70.5% of those surveyed. Participants cited comfort (48%) and odor prevention (33%) as the most common reasons for hair removal, while sexual image (14%) and religious reasons (8%) were noted as the least important

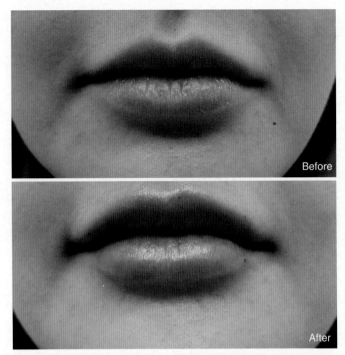

Fig. 6.2. Volumization of the lips with 1 ml of hyaluronic acid filler. This is a commonly sought treatment in patients from the Middle East.

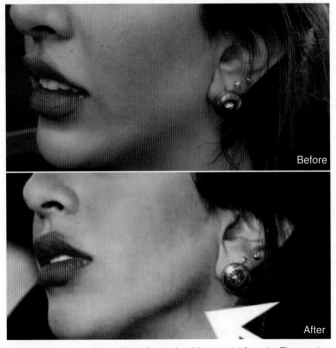

Fig. 6.3. Augmentation of the lower-third of the face of a 29-year-old female. The angle of the jaw, jawline, and chin were injected with 4 ml of a hyaluronic acid filler.

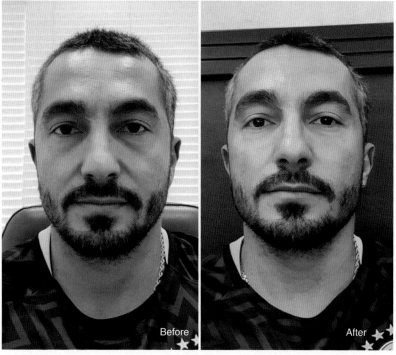

Fig. 6.4. Augmentation of the midface of a 42-year-old male. Both cheeks and tear troughs were injected with a hyaluronic acid filler.

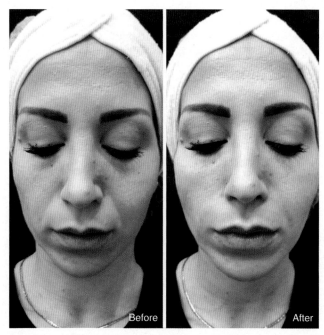

Fig. 6.5. Augmentation of the midface of a 37-year-old female with hyaluronic acid. Note the positive effects on the tear troughs.

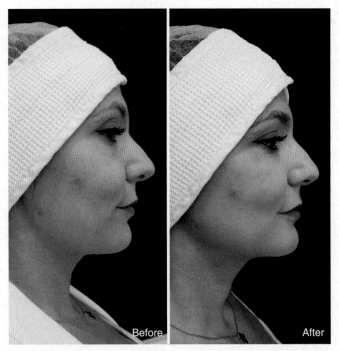

Fig. 6.6. Augmentation of cheeks, marionette lines, chin, and mental crease were performed.

reasons. This study highlighted that despite newly available treatments, traditional methods such as waxing and shaving were still favored. Adverse effects from these treatments including burns and dyspigmentation. Folliculitis in this population should be kept in mind when evaluating a patient with these complaints in their pubic area.[24]

Given the higher prevalence of skin types III–V, dyspigmentation and scarring are potential concerns when using laser technologies for hair removal. In one 2004 study, the use of intense pulsed light as a hair removal device was found to be safe in the 210 Egyptian men and women treated. Those who underwent 3 to 5 treatments noted an average of 80% hair reduction, with the other 20% to 30% of hairs attributed to vellus hairs. While no postinflammatory changes were noted in the study group, it is important to note that like laser hair removal methods, the risks of dyspigmentation, leukotrichia, and paradoxical hair growth are also present with intense pulsed light.[25] Particularly when removing vellus hairs on the lateral face and chin, the Middle Eastern population has a higher incidence of paradoxical hair growth.[26]

In addition to the hair removal methods mentioned above, a method unique to the Middle East that dermatologists should be aware of is threading. It is offered by barbers or beauticians and is used by both men and women for the removal of facial hair. Cotton threads roughly 50 to 70 cm are preferred to prevent cuts to the operator as the thread is held by the operator's hand as well as teeth with a loop encircling hair that is trapped in this area and then removed. It is noted to be painful and potential adverse effects include folliculitis and dyspigmentation.[27] The benefits of this removal technique may go beyond removing hair. A 2019 study evaluating facial threading (with application of powder prior) found significant improvements in perceived facial skin roughness in various areas of the face treated, likely sue to the removal of vellus hairs.[28]

ALOPECIA

Hair loss is an important aesthetic concern among the Middle Eastern population. Despite the term "hair transplant" being most searched among the Middle Easterns and South Asians on YouTube, there is a relative paucity of articles regarding hair loss in the Middle Eastern community. According to the International Society of Hair Restoration Surgery, the Middle East accounted for 188,360 of the 735,312 surgical hair restoration procedures performed in 2019.[29] It is important to delineate the true cause of hair loss that is perceived by patients—mainly hair shaft breakage versus true alopecia. Of note, our literature review yielded minimal data specifically addressing alopecia in the Middle Eastern populations. A cross-sectional study evaluating the frequency of androgenic alopecia in men and women in a hospital-based setting in Turkey found a prevalence of 67% in men and 23.9% in women. The mean age of onset of androgenic alopecia was 31 in men and 40 in women.[30] The following text will be based on findings of African hair as this is most similar in texture. In a survey of over 700 African women, 64% noted breakage; however, where exactly the breakage occurred was not as discernable from those surveyed. Activities associated with increased breakage included more manipulation, the use of small tooth combs, using brushes, and combing with high force. These same patients provided hair samples for analysis and break stress or the amount of force needed to break a hair. In that sample, it was found that the further the hair was from the scalp, the less force would be needed to break it, resulting in perceived hair loss.[22] While not a complete reflection of the Middle Eastern population, hair texture similarity allows us to extrapolate that less processing to the naturally curlier Middle Eastern hair can prevent breakage and thus perceived hair loss. This may prove difficult as hair straightening and coloring are popular aesthetic treatments in the Middle East to westernize appearances. With current opinion regarding curly hair changing, a favorable outcome may be seen in hair breakage.[4]

Despite an Internet presence and a documented interest in hair transplantation, articles specifically about alopecia in Middle Eastern patients were limited.[29] This area represents a significant knowledge gap and further information regarding the types of hair loss experienced in Middle Eastern populations is needed to further tailor treatment.

PREMATURE GRAYING

Premature graying is a noticeable problem in the Middle East population. The exact prevalence is unknown. However, efforts have been taken to uncover why this is the case. One theory includes the connection between smoking and premature graying. Smoking is much more socially acceptable in Middle Eastern cultures with some areas reporting greater than 50% of adults regularly smoking.[5] In a 2013 study of Jordanians, those with premature graying defined as white hair before the age of 30 were more likely to identify as smokers. Smoking placed subjects at 2.5 times greater risk of having premature graying. It is important to note that smokers were anyone who ever smoked, and the amount smoked ranged anywhere from zero to 70 cigarettes.[31]

TREATMENT APPROACHES

While many of the available products are similar to those available in the United States, there are notable differences. We will review these below.

Filler

Compared to products in the United States, there are some similarities, distinct products, as well as products with a different brand name. Merz Aesthetics calcium hydroxyapatite filler Radiesse is available in addition to their Belotero line. The Belotero hyaluronic acid fillers are divided up into four subgroups—soft, balance, intense, and volume—that are available in the Middle East. Differences between them include optimal depth of filling and volume loss restoration. Similar to the United States, Allergan's hyaluronic acid fillers Juvederm Volbella, Vollure, and Voluma are available in the Middle East. Allergan's Juvederm Volux is currently available in the Middle East and as of 2021 is pending release in the United States. Galderma's Restylane line parallels those available in the United States and include Restylane, Restylane Lyft, Refyne, Defyne, Kyesse, and Volyme. Teoaxane's Swiss-patented resilient hyaluronic acid technology is available in the Middle East with RHA 1,2,3,4; fillers that differ from those available in the United States include Global Action, Ultra deep, Kiss, and Redensity 1 and 2. Neuvia hyaluronic acid fillers available in the Middle East include Intense, Intense Volume, Stimulate, Rheology, and Hydrodeluxe. French-based Sinclair Perfectha filler is also available in addition to Ellanse, a polycaprolactone dermal filler. Hyaluronic acid body fillers are also available in the Middle East under the brand Hyacorp Body.

Toxin

Neurotoxins available in the Middle East include Onabotulinum toxin (Botox), prabotulinumtoxin A marketed as Nabota (known as Jeuveau in the United States), abotulinumtoxin A (Dysport), and incobotulinum toxin (Xeomin).

CONCLUSION

Populations of Middle Eastern ancestry are a diverse populations represented by a broad range of skin phototypes and cultural backgrounds. Common cosmetic dermatological concerns in these populations include dyspigmentation, facial lines, volume loss, unwanted hair, and alopecia. Enhancement of the nasal dorsum and chin are among the leading reasons for cosmetic consultation in Middle Eastern populations.

REFERENCES

1. Middle East. *Encyclopædia Britannica*. Published February 9, 2021. Available at: https://www.britannica.com/place/Middle-East. Accessed March 20, 2021.
2. Kashmar M, Alsufyani MA, Ghalamkarpour F, et al. Consensus opinions on facial beauty and implications for aesthetic treatment in Middle Eastern women. *Plast Reconstr Surg Glob Open*. 2019;7(4):e2220. doi:10.1097/gox.0000000000002220.
3. Aldhaheri AS, Galadari H, Hashim MJ, Joly P. Tanning practice, perception, and sunburn among Emirati youth. *Int J Dermatol*. 2017;56(3):354-357. doi:10.1111/ijd.13447.
4. Yee V. *The Freedom of Natural Curls: Egypt's Quiet Rebellion*. The New York Times; Published March 11, 2021. Available at: https://www.nytimes.com/2021/03/11/world/middleeast/egypt-hair-curls-natural.html. Accessed March 20, 2021.
5. Khattab A, Javaid A, Iraqi G, et al. Smoking habits in the Middle East and North Africa: Results of the BREATHE study. *Respir Med*. 2012;106(suppl 2):S16-S24. doi:10.1016/s0954-6111(12)70011-2.
6. Vashi NA, BuainainI de Castro Maymone M, Kundu RV. Aging differences in ethnic skin. *J Clin Aesthet Dermatol*. 2016;9(1):31-38.
7. Kuttab JA. *Plastic Surgery on The Rise in UAE. Khaleej Times*; Published May 1, 2016. Available at: https://www.khaleejtimes.com/nation/uae-health/plastic-surgery-on-the-rise-in-uae. Accessed March 20, 2021.
8. Parthasaradhi A, Al Gufai AF. The pattern of skin diseases in Hail Region, Saudi Arabia. *Ann Saudi Med*. 1998;18(6):558-561. doi:10.5144/0256-4947.1998.558.
9. El-Essawi D, Musial JL, Hammad A, Lim HW. A survey of skin disease and skin-related issues in Arab Americans. *J Am Acad Dermatol*. 2007;56(6):933-938. doi:10.1016/j.jaad.2007.01.031.
10. Lahiri K, Galadrai H. Topical corticosteroid use in the Middle East. In: *A Treatise on Topical Corticosteroids in Dermatology Use*, Misuse and Abuse. Singapore: Springer; 2018:205-207.
11. Sarkar R, Ranjan R, Garg S, et al. Periorbital hyperpigmentation: A comprehensive review. *J Clin Aesthet Dermatol*. 2016;9(1):49-55.
12. Abuyassin B, Laher I. Diabetes epidemic sweeping the Arab world. *World J Diabetes*. 2016;7(8):165. Available at: https://doi.org/10.4239/wjd.v7.i8.165.
13. Al-Samary A, Al Mohizea S, Bin-Saif G, Al-Balbeesi A. Pigmentary demarcation lines on the face in Saudi women. *Indian J Dermatol Venereol Leprol*. 2010;76:378-381.
14. Yates B, Que SK, D'Souza L, Suchecki J, Finch JJ. Laser treatment of periocular skin conditions. *Clin Dermatol*. 2015;33(2):197-206. Available at: https://doi.org/10.1016/j.clindermatol.2014.10.011.
15. Vrcek I, Ozgur O, Nak T. Infraorbital dark circles: A review of the pathogenesis, evaluation and treatment. *J Cutan Aesthet Surg*. 2016;9(2):65-72. Available at: doi:10.4103/0974-2077.184046.
16. Abanmi A, Al-Enezi M, Al Hammadi A, Galadari I, Kibbi A-G, Zimmo S. Survey of acne-related post-inflammatory hyperpigmentation in the Middle East. *J Dermatolog Treat*. 2018;30(6):578-581. doi:10.1080/09546634.2018.1542807.
17. AlShahwan MA. Prevalence and characteristics of body dysmorphic disorder in Arab dermatology patients. *Saudi Med J*. 2020;41(1):73-78. doi:10.15537/smj.2020.1.24784.
18. Hamed SH, Tayyem R, Nimer N, AlKhatib HS. Skin-lightening practice among women living in Jordan: Prevalence, determinants, and user's awareness. *Int J Dermatol*. 2010;49(4):414-420. doi:10.1111/j.1365-4632.2010.04463.x.
19. Al Taki A, Guidoum A. Facial profile preferences, self-awareness and perception among groups of people in the United Arab Emirates. *J Orthod Sci*. 2014;3(2):55. doi:10.4103/2278-0203.132921.
20. Rohrich RJ, Ghavami A. Rhinoplasty for Middle Eastern noses. *Plast Reconstr Surg*. 2009;123(4):1343-1354. doi:10.1097/prs.0b013e31817741b4.
21. Sherrow, V. *Encyclopedia of Hair*: A Cultural History. Santa Barbara: Greenwood; 2019.
22. Bryant H, Porter C, Yang G. Curly hair: Measured differences and contributions to breakage. *Int J Dermatol*. 2012;51:8-11. doi:10.1111/j.1365-4632.2012.05555.x.

23. Mimoto MS, Oyler JL, Davis AM. Evaluation and treatment of hirsutism in premenopausal women. *JAMA.* 2018;319(15):1613-1614. doi:10.1001/jama.2018.2611.

24. Muallaaziz D, Yayci E, Atcag T, Kaptanoglu AF. Pubic hair removal practices in Muslim women. *Basic Clin Sci.* 2014;3:39-44. doi:10.12808/bcs.v3vi4i.5000083958.

25. El Bedewi AF. Hair removal with intense pulsed light. *Lasers Med Sci.* 2004;19(1):48-51. doi:10.1007/s10103-004-0298-6.

26. Ibrahimi OA, Avram MM, Hanke CW, Kilmer SL, Anderson RR. Laser hair removal. *Dermatol Ther.* 2011;24(1):94-107. Available at: https://doi.org/10.1111/j.1529-8019.2010.01382.x.

27. Abdel-Gawad MM, Abdel-Hamid IA, Wagner RF. Khite: A non-Western temporary hair removal technique. *Int J Dermatol.* 1997;36(3):217. doi:10.1046/j.1365-4362.1997.00189.x.

28. Lin LY, Chiou SC, Wang SH, Ching CC. Effects of facial threading on female skin texture: A prospective trial with physiological parameters and sense assessment. *Evid Based Complement Alternat Med.* 2019;2019:1535713. doi:10.1155/2019/1535713.

29. *Worldwide Demand for Effective Hair Restoration Procedures Continues to Increase.* ISHRS; July 21, 2020. Available at: https://ishrs.org/2020/06/03/worldwide-demand-for-effective-hair-restoration-procedures-continues-to-increase/#:~:text=A%20total%20of%20735%2C312%20surgical,decrease%20from%202016%2C%20and%20Dr.

30. Salman KE, Altunay IK, Kucukunal NA, Cerman AA. Frequency, severity and related factors of androgenetic alopecia in dermatology outpatient clinic: Hospital-based cross-sectional study in Turkey. *An Bras Dermatol.* 2017;92(1):35-40.

31. Zayed AA, Shahait AD, Ayoub MN, Youssef Am. Smokers' hair: Does smoking cause premature hair graying? *Indian Dermatol Online J.* 2013;4(2):90-92. doi:10.4103/2229-5178.110586.

7

Populations of South Asian Ancestry

Malcolm Pyles, Sokhna Seck, Shilpi Khetarpal

SUMMARY AND KEY FEATURES

- Within each region of South Asia, there are varying perceptions of beauty. It is important to understand these differences when performing cosmetic treatments on each individual population.
- Hyperpigmentation and uneven skin tone are common concerns among those of South Asian descent, most commonly melasma and postinflammatory hyperpigmentation.
- It is essential to consider cultural viewpoints and underlying biological attributes in patients of South Asian origin.

INTRODUCTION

South Asia is defined as the region southwest of China and consists of the countries of Bangladesh, Bhutan, India, Nepal, Pakistan, and Sri Lanka; Afghanistan and the Maldives are also often considered part of this region. As one of the most populated regions in the world, it is characterized by significant social and cultural variation. The region's ethnic diversity is also wide ranging, with many of these groups having distinct religious beliefs and cultural practices.[1] Such diversity is of considerable significance as it gives rise to contrasting views of beauty standards and unique dermatological needs. Dermatologists must be aware of, and responsive to, the religious and cultural practices of these populations in order to provide optimal patient-centered and culturally competent care.[2] Broad generalizations about this diverse population may hinder patients' therapeutic relationship with their physician and contribute to racial and ethnic healthcare disparities. Thus care must be taken to incorporate individual patient values and cultural preferences in our approach to dermatologic care.

Although the facial triangle of beauty with prominence of the upper two-thirds of the face relative to the lower one-third is considered to be the ideal aesthetic, beauty canons greatly vary by culture and geographic region.[3] British colonial influence and Western media play a major role in the portrayal of ideal beauty in many regions in South Asia; however, perceptions of beauty are changing within ethnic groups and in mass culture.[4] While some South Asian patients may strive for more Eurocentric beauty features, a significant portion of patients aspire to look more attractive within their ethnic anthropometric parameters.[5] Several studies have shown that familiarity and typicality influence aesthetic preferences.[6–8] Consequently, concerns of aging skin and facial rejuvenation also differ by region and cultural surroundings. The objective of this chapter is to describe beauty standards and aging patterns of the South Asian face and to discuss various aesthetic procedures with a specific focus on common concerns within this demographic. There is a paucity of literature on this diverse population; thus this chapter is based on limited published evidence and the authors' clinical experience.

AESTHETIC GOALS AND CONCERNS IN SOUTH ASIAN POPULATIONS

Skin Discoloration

Studies on skin color and texture have shown that discoloration and ultraviolet-related sun changes can account for up to 20 years of perceived age and have a greater effect than other forms of aging such as volume loss and wrinkles.[9,10] The increased epidermal melanin and distribution of melanosomes in skin of color provides an inherent photoprotection and thus decreased susceptibility to photodamage. However, this increased melanin makes skin of color more vulnerable to pigmentary change, a prominent feature of photoaging in this group. Overall, uneven skin tone is a great concern and studies have shown that visible skin color distribution plays an important role in the perception of attractiveness.[10–12] Given that ultraviolet radiation and heat both alter pigmentation (e.g., in the context of melasma), we counsel patients to avoid excessive exposure to both sun and heat. Patients should also be advised to practice safe skincare routines to minimize postinflammatory hyperpigmentation such as avoiding abrasives on the skin and not combining multiple skincare products with potentially irritating ingredients.[13] Use of broad-spectrum sunscreens is strongly advocated regardless of skin type and ethnicity to prevent any further darkening of lesions.

Common skin discoloration concerns are related to postinflammatory pigmentary changes, melasma, and facial pigmentary demarcation lines. Other pigmentary conditions that are common in South Asians include nevus of Ota, Hori's nevus, erythema dyschromicum perstans, and lichen planus pigmentosus. These are chronic, often recalcitrant pigmentary disorders. Melasma, a cosmetically disfiguring and troubling disorder with limited treatment options, has a higher prevalence in people with darker Fitzpatrick skin types and is estimated to occur in approximately 40% of patients of South Asian ethnicity.[14–16] Successful topical treatments have included a triple-combination cream containing fluocinolone acetonide 0.01%, tretinoin 0.05%, and hydroquinone 4% once daily.[17,18] There has also been reported success in combining this treatment with oral tranexamic acid 250 mg twice daily.[19] Other modalities include chemical peels, laser/light-based options, and microneedling, which will be discussed later in this chapter. These are typically reserved for cases that are not responsive to topical management due to the increased risk of postinflammatory hyperpigmentation, melasma exacerbation, and scarring (as well as cost considerations). Strict avoidance of sun and heat should be stressed in all patients with melasma. Ultimately, although melasma cannot be cured, treatments can put it into remission. Because the etiology is multifactorial, a combination treatment approach should be used for optimal outcomes.

Periorbital hyperpigmentation is another frequent concern of South Asian populations. This often occurs before middle age and sometimes in teenagers as well. In comparison to East Asian groups, South Asians are more likely to have excessive constitutional pigmentation with a velvety texture as opposed to more vascular types.[20] Various treatment regimens have been reported in the literature ranging from topical regimens such as vitamins K, C, and E and topical retinoids. Other options reported include chemical peeling, fillers, infrared, intense pulsed light (IPL), erbium-doped yttrium aluminum garnet and carbon dioxide laser resurfacing, autologous fat transplant, and blepharoplasty.[21,22]

Skin Lightening

In many South Asian languages, the term "fairness" is used to imply beauty and virtue.[23] Notions of beauty and fairness are interlinked and fair skin is commonly seen as the beauty ideal. Historically, the caste system created status hierarchies on a hereditary basis and those with light skin were associated with the highest caste, which meant high status and religious purity.[13,24] Despite having normally pigmented skin at baseline, skin lightening is a commonly sought procedure in South Asians with half of all spending in the skincare industry in that region being for skin lightening creams.[25] Efforts have been made by many South Asian government regulatory agencies to prohibit the use of skin lightening agents such as hydroquinone, mercury salts, hydrogen peroxide, and magnesium peroxide among others in cosmetics and toiletries.[26] To circumvent these regulatory efforts many manufacturers have introduced new chemicals of unknown safety. Many preparations are unregulated, have no or misleading ingredient labeling, and contain misbranded toxic products.[26,27]

Procedures for skin lightening can range from noninvasive treatments such as creams and facials to invasive treatments such as oral or intravenous glutathione.

The current evidence for glutathione injections is inconclusive with existing studies being of poor quality with inconsistent findings.[28–31] Additionally, serious adverse outcomes of intravenous glutathione have been reported.[32,33] Skin lightening creams are also known to cause various complications including irritant and allergic contact dermatitis, acne, and exogenous ochronosis.[34] Exogenous ochronosis is a cutaneous disorder characterized by blue-black pigmentation and is the complication of long-term application of skin creams containing hydroquinone, phenol, or rescorcinol. Dermoscopy reveals caviar-like hyperpigmentation with bluish-grey amorphous structures and obliterating follicular openings, which can help distinguish it from melasma. Even at low concentrations of hydroquinone, ochronosis can still occur with overuse. It is important to counsel patients against the use of skin lightening products and advise acceptance of normal skin complexion in combination with photoprotection. Dermatologists must also recognize the cultural pressures driving the patient to want to lighten their skin and provide culturally sensitive management of complications that may arise.[13]

Volume Loss

The Indian Facial Aesthetics Expert Group (IFAEG) aimed to present unique aspects of Indian facial structure and aging in those with Indian ancestry.[35] This article presents some stereotypes and challenges from an evidence-based perspective, but due to the paucity in the medical literature on patients from the Indian subcontinent, the article provides much needed insight in aesthetic concerns in this population. According to this survey by IFAEG, infraorbital hollowing is the number-one aesthetic concern for Indian patients under 40.[35] For patients older than 40, the number-one concern is malar volume loss. Structural aging is the result of volumetric loss from all hard and soft tissues including bone, dentition, fat, muscle, ligaments, and dermal components. Loss of these structures causes irregular changes on the face. All of these factors contribute to sagging of the overlying skin. Multiple studies suggest that changes in the nasolabial folds, jowls, buccal areas, and submental regions are more marked in Asians as compared to White individuals of a similar age group.[36–38] This is believed to be in part due to a weaker facial skeletal framework that results in greater gravitational soft-tissue descent of the midface, malar fat pads, ptosis, and tear

trough formation.[35,36] South Asians tend to have fuller lips and higher cheekbones with more buccal fat, often giving the lower cheek a more rounded contour.[9] These features can provide physical support for the aging face and loss of these structures lead to sagging contours and deepening of wrinkles. Chin retrusion can be seen in some which can cause submental fullness earlier than in other ethnicities. Tear trough deficiency is the most common midface indication in Indian women aged 20 to 40 years.[35] In older women, malar volume loss and jowls are the most common aesthetic concerns. Excess medial soft tissue on a relatively smaller midface precedes age-related sagging. Hence, in older Indians, fillers should be used peripherally to achieve lift and conservatively in the medial zones to avoid adding bulk. The one exception to this rule is the chin where additional volume is needed to correct chin retrusion.

Regional variations in facial morphology significantly influence aging. In a study by Shome et al., the mean age for deepening of the nasolabial folds in an Indian population was 40 to 45 years old.[36] East and West Indian ethnicities developed the folds earlier than North and South Indians. In contrast, mandibulo-labial folds were found to occur earliest in North Indians in the 40-to-45 age group. A significant increase in the neck volume was noted in the fourth to fifth decade of life in the East Indian ethnic group, followed by North, West, and South Indians. Loss of definition of jawline was noted to be prominent by the fifth to sixth decade, which is much later than in the White population.

Facial Lines

The larger melanosomes and increased melanin in skin of color allows for less UV penetration, reducing the impact of photoaging, and delaying the development of wrinkles. The increased pigment in South Asian skin allows for later development of lines and wrinkles compared to those with light skin. Cultural practices may also discourage skin exposure, further decreasing UV penetration. As noted above, due to the downward and medial shifting of fat compartments within the face, folds are typically a more worrisome concern than static lines in middle age. Forehead wrinkles are typically not a concern for patients until over the age of 60 although the appearance of forehead wrinkles is noted to be more prominent in ethnicities in the Western part of India. Perpendicular glabellar lines across the forehead due to the corrugators is the most common pattern second to a U pattern causing both perpendicular and transverse glabellar lines involving both the corrugators and the procerus. Lateral canthus crow's feet wrinkles have been demonstrated to occur earlier than in White individuals, frequently appearing by the fourth decade of life.[39] This is believed to be due to greater ptosis and laxity of the lateral orbicularis oculi muscle. Other static lines that are less common include bunny lines, dimpled chin, and platysmal bands.

Facial Augmentation

Because South Asian ethnicity and facial morphology manifest in differences in the aging process, it is important to discuss considerations in providing facial rejuvenation procedures to this group and commonly encountered aesthetic preferences.

Eyebrow reshaping is one of the more commonly requested features of the upper face and this is typically done with botulinum toxin targeting both glabellar and crow's feet areas. A high-arched brow without lateral flare is generally preferred.[35,40] In the midface, tear trough deformity is a very common aesthetic concern in combination with periorbital hyperpigmentation. In younger patients, there is often increased orbital hollowness that can be filled to correction. In older patients, deep malar fat pad reduction, maxillary bone, and orbital bone resorption in addition to thinning of the skin overlying the orbital rim leads to a deep infraorbital hollow. Postseptal fat herniation increases this effect and is more commonly seen above age 50. Therefore, a multimodal approach is often required to correct orbital hollowing in older patients. In the lower face, South Asians frequently have a relatively smaller bony framework.[35] Bone loss and ligament laxity, on top of congenital chin retrusion, lead to the development of pre-jowl sulci and marionette lines forming at an earlier age.

Compared to the White population, South Asians have a greater inter-alar distance, a wider alar base, and less tip projection.[41] Together, these features contribute to a wider nose appearance and patients will often seek to narrow its appearance. Other common concerns that pertain to the nose include humps, supratip deformities, and recessed radix.

South Asian lips are generally naturally full and have ample projection; thus excessive volumization is not often sought after. When it is, younger patients tend to seek increased definition whereas older patients seek to correct what has been lost through age-related atrophic changes.[42] Older patients will also require filling of the perioral compartments in addition to lip-body volumization. The lips should be in balance with surrounding soft tissue and the skeleton of the midface for a more natural appearance.

Increased facial height and oval facial shape is a desired characteristic. In individuals with low-set brows or mild brow ptosis, frontalis injections may be contraindicated as injections that are too low or potent may easily result in ptosis.[43,44] This effect should be discussed with the patient and injection of the brow depressors should also be performed. Chin augmentation is a technique that may be used to enhance these features and correct congenital retrusion. Mandibular retrusion is more commonly seen in some Indian morphotypes that can lead to reduced chin projection, particularly in patients with shorter and wider lower faces.[41,45] This should first be corrected with filler. A retruded chin can also create mentalis hypertrophy that is undesired and can be corrected with a minimum amount of botulinum toxin. Care should be taken when correcting and filling the chin as a shorter chin naturally gives rise to a more rounded facial shape that some patients may desire to maintain.

Excess Hair

Excess facial hair as a result of hirsutism or naturally occurring unwanted facial hair is noted to be psychologically disturbing and is of particular concern in South Asian populations. In addition to facial hair, reduction of excess body hair is a popular request. Due to the increased pigmentation, laser hair removal can present a challenge. When counseling patients, it is important to explain that more sessions at lower energy levels will be needed compared to patients with lighter skin phototypes to minimize unwanted side effects of pigmentary alteration. Skin cooling and test spots prior to full treatment can additionally help to minimize complications.

TREATMENT APPROACHES IN SOUTH ASIAN POPULATIONS

Chemical Peels

Chemical peels are an established, safe, and cost-effective option for South Asian skin. The most common indications for chemical peels in these populations are melasma, periorbital hyperpigmentation, postinflammatory hyperpigmentation, acne scarring, and facial rejuvenation. Chemical peels allow for controlled exfoliation of the skin with subsequent regeneration and resurfacing of the epidermis. A well-known side effect of chemical peels is postinflammatory hyperpigmentation, more commonly seen in darker skin types and with medium and deep peels carrying the largest risks. The superficial chemical peels are very safe when used properly but can cause itching, erythema, and allergic and irritant contact dermatitis.[46] Medium and deep peels are not popular in South Asian skin because they can cause milia, dyspigmentation, and scarring. Proper patient selection and priming of the skin can prevent poor outcomes.

Priming agents enhance the peel penetration and accelerate the postpeel healing process. For many pigmentary conditions, priming the skin for at least 4 weeks prior to a peel is essential to reduce the risk of postpeel hyperpigmentation and scarring. The gold standard for priming is hydroquinone at a concentration of 2% to 4%. In patients who cannot tolerate hydroquinone due to irritation or exogenous ochronosis, retinoids (used alone or in combination with kojic acid), azelaic acid, and glycolic acids can be used. Tretinoin is most commonly used; however, adapalene or bakuchiol may be preferred by some patients because it is less irritating. Tretinoin 0.025% to 0.05% is found useful for darker Asian skin whereas 0.1% is more commonly used in lighter skin types.[47] In this author's experience, topical retinoids are held one day prior to the peel with resumption one day after (however, recommendations for this vary in the literature and include discontinuation of retinoids/other exfoliating treatments 7 days prior to peeling). Treatment should be continued for 2 to 3 months, followed by a 4-week pause before engaging in the next round of treatments. In general, emollients are recommended when retinoids are used as primers. If a patient has experienced any retinoid dermatitis, it is advisable to initiate the peel after inflammation has subsided. When glycolic acids are used as a primer, a low concentration between 6% and 12% is preferred and it is recommended to discontinue these at least 1 week prior to a chemical peel. Kojic acid is often more effective as a primer in concert with other priming methods as opposed to being used alone. No matter which method is used, strict photoprotection is required to ensure proper suppression of melanogenesis.

Glycolic acid is the most widely used alpha-hydroxy acid for chemical peeling and there is good evidence to support its use in skin of color.[48,49] Patients who are chemical peel naïve should be started at lower concentrations of around 30% with slow upward titration of concentration to a maximum of 50%. Glycolic acid peels should be spaced 3 to 4 weeks apart for a total of 4 to 6 sessions depending on the patient's goals and ability to tolerate peels. Other superficial peels include the beta-hydroxy acid salicylic acid, Jessner's solution, and trichloroacetic acid. There have been prior reports of success when combining serial glycolic acid peels with a modified Kligman formula consisting of 0.05% tretinoin, 5% hydroquinone, and 1% hydrocortisone in a cream base.[49]

Chemical peels are a useful adjuvant in the management of acne and as a first-line therapy for acne scars in South Asian populations. As part of a regimen, peels can result in a rapid decrease in lesional count, improve skin texture, and have a lightening effect on scars. Salicylic acid 30% peels and glycolic acid 35% to 70% have been used with much success reducing both inflammatory and noninflammatory lesions of acne in Asian skin.[50] New reports also suggest that mandelic acid 45% peels have a similar efficacy and might be more well tolerated in South Asian skin.[51]

Botulinum Toxin

Another popular nonsurgical aesthetic procedure that requires an individualized approach to assessment given variations in South Asian ideals of beauty is botulinum toxin injection. Botulinum toxin in combination with fillers is used to result in an overall more natural and aesthetically harmonious result. If excessive muscular contraction is the primary cause of what is being addressed, botulinum toxin type A is indicated as the primary treatment. If volume loss is the primary cause, soft tissue fillers is the appropriate first intervention.[52]

As has been mentioned above, due to increased photoprotection and thicker skin, South Asian populations tend to require less botulinum toxins to treat forehead lines. In our experience, there is also a preference for a more natural appearance in the upper face. The key is to recognize and correct volume loss first rather than add excessive toxins that create a frozen look. In general, men will require more units than women due to increased muscle mass.

Women have a preference for an eyebrow lift featuring a highly arched brow without lateral flare. Assessment of the resting brow position is important and can be achieved by having the patient close their eyes for 10 to 15 seconds prior to the examination. The ideal female brow position has been stated as medially at the level of an imaginary vertical line drawn through the alar base and medial canthus arch, superiorly 1 cm above the supraorbital rim, and terminating laterally at a point on the line drawn from the alar base to the lateral canthus.[53] In males, the arch of the brow is described as a more leveled appearance positioned at or slightly above the level of the supraorbital rim. Therefore, targeting the procerus in addition to the corrugator and orbicularis oculi muscles will help to ensure an ideal eyebrow contour. Injection of toxin into the pretarsal orbicularis oculi can also create a welcomed eye-opening effect.

To achieve ideal brow lift with arching, treat the brow depressors on the medial and lateral parts of the eyebrow and the medial frontalis for a complete and more natural appearing lift. The current approach is with 0.5 to 1.5 units of onabotulinumtoxinA (onabotA), incobotulinumtoxinA (incobotA), or prabotulinumtoxinA (prabotA). For abobotulinumtoxinA, (abobotA) an estimated dose ratio of 1:2.5 (onabotA: abobotA) may be assumed.[54] Injection points should be based on the patient's anatomy, goals, and preferences, as well as the physician's professional experience. General injection recommendations for brow lift are the lateral aspect of the orbital section of the orbicularis oculi muscle, at a point at the lateral canthus, just above the supraorbital ridge and along the superior temporal line, which can be just above or below the hairs of the eyebrows. It is important to take note of any preexisting brow asymmetry and attempt to diminish this as best as possible with a forewarning to the patient that it may become accentuated. If this is due to volume loss, it must first be corrected before the filling of toxin.

For the midface, common indications for botulinum toxin include bunny lines, nasal tip elevation, and a gummy smile. For transverse nasal rhytids (bunny lines), we recommend intramuscular injections 1 cm below the medial canthus on the lower half of the nasal bones. There should be one to two injection points per side with a typical total dose of 3 to 4 units of incobotA.[52] Nasal tip elevation can be achieved by one injection with typical total dose of 2 to 4 units of incobotA into the anterior nasal spine perpendicular to the columella targeting the depressor nasi septi.[52] To correct excessive gingival display (gummy smile), the standard injection point is at the convergence point of levator labii superioris, levator labii superioris alaeque nasi, and zygomaticus minor. There should be at least two injection points, one per side, with a typical total dose of 2 to 4 units of incobotA.

The lower face does not differ as dramatically in its approach to treatment. What is more of a concern is knowing what not to treat. For example, while masseter hypertrophy is less common than in other East Asian groups, botulinum toxin can help to narrow the lower face. Aggressive treatment to this area, however, can cause increased signs of aging and contribute to jowl formation. For example, misdiagnosis of masseteric prominence can be overtreated as hypertrophy rather than understanding it as due to overall volume loss in the cheeks.

Soft Tissue Augmentation

As mentioned in the previous section, soft tissue augmentation is recommended in concert with botulinum toxin to achieve the most optimal and natural-looking results. Volume loss as a critical component of facial aging, hence volume replacement contributes significantly to facial rejuvenation. In the same way that less botulinum toxin is required to achieve good outcomes, so too is the case in filler administration. This is especially true of the forehead given that the forehead takes up a larger proportion of facial height and tends to be well projected, though this is not always true in Indians and those with a lower hairline. It is important to start by filling the facial frame to slim the face with injections in the lateral midface, temples, and lateral mandibular line. This is followed by correction of chin retrusion if present and enhancement of the forehead if needed. It is then appropriate to work inwards to the nose, chin, medial malar, and perioral region. To enhance the brow shape, filler can be added lateral to the mid-pupillary line and superior to the orbital rim.

Fillers are the preferred method for correcting tear trough deformity. Treatment varies with age with younger patients requiring treatment of medial hollowness through filling the medial suborbicularis oculi fat pad, whereas in older patients, lifting and filling the lid-cheek junction helps to counteract loss of lateral suborbicularis oculi fat that occurs as part of the aging process.[55] Both of these techniques reduce the amount of filler needed in the actual tear trough and undercorrection of the deep malar fat pad is recommended due to excess soft tissue below this area that is responsible for the relative fullness of Indian faces. While needle injection is common, cannulas can be used to limit procedure pain and subsequent bruising and allows for more precise injection above the periosteum. For younger tissue, use of a thicker viscosity and for older tissues, use of a thinner viscosity can avoid contour irregulation. Patients with a shallow orbit, retrusive anterior maxilla, and inferior orbital rim often have a deep tear trough. In such cases, treating the prezygomatic space, pyriform aperture, and the deep midfacial fat before treating the tear trough will give a natural and better outcome.[55] Avoid correction of the medial part of the tear trough to avoid the proximal angular artery or use a cannula. As patients often have concerns of both tear trough deformity and periorbital hyperpigmentation, care must be taken to inform patients that while the shadowing effect will decrease, other treatment modalities may be needed, otherwise hyperpigmentation will persist.

South Asians are observed to have high amounts of soft tissue in the medial part of the midface. Age-associated volume loss is a common target for filler in older patients. Younger patients prefer augmented contouring in the lateral cheeks. In either group, filler injected into the lateral cheeks lifts and reduces the nasolabial folds and thus injections here should be performed integratively with the midface fat compartments. To correct a malar groove, filler should be injected into the groove using a layering technique, starting supraperiosteally and then more superficially in the deep dermis. Care should be taken not to inject above the groove as it would make the malar mound more prominent. Injection in the vicinity of the malar mound should be supraperiosteal or just subdermal to avoid the lymphatic vessels in the subcutaneous plane. After the lateral cheeks have been filled, if there is still a nasolabial fold, care should be taken as to not overfill this area to avoid adding to the central soft-tissue fullness. Similarly, filling the lateral midface fat compartment with the appropriate volume of filler decreases the appearance of jowls and marionette lines so that less filler is required in the actual lines and prejowl sulcus. Any remaining marionette lines or the prejowl sulcus itself can then be minimally filled.

It has been discussed earlier in this chapter that South Asians have a wider nose appearance compared to other Asian ethnicities such as Vietnamese and Southeast Asians. The opinion group IFAEG suggests that the wide alar span in Indians can be corrected with filler injections in the alar base/piriform fossa to narrow the base of the nose, in the columella as a bolus on the anterior nasal spine, and as a pillar to support the tip. The nose is a high-risk cosmetic unit due to its high vascularity, thus a 23G or 22G cannula should be used. The authors recommend using small volumes, no more than 0.4 ml, and a perpendicular approach or a 22G cannula to the nasolabial fold when injecting near the piriform fossa as to avoid vascular compromise with the angular artery. In general, filler in the nasal dorsum of Indians is used mainly in low volumes to camouflage a hump, correct supratip deformity, or to augment low-profile noses or a recessed radix. Nonsurgical correction for a drooping/less-projected nasal tip with botulinum toxin in the depressor septi muscle is also very effective in Indians if any remaining deformity exists after correction with filler. It is important to stay midline above the periosteum and cartilage to avoid the lateral and dorsal nasal arteries. Filling of the chin and lower jaw can help create a longer facial height, increase projection of the chin, and correct the appearance of any mandibular retrusion.

Lasers and Light

It has been well documented that in skin of color, laser therapies are safest with longer wavelengths between 600 and 1200 nm such as neodymium-doped yttrium aluminum garnet (Nd:YAG), long-pulsed diode (810 nm), long-pulsed alexandrite (755 nm), and ruby lasers (694 nm), as well as certain intense pulsed light sources.[56–58] Long-pulse 1064 nm Nd:YAG laser has over the years proven to be the preferred laser for darker skin types. There are also recent studies that demonstrate that short pulse (0.6–1.6 ms) may be more effective in these skin types as well.[59] In general, it is recommended to use lower fluence, longer pulse duration, and multiple treatments to minimize side effects.

For laser hair removal, the target of the laser is the chromophore of melanin in the hair bulb in the hair shaft. In darker skin types, melanin in the epidermis is a competing chromophore that leads to higher rates of adverse effects of unwanted postprocedure pigmentary alteration. For traditional lasers with pulsed durations in the millisecond range, lower fluences, longer pulsed durations, and skin cooling are employed to minimize the risk of burns or postinflammatory hyperpigmentation. The two safest wavelengths for laser hair reduction on darker skin types including the South Asian population are the diode (810 nm) and Nd: Yag (1064 nm). A microsecond pulsed (650 microseconds) 1064 Nd:YAG laser has also been used successfully in skin of color (including South Asian skin types). Melanin has a higher absorption value that decreases with longer wavelengths, and with a longer wavelength laser, scatter is reduced and deeper penetration allows for better targeting of the hair follicle. Permanent and complete hair removal is not likely but that, with multiple treatments, significant long-term reduction can be achieved and patients should be counseled of this to manage expectations. Paradoxical hypertrichosis, the conversion of vellus hairs to thicker, more obvious terminal hairs is most associated with intense pulsed laser and long-pulse alexandrite laser.[60] Although it has an unknown prevalence and varying incidence rates, it more frequently affects those with darker skin (Fitzpatrick III–VI) and darker hair color.[61]

Lasers to target pigment alteration are frequently used in South Asian skin. FDA-approved laser treatments for melasma include the fractional 1550/1540 nm nonablative laser that has demonstrated promising results. Because of the concern for hyperpigmentation, we recommend using lower fluences, variable pulses, and cooling, especially in patients with a history of postinflammatory hyperpigmentation. Brauer et al., studied a low-energy, low-density, nonablative fractional 1927-nm laser for melasma, postinflammatory hyperpigmentation, and photodamage.[62] In this study, favorable outcomes were demonstrated and results were maintained at the 3-month follow up. It should be noted, however, that for such a chronic condition, longer follow-up studies are needed.

A randomized control trial by Garg et al., demonstrated that epidermal melasma had the best results with super skin rejuvenation (540 nm) and pixel Q-switched Nd-YAG (1064) while recalcitrant cases of dermal and mixed melasma were successfully treated with pixel-erbium YAG laser (2940 nm).[63] Fractional CO_2 laser (Qray-FRX device) at a fluence of 5 J/cm2, Dot cycle of 6, and Pixel pitch of 2 has been used with some success as well when combined with topical therapy of hydroquinone 4% or the modified Kligman-Willis formula.[64] Low-fluence Q-switched Nd:YAG laser at 1064 nm utilizing the multi-pass technique with a large spot size has been suggested as another modality to treat melasma.[65] Varying degrees of success have been reported but recurrences are common on discontinuing laser therapy. Most recently, picosecond lasers (e.g., the 755-nm picosecond laser) have been used successfully in the treatment of melasma.

In general, topical treatments are required to maintain long-term results, particularly in cases of recalcitrant melasma. Although lasers and light devices have shown to be helpful in melasma, the authors prefer a tiered treatment approach. All patients should be counseled on daily topical antioxidant use along with broad-spectrum iron oxide containing sunscreen. Topical therapies are first line including hydroquinone alone or in combination with other skin lightening and brightening agents. If after 3 months of topical therapy pigment remains, these authors prefer using a combination of glycolic acid chemical peels and oral tranexamic (TXA) acid 650 mg daily for 4 to 6 months. Given it is a plasmin inhibitor, it is important to not use it in patients with a history of vasculopathy or thrombotic events. Its use should also be limited in patients on hormonal contraception as it can increase the chances of blood clots or stroke, particularly in patients who smoke, are overweight, and are over the age of 35. If patients fail oral TXA, only then are laser and light devices considered.

Microneedling, Microfocused Ultrasound and Platelet-rich Plasma Injections

Microneedling has become an increasingly popular choice for patients with skin of color to address concerns such as facial recalcitrant melasma, acne scarring, reversal of photoaging, skin tightening, skin volumization, and dyspigmentation. The main benefit of microneedling is the stimulation of fibroblasts, release of growth factors, and upper dermal collagen production. The epidermis remains partially intact, which allows for a fast recovery and limits the risks of infection and scarring. Because there is no chromophore, this limits unwanted adverse effects such as postinflammatory pigment alteration. Microneedling has also been used in combination with other therapeutics such as platelet-rich plasma and radiofrequency. When combined with radiofrequency, short-pulse duration is preferred to long-pulse duration. Multiple passes and multiple treatments are required; however, this allows for minimal downtime between sessions. Care should be taken in selecting patients to minimize risk of postinflammatory pigment alteration. This risk is increased if the needle depth is too superficial. Correct posttreatment products are paramount to limit foreign body granulomatous reactions.

Microfocused ultrasound is another noninvasive option for skin tightening and lifting in the facial and neck areas. Because ultrasound is chromophore-insensitive it has a low risk of causing postinflammatory pigment alteration.[66] The creation of thermal microcoagulation in the deeper reticular layers of the dermis and the subdermis creates neocollagenesis and remodeling that causes the lifting and tightening of the skin. This procedure has also been used to lift the eyebrow in addition to the neck. Most adverse effects are limited to mild erythema, edema,

bruising, and dysethesia that resolves without further sequelae. This treatment can be combined with ultrasound imaging to ensure proper acoustic coupling that can help to minimize these effects.

Androgenetic alopecia or pattern alopecia affects both men and women and platelet-rich plasma therapy has been shown to be an effective treatment modality. Ideal patients are those who are either nonresponsive or minimally responsive to traditional treatments, such as topical minoxidil, after 6 months to 1 year of consistent treatment. The activated platelets release growth factors and cytokines that stimulate hair growth and decrease shedding (Fig. 7.1). Fresh blood is spun down with an

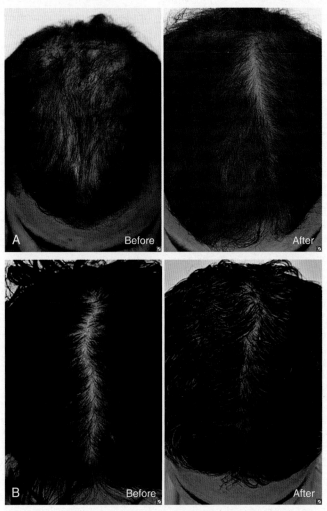

Fig. 7.1 (A) 33-year-old Indian male treated with three sessions of PRP and topical 5% minoxidil (7 months later). (B) 39-year-old Indian male treated with three sessions of PRP and topical 5% minoxidil (9 months later).

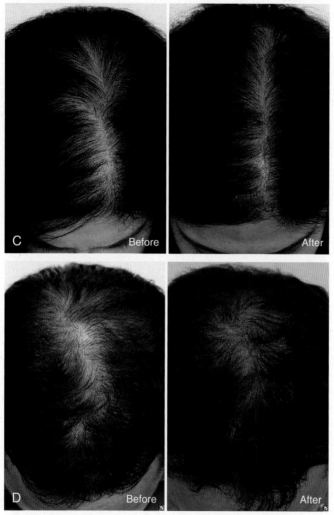

Fig. 7.1, cont'd   (C) 44-year-old Indian female with 50 mg of spironolactone and topical 5% minoxidil plus two sessions of PRP (5 months later). (D) 40-year-old Indian male treated with three sessions of PRP and topical 5% minoxidil (12 months later).

initial soft spin followed by a hard spin followed by extraction of the lower-level platelet-rich plasma concentrate. This concentrate is then combined with an activator and then injections of 0.2 ml to 0.3 ml are placed every 1 cm in the affected areas. A typical treatment regimen would be monthly treatments for 3 months with follow up after 6 months and annual maintenance treatments thereafter. Patients should continue medical therapy during the treatment period.

Microneedling can be combined with platelet-rich plasma therapy for both atrophic acne and androgenetic alopecia and has been shown to be more effective than either treatment in isolation. The benefit of this combination includes faster healing with decreased erythema and edema as well as increased patient satisfaction. For atrophic acne, studies demonstrate increased scar remodeling and cellular regeneration and for androgenetic alopecia, there is increased mean hair diameter, increased root strength, and less shedding.

CONCLUSION

In conclusion, there are many considerations for the management of aesthetic concerns in patients of South

Asian origin including nuances in cultural viewpoints and underlying biological attributes. Like in all populations, there is an increasing interest in cosmetic procedures within this demographic. Given this changing landscape, it is paramount that providers have familiarity with the cultural concerns and desires that each ethnic group has and educate patients that there are many safe and effective treatment options available. Additionally, a vital understanding of the various cosmetic subunits is required to adequately address patient concerns from a global perspective. As we have discussed here, many desires of patients will require a multimodal and multifactorial approach for optimal patient satisfaction. With so many treatment options available, it is advisable that clinicians use their clinical expertise in combination with well-researched studies and data to achieve appropriate treatment endpoints in the appropriate patients.

REFERENCES

1. Vatsyayan K. Pluralism and diversity in South Asia. In: Hussain A, Dubey M, eds. *Democracy, Sustainable Development and Peace: New Perspectives on South Asia.* New Delhi: Oxford University Press; 2014.
2. Hussain A. Recommendations for culturally competent dermatology care of Muslim patients. *J Am Acad Dermatol.* 2017;77(2):388-389.
3. Hashim PW, Nia JK, Taliercio M, Goldenberg G. Ideals of facial beauty. *Cutis.* 100(4):222-224.
4. Hicks KE, Thomas JR. The changing face of beauty: A global assessment of facial beauty. *Otolaryngol Clin North Am.* 2020;53(2):185-194.
5. Hwang WC. Demystifying and addressing internalized racism and oppression among Asian Americans. *Am Psychol.* 2021;76(4):596.
6. Langlois JH, Roggman LA. Attractive faces are only average. *Psychol Sci.* 1990;1(2):115-121.
7. Langlois JH, Roggman LA, Musselman L. What is average and what is not average about attractive faces? *Psychol Sci.* 1994;5(4):214-220.
8. Vokey JR, Read JD. Familiarity, memorability, and the effect of typicality on the recognition of faces. *Mem Cognit.* 1992;20(3):291-302.
9. Vashi NA, Maymone MBDC, Kundu RV. Aging differences in ethnic skin. *J Clin Aesthet Dermatol.* 2016;9(1):31.
10. Fink B, Grammer K, Matts PJ. Visible skin color distribution plays a role in the perception of age, attractiveness, and health in female faces. *Evol Hum Behav.* 2006;27(6):433-442.
11. Stephen ID, Law Smith MJ, Stirrat MR, Perrett DI. Facial skin coloration affects perceived health of human faces. *Int J Primatol.* 2009;30(6):845-857.
12. Fink B, Grammer K, Thornhill R. Human (Homo sapiens) facial attractiveness in relation to skin texture and color. *J Comp Psychol.* 2001;115(1):92.
13. Sommerlad M. Skin lightening: Causes and complications. *Clin Exp Dermatol.* 2022;47(2):264-270.
14. Doolan BJ, Gupta M. Melasma. *Aust J Gen Pract.* 2021; 50(12):880-885.
15. Sarkar R, Gokhale N, Godse K, et al. Medical management of melasma: A review with consensus recommendations by Indian pigmentary expert group. *Indian J Dermatol.* 2017;62(6):558.
16. Sivayathorn A. Melasma in Orientals. *Clin Drug Investig.* 1995;10(2):34-40.
17. Torok HM, Jones T, Rich P, Smith S, Tschen E. Hydroquinone 4%, tretinoin 0.05%, fluocinolone acetonide 0.01%: A safe and efficacious 12-month treatment for melasma. *Cutis.* 2005;75(1):57-62.
18. Nasrollahi SA, Nematzadeh MS, Samadi A, et al. Evaluation of the safety and efficacy of a triple combination cream (hydroquinone, tretinoin, and fluocinolone) for treatment of melasma in Middle Eastern skin. *Clin Cosmet Investig Dermatology.* 2019;12:437.
19. Del Rosario E, Florez-Pollack S, Zapata Jr L, et al. Randomized, placebo-controlled, double-blind study of oral tranexamic acid in the treatment of moderate-to-severe melasma. *J Am Acad Dermatol.* 2018;78(2):363-369.
20. Ranu H, Thng S, Goh BK, Burger A, Goh CL. Periorbital hyperpigmentation in Asians: An epidemiologic study and a proposed classification. *Dermatol Surg.* 2011;37(9):1297-1303.
21. Michelle L, Foulad DP, Ekelem C, Saedi N, Mesinkovska NA. Treatments of periorbital hyperpigmentation: A systematic review. *Dermatol Surg.* 2021;47(1):70-74.
22. Sarkar R, Parmar NV, Kapoor S. Treatment of postinflammatory hyperpigmentation with a combination of glycolic acid peels and a topical regimen in dark-skinned patients: A comparative study. *Dermatol Surg.* 2017;43(4):566-573.
23. Pollock S, Taylor S, Oyerinde O, et al. The dark side of skin lightening: An international collaboration and review of a public health issue affecting dermatology. *Int J Womens Dermatol.* 2021;7(2):158-164.
24. Sankaran S, Sekerdej M, Von Hecker U. The role of Indian caste identity and caste inconsistent norms on status representation. *Front Psychol.* 2017;8:487.
25. Shroff H, Diedrichs PC, Craddock N. Skin color, cultural capital, and beauty products: An investigation of the use of skin fairness products in Mumbai, India. *Front Public Health.* 2018;5:365.

26. Olumide YM. Use of skin lightening creams. *BMJ*. 2010; 341:c6102.

27. Shankar PR, Subish P. Fair skin in South Asia: An obsession? *J Pakistan Assoc Dermatologists*. 2007;17(2): 100-104.

28. Sonthalia S, Jha AK, Lallas A, Jain G, Jakhar D. Glutathione for skin lightening: A regnant myth or evidence-based verity? *Dermatol Pract Concept*. 2018;8(1):15.

29. Zubair S, Hafeez S, Mujtaba G. Efficacy of intravenous glutathione vs. placebo for skin tone lightening. *J Pakistan Assoc Dermatologists*. 2016;26(3):177-181.

30. Dadzie OE. Unethical skin bleaching with glutathione. *BMJ*. 2016;354:i4386.

31. Sonthalia S, Sarkar R. Glutathione for skin lightning: An update. *Pigment Int*. 2017;4(1):3.

32. Juhasz ML, Levin MK. The role of systemic treatments for skin lightening. *J Cosmet Dermatol*. 2018;17(6): 1144-1157.

33. Davids LM, Van Wyk JC, Khumalo NP. Intravenous glutathione for skin lightening: Inadequate safety data. *S Afr Med J*. 2016;106(8):782-786.

34. Dadzie OE, Petit A. Skin bleaching: Highlighting the misuse of cutaneous depigmenting agents. *J Eur Acad Dermatol Venereol*. 2009;23(7):741-750.

35. Kapoor KM, Chatrath V, Anand C, et al. Consensus recommendations for treatment strategies in Indians using botulinum toxin and hyaluronic acid fillers. *Plast Reconstr Surg Glob Open*. 2017;5(12):e1574.

36. Shome D, Vadera S, Khare S, et al. Aging and the Indian face: An analytical study of aging in the Asian Indian face. *Plast Reconstr Surg Glob Open*. 2020;8(3):e2580.

37. McCurdy JA, Falces E. Cosmetic surgery of the Asian face. *Plast Reconstr Surg*. 1993;91(6):1167.

38. Shiffman MA, Mirrafati S, Lam SM, Cueteaux CG, eds. *Simplified Facial Rejuvenation*; Berlin, Heidelberg: Springer Science & Business Media; 2007.

39. Alexis AF, Grimes P, Boyd C, et al. Racial and ethnic differences in self-assessed facial aging in women: Results from a multinational study. *Dermatol Surg*. 2019;45(12): 1635-1648.

40. Nanda S, Bansal S. Upper face rejuvenation using botulinum toxin and hyaluronic acid fillers. *Indian J Dermatol Venereol Leprol*. 2013;79(1):32-40.

41. Farkas LG, Katic MJ, Forrest CR. International anthropometric study of facial morphology in various ethnic groups/races. *J Craniofac Surg*. 2005;16(4):615-646.

42. Thomas M, D'Silva J, Kohli S, Sarkar S. Lip designing: The need for a beautiful smile: An Indian perspective. *Indian J Dent Res*. 2014;25(4):449.

43. Keaney TC, Alster TS. Botulinum toxin in men: Review of relevant anatomy and clinical trial data. *Dermatol Surg*. 2013;39(10):1434-1443.

44. Carruthers A, Carruthers J. Clinical indications and injection technique for the cosmetic use of botulinum A exotoxin. *Dermatol Surg*. 1998;24(11):1189-1194.

45. Jagadish Chandra H, Ravi MS, Sharma SM, Rajendra Prasad B. Standards of facial esthetics: An anthropometric study. *J Maxillofac Oral Surg*. 2012;11(4):384-389.

46. Resnik SS, Resnik BI. Complications of chemical peeling. *Dermatol Clin*. 1995;13(2):309-312.

47. Sarkar R. How to choose the best peeling agent for the patient: Asian skin. In: *Color Atlas of Chemical Peels*. Berlin, Heidelberg: Springer; 2011:185-192.

48. Sehgal VN, Luthra A, Aggarwal AK. Evaluation of graded strength glycolic acid (GA) facial peel: An Indian experience. *J Dermatol*. 2003;30(10):758-761.

49. Sarkar R, Kaur C, Bhalla M, Kanwar AJ. The combination of glycolic acid peels with a topical regimen in the treatment of melasma in dark-skinned patients: A comparative study. *Dermatol Surg*. 2002;28(9):828-832.

50. Handog EB, Datuin MSL, Singzon IA. Chemical peels for acne and acne scars in Asians: Evidence based review. *J Cutan Aesthet Surg*. 2012;5(4):239.

51. Dayal S, Kalra KD, Sahu P. Comparative study of efficacy and safety of 45% mandelic acid versus 30% salicylic acid peels in mild-to-moderate acne vulgaris. *J Cosmet Dermatol*. 2020;19(2):393-399.

52. Sundaram H, Huang PH, Hsu NJ, et al. Aesthetic applications of botulinum toxin A in Asians: An international, multidisciplinary, pan-Asian consensus. *Plast Reconstr Surg Glob Open*. 2016;4(12):e872.

53. Sedgh J. The aesthetics of the upper face and brow: Male and female differences. *Facial Plast Surg*. 2018;34(02): 114-118.

54. Carruthers J, Fournier N, Kerscher M, et al. The convergence of medicine and neurotoxins: a focus on botulinum toxin type A and its application in aesthetic medicine—A global, evidence-based botulinum toxin consensus education initiative: Part II: Incorporating botulinum toxin into aesthetic clinical practice. *Dermatol Surg*. 2013;39(3 Pt 2):510-525.

55. Sharad J. Treatment of the tear trough and infraorbital hollow with hyaluronic acid fillers using both needle and cannula. *Dermatol Ther*. 2020;33(3):e13353.

56. Alster TS, Bryan H, Williams CM. Long-pulsed Nd: YAG laser-assisted hair removal in pigmented skin: A clinical and histological evaluation. *Arch Dermatol*. 2001;137(7): 885-889.

57. Tanzi EL, Alster TS. Long-pulsed 1064-nm Nd: YAG laser-assisted hair removal in all skin types. *Dermatol Surg*. 2004;30(1):13-17.

58. Garcia C, Alamoudi H, Nakib M, Zimmo S. Alexandrite laser hair removal is safe for Fitzpatrick skin types IV-VI. *Dermatol Surg*. 2000;26(2):130-134.

59. Jane SD, Mysore V. Effectiveness of short-pulse width Nd: YAG in laser hair reduction. *J Cosmet Dermatol.* 2018;17(6):1046-1052.

60. Town G, Bjerring P. Is paradoxical hair growth caused by low-level radiant exposure by home-use laser and intense pulsed light devices? *J Cosmet Laser Ther.* 2016;18(6): 355-362.

61. Baah N, Chacon AH. A paradoxical phenomenon: Intense pulsed light-induced hypertrichosis, a brief review. *Dermatol Rev.* 2021;2(2):106-110.

62. Brauer JA, Alabdulrazzaq H, Bae YS, Geronemus RG. Evaluation of a low energy, low density, non-ablative fractional 1927 nm wavelength laser for facial skin resurfacing. *J Drugs Dermatol.* 2015;14(11):1262-1267.

63. Garg S, Vashisht KR, Makadia S. A prospective randomized comparative study on 60 Indian patients of melasma, comparing pixel Q-switched NdYAG (1064 nm), super skin rejuvenation (540 nm) and ablative pixel erbium YAG (2940 nm) lasers, with a review of the literature. *J Cosmet Laser Ther.* 2019;21(5):297-307.

64. Abadchi SN, Naeini FF, Beheshtian E. Combination of hydroquinone and fractional CO2 laser versus hydroquinone monotherapy in melasma treatment: A randomized, single-blinded, split-face clinical trial. *Indian J Dermatol.* 2019;64(2):129.

65. Choi JE, Lee DW, Seo SH, Ahn HH, Kye YC. Low-fluence Q-switched Nd: YAG laser for the treatment of melasma in Asian patients. *J Cosmet Dermatol.* 2018;17(6): 1053-1058.

66. Bader KB, Makin IRS, Abramowicz JS, Bioeffects Committee of the American Institute of Ultrasound in Medicine. Ultrasound for aesthetic applications: A review of biophysical mechanisms and safety. *J Ultrasound Med.* 2022;41(7):1597-1607.

8

Topical Treatments for Melasma

Heather Woolery-Lloyd, Kiyanna Williams, Janeth R. Campbell

SUMMARY AND KEY FEATURES

- Melasma is a disorder of pigmentation characterized by well-demarcated hyperpigmented patches on the face. It is one of the most challenging conditions to treat in a dermatology practice.
- Hydroquinone is the "gold standard" to which all other topical melasma therapies are compared. Modified versions of the Kligman-Willis formula, which includes a combination of hydroquinone, a retinoid, and a topical steroid, have shown efficacy and are frequently utilized as the first-line therapy when initiating a melasma treatment plan.
- Although effective, hydroquinone may be irritating for some patients and carries a risk of ochronosis

with long-term use. For this reason, many clinicians will start therapy with a modified Kligman-Willis formula and then switch to alternative therapies for maintenance.
- Many alternatives to hydroquinone have been used as adjunctive therapy to manage melasma including retinoids, cortical steroids, vitamin C, azelaic acid, cysteamine, tranexamic acid, niacinamide, and licorice extract.
- Utilizing combination therapy, including an emphasis on sun protection and sun avoidance, offers patients a comprehensive and effective approach to the management of melasma.

Melasma is a disorder of pigmentation characterized by well-demarcated hyperpigmented patches on the face. Although melasma can occur in all skin types, it is most common in patients with skin of color. Women are most commonly affected, representing the vast majority of cases.[1] The two most common clinical presentations are the malar and the centrofacial patterns.[2,3] Other affected areas include the mandible, neck, and brachial arms. The etiology of melasma remains unclear but UV radiation, visible light, family history, air pollution, and hormonal factors have been implicated in the pathogenesis of melasma.[4,5] Melasma can be treated with both topical and procedural therapies. For most clinicians, topical therapy remains the first-line treatment. This chapter will focus on topical therapies to treat melasma.

TOPICAL THERAPIES

Hydroquinone

Hydroquinone is considered one of the most effective agents for the treatment of pigmentary disorders including melasma. Hydroquinone is a potent tyrosinase inhibitor and is often used as the "gold standard" to which all other topical melasma therapies are compared. Formulations of 4% are commercially available by prescription. In patients with skin of color that do not respond adequately to 4% hydroquinone, higher concentrations can be compounded (e.g., 6%–10%). Monotherapy with hydroquinone has been reported in the treatment of melasma.[6] However, the Kligman-Willis formula, which includes a combination of hydroquinone, a retinoid, and a topical steroid, is often used in the treatment of melasma.[7] The original Kligman-Willis formula included 0.1% tretinoin, 5.0% hydroquinone, and 0.1% dexamethasone in a hydrophilic ointment and revolutionized the treatment of hyperpigmentation. This unique combination of ingredients was found to work synergistically and was reported to be more efficacious than the individual ingredients when used alone in the treatment of hyperpigmentation. The first FDA-approved treatment for melasma was a modified Kligman-Willis formula.[8] In the randomized investigator-blinded phase III trial of 641 subjects with melasma, the triple combinations of tretinoin 0.05%, hydroquinone 4.0%, and fluocinolone acetonide 0.01% was compared to the dual combinations of tretinoin plus hydroquinone, tretinoin plus fluocinolone acetonide, and hydroquinone plus fluocinolone acetonide. In this pivotal trial, 26.1% of subjects in the triple-combination treatment group achieved complete clearing compared to 4.6% of subjects in the other treatment groups at week 8 ($P = 0.0001$). Additionally, at week 8, a 75% reduction in melasma pigmentation was observed in more than 70% of patients treated with the triple-combination therapy compared to 30% of subjects treated with the dual-combination agents.[8] Kligman-Willis formulations may be particularly effective in melasma for many reasons. The individual ingredients—hydroquinone and retinoids—have been established as effective agents to treat melasma, while topical corticosteroids suppress melanocyte secretory function.[6,9,10] However, potent topical corticosteroids have limitations due to the significant risk of atrophy. Kligman proposed that the addition of a retinoid may reduce or prevent atrophy caused by topical steroids when treating melasma.[11] Modified versions of the Kligman-Willis formula remain the mainstay of treatment for melasma and are frequently utilized as the first-line therapy when initiating a melasma treatment plan.

Although effective, hydroquinone has limitations as a long-term therapy for melasma. For some patients, hydroquinone can be irritating and is poorly tolerated. This irritation may be due to the hydroquinone itself or may be caused by allergic contact dermatitis to a common preservative in hydroquinone formulations, sodium metabisulfite.[12] However, the main risk of long-term hydroquinone use is ochronosis, which is a paradoxical darkening of the skin caused by homogentisic acid accumulation in the dermis.[13] For this reason, many clinicians will start therapy with a modified Kligman-Willis formula and then switch to alternative therapies for maintenance.

With this approach, hydroquinone is reserved for initiation of therapy and used intermittently throughout the course of melasma treatment on an as-needed basis. There is no clearly established maximum length of time for hydroquinone use in melasma but many clinicians try to limit treatment duration to less than 3 months of continued use. Two studies have specifically examined 6-month safety data for the FDA-approved modified Kligman-Willis melasma therapy. The first study examined the atrophogenic potential of this formula in 62 subjects using serial skin biopsies. No statistically significant histopathologic signs of atrophy were noted. The authors concluded that the risk of skin atrophy with this treatment is very low with 6 months of use.[14]

A second study of 25 subjects looked at safety with intermittent and continuous use of the same formula. This study reported a significant increase in telangiectasias in one cohort at 6 months, but the severity was mild. The authors concluded that the treatment was safe for moderate to severe melasma up to 6 months.[15]

Intermittent use of hydroquinone is widely utilized by many clinicians. This approach may also reduce the risk of ochronosis while offering patients the benefits of hydroquinone as a highly effective treatment agent. Many alternatives to hydroquinone have been used as adjunctive therapy to manage melasma and these options will later be covered (Table 8.1).

RETINOIDS

Retinoids have been used for decades for their cosmetic benefits and tretinoin is one of the earliest treatments published in the management of melasma.[16,17] Retinoids may work to treat hyperpigmentation by increasing epidermal turnover and decreasing melanosome transfer.[18] Although effective as a monotherapy, tretinoin is now more commonly used in combination with other ingredients when treating melasma. The most common use of tretinoin in melasma is in the modified Kligman-Willis formula. However, tretinoin has also been reported as an effective melasma treatment in combination with other skin-lightening agents including azelaic acid and mequinol.[19,20]

TOPICAL CORTICOSTEROIDS

Topical corticosteroids have been utilized to treat melasma. Topical corticosteroids may influence melanogenesis

TABLE 8.1   Review of Melasma Studies

Author (Year)	Ingredient(s)	Comparison Treatment	Number of Subjects (n)	Study Design	Results
Pathak (1986)	Tretinoin .05% or .1% and hydroquinone 2%–5%	Hydroquinone 2%–5%	n = 300	CCT[a]	Superior
Griffiths (1993)	Tretinoin .1%	Vehicle cream	n = 38	RCT[b]	Superior
Graupe (1996)	20% Azelaic acid cream and 0.05% tretinoin cream	20% azelaic acid cream	n = 50	RCT	Superior
Keeling (2008)	Mequinol 2% and tretinoin 0.01% solution	N/A	n = 5	Case series	Complete (4/5) to moderate clearance (1/5) (clinician assessment)
Neering (1975)	Betamethasone 17-valerate in a cream base containing DMSO	N/A	n = 17	Case series	Good improvement (clinician assessment)
Kanwar (1994)	Clobetasol propionate 0.05%	N/A	n = 10	Case series	80%–90% clearance (clinician assessment)
Taylor (2003)	Tretinoin .05%, hydroquinone 4%, and fluocinolone acetonide 0.01%	Tretinoin .05% and hydroquinone 4% tretinoin .05% and fluocinolone acetonide .01% hydroquinone 4% and fluocinolone acetonide .01%	n = 641	RCT	Superior
Espinal-Perez (2004)	L-ascorbic acid 5%	Hydroquinone 4%	n = 16	RCT	Inferior (patient subjective assessment) Equivalent (colorimetric assessment with melanin index difference)
Huh (2003)	Vitamin C iontophoresis	Distilled water iontophoresis	n = 29	RCT	Superior
Ismail (2019)	Microneedling with topical vitamin C	N/A	n = 30	Case series	Decrease in melasma area and severity index (MASI) score
Garcia-Lopez (1989)	Azelaic acid 20% cream	Hydroquinone 2% cream	n = 155	RCT	Superior
Baliña (1991)	Azelaic acid 20% cream	Hydroquinone 4%	n = 329	RCT	Equivalent
Kakita (1998)	Azelaic acid 20% cream and glycolic acid 15% or 20% lotion	Hydroquinone 4%	n = 65	RCT	Equivalent
Nguyen (2020)	Cysteamine 5%	Hydroquinone 4%	n = 20	RCT	Equivalent
Lima (2020)*	Cysteamine 5%*	Hydroquinone 4%	n = 40	RCT	Inferior

Continued

TABLE 8.1   Review of Melasma Studies—cont'd

Author (Year)	Ingredient(s)	Comparison Treatment	Number of Subjects (n)	Study Design	Results
Karrabi (2020)	Cysteamine 5%	4% hydroquinone, 0.05% retinoic acid, and 0.1% betamethasone (modified Kligman)	n = 50	RCT	Superior
Ebrahimi (2014)	Tranexamic acid 3% solution	Hydroquinone 3% and dexamethasone 0.01% solution	n = 50	CCT	Equivalent
Lee (2006)	Tranexamic acid (4 mg/mL) injected intradermally	N/A	n = 100	OLP[c]	Decrease in MASI score from baseline
Del Rosario (2018)	250 mg of tranexamic acid capsules twice daily	Placebo capsules	n = 44	RCT	Superior
Atefi (2017)	Tranexamic acid 5%	Hydroquinone 2%	n = 60	RCT	Equivalent
Banihashemi (2015)	Liposomal tranexamic acid 5%	Hydroquinone 4%	n = 30	CCT	Equivalent
Navarrete – Solis (2011)	Niacinamide 4% cream	Hydroquinone 4% cream	n = 27	RCT	Equivalent
Zubair (2009)	Liquiritin 2% and liquiritin 4%	Hydroquinone 4%	n = 90	RCT	Superior
Monteiro (2013)	0.75% kojic acid and 2.5% vitamin C	Hydroquinone 4% cream	n = 60	CCT	Inferior
Garcia (1996)	Kojic acid 2% (and padimate O 4%, glycolic acid 5% propylene glycol 10%)	Hydroquinone 2% and sodium bisulfite .1% (and padimate O 4%, glycolic acid 5% propylene glycol 10%)	n = 39	CCT	Equivalent
Gheisari (2020)	5% Methimazole	Hydroquinone 4%	n = 50	RCT	Inferior
Nofal (2019)	Silymarin 0.7% and 1.4%	Hydroquinone 4%	n = 42	CCT	Equivalent
Katoulis (2014)	Undecylenoyl phenylalanine 2%	Vehicle cream	n = 40	RCT	Superior
Lyons (2018)	Epidermal growth factor	Placebo	n = 15	RCT	Superior
Draelos (2015)	Lignin peroxidase	Hydroquinone 4%	n = 60	RCT	Equivalent
Alvin (2011)	75% Mulberry extract oil	Placebo	n = 50	RCT	Superior
Mendoza (2014)	3% Rumex occidentalis	Hydroquinone 4%	n = 45	RCT	Equivalent
Huh (2010)	Liposome-encapsulated 4-n-butylresorcinol 0.1% cream	Vehicle cream	n = 23	RCT	Superior
Ibrahim (2015)	10% glycolic acid and 4% hydroquinone 10% glycolic acid, 4% hydroquinone, and 0.01% hyaluronic acid	4% Hydroquinone or hydroquinone and 0.01% hyaluronic acid	n = 100	CCT	Equivalent

TABLE 8.1	Review of Melasma Studies—cont'd				
Author (Year)	Ingredient(s)	Comparison Treatment	Number of Subjects (n)	Study Design	Results
Ghafarzadeh (2017)	Liposome-encapsulated aloe vera leaf gel extract	Aloe vera leaf gel extract	n = 180	RCT	Superior
Tirado-Sánchez (2009)	1% dioic acid cream	hydroquinone 2%	n = 96	RCT	Equivalent
Ertam (2008)	Synthetic ellagic acid 1% Natural ellagic acid 1%	Arbutin (1%)	n = 30	RCT	Equivalent
Adalatkhah (2015)	1% Flutamide cream	Hydroquinone 4%	n = 74	RCT	Superior
Khosravan (2017)	Petroselinum crispum (parsley)	Hydroquinone 4%	n = 70	RCT	Equivalent
Desai (2019)	3% tranexamic acid, 1% kojic acid, 5% niacinamide, and 5% hydroxyethylpipera-zineethane sulfonic acid (HEPES)	N/A	n = 55	OLP	Decrease in modified MASI score from baseline
Makino (2013)	Multimodality skin brightener composition containing SMA-432 (prostaglandin E2 inhibitor)	Hydroquinone 4%	n = 75	RCT	Equivalent *in two of three formulations*

[a]Controlled Clinical Trial
[b]Randomized Control Trial
[c]Open Label Pilot
*Note: A follow-up letter reported the concentration of the tested product to be .56% of cysteamine, rather than 5% as originally reported.

through their effects on prostaglandin and leukotriene synthesis.[21] Original reports of topical corticosteroids for melasma included fluorinated corticosteroids as monotherapy.[22,23] Potent topical corticosteroids are now used less frequently since safer alternatives are available. The main concerns with the use of fluorinated corticosteroids in melasma are atrophy and telangiectasias. Currently, the most common use of topical corticosteroids in melasma is in commercially available and compounded versions of the modified Kligman-Willis formula.[8] In current practice, topical corticosteroids and other antiinflammatory medications are also sometimes utilized to mitigate irritation from other agents to treat melasma.[24]

VITAMIN C

Vitamin C is another ingredient that has been used for decades for its cosmetic benefits and it is a well-established adjunctive therapy in the management of melasma. Vitamin C is a potent antioxidant and may influence melanogenesis by reduction of melanin and melanin intermediates such as dopaquinone.[25] A double-blind randomized split-face trial compared ascorbic acid 5% to hydroquinone 4% in 16 women with melasma.[26] In this study, the best subjective improvement was observed on the hydroquinone side with 93% achieving good and excellent results, compared with 62.5% on the ascorbic acid side. Although hydroquinone was more effective, side effects were noted in 68.7% of subjects on the hydroquinone-treated side versus only 6.2% of subjects on the ascorbic acid-treated side. The skin-lightening benefits and tolerability of vitamin C are well-established; however, it is rarely used as a monotherapy in the treatment of melasma. Many published studies on vitamin C for melasma combine vitamin C with procedures such as iontophoresis and microneedling.[27,28] As a topical agent, vitamin C is most helpful as an adjunct in a comprehensive melasma treatment plan.

AZELAIC ACID

Azelaic acid acts as a tyrosinase inhibitor and large randomized trials have been published on its use in melasma. In a Filipino study of 155 subjects of Indo-Malay-Hispanic origin with Fitzpatrick Skin Type (FST) III-V, azelaic acid (AZA) 20% cream twice daily was compared to hydroquinone (HQ) 2% cream twice daily. At 24 weeks, 73% of AZA subjects and 19% of the HQ subjects had good to excellent results ($P < 0.001$). Local irritation was reported in 11/77 in the AZA group and 9/78 in the HQ group. In this study, AZA 20% cream was found to be superior in efficacy to HQ 2% cream with similar tolerability.[29]

A larger multicenter controlled double-blinded study of 329 women with melasma compared azelaic acid 20% cream twice daily to hydroquinone 4% cream twice daily. The study took place at multiple sites in South America (Brazil, Peru, Uruguay, Venezuela, Argentina) with over 75% of subjects described as either "Hispanic," "American Indian," or "Other." At 24 weeks, 64.8% of patients treated with AZA and 72.5% of patients treated with HQ had achieved good or excellent overall results. The difference in response rate was not statistically significant.[30]

Topical azelaic acid can be drying for some patients and in this study, local irritation was noted more frequently in the azelaic acid group (18 subjects in AZA group vs. 1 subject in the HQ group). Allergic sensitization was observed in one subject in the hydroquinone group.[30] It is important to consider the risk of local irritation when treating melasma patients with 20% azelaic acid. Generous use of moisturizers and the addition of an antiinflammatory agent are particularly helpful if irritation occurs. With this approach, azelaic acid is well tolerated as a topical skin-lightening agent. Azelaic acid can be used alone or in combination formulas with other skin lightening agents such as glycolic acid[31] and retinoids.[19] Used alone, or in combination with other agents, azelaic acid is an effective and well-established treatment option for patients with melasma. While studies are lacking, 15% azelaic foam or gel is frequently used in clinical practice as an alternative to 20% cream.

CYSTEAMINE

Cysteamine is a newer agent that has demonstrated efficacy in randomized controlled trials for melasma.

The mechanism of cysteamine in treating hyperpigmentation is not clearly understood. However, cysteamine is a thiol compound and thiolic agents can inhibit both tyrosinase and peroxidase, two key enzymes involved in melanin synthesis.[32,33]

In a double-blinded randomized controlled trial cysteamine 5% was compared to HQ 4% in 20 subjects with melasma in Australia. The trial included five subjects with FST II, ten subjects with FST III, four subjects with FST IV, and one subject with FST V. In this 16-week trial, cysteamine was applied for 15 minutes and then rinsed, and HQ was applied once daily. Six subjects did not complete the trial. The statistical analysis was conducted on the 14 remaining subjects (cysteamine, n = 5; hydroquinone, n = 9). At week 16 there was a 21.3% reduction in mMASI for the cysteamine group and a 32% reduction in the hydroquinone group. The reduction in mMASI between the two groups was not statistically significant ($P = 0.3$). In this trial, HQ 4% cream was better tolerated than cysteamine 5% cream with lower rates of local skin irritation.[34]

Another multicenter, evaluator-blinded clinical trial of 40 Brazilian women with melasma compared cysteamine 5% cream to HQ 4% cream. In this 120-day trial, cysteamine was applied from 15 minutes up to 2 hours at night, and hydroquinone was applied once daily at bedtime. The trial included 36 subjects with FST II-III and 44 subjects with FST IV-V. At 120 days the mean reduction of the mMASI was 38% for cysteamine and 53% for HQ ($P = 0.017$). Tolerability was similar between the two groups.[35] It is important to note that in a follow-up letter to the editor, the manufacturers of a commercially available cysteamine product analyzed the percentage of cysteamine in the product used in this study and reported a cysteamine concentration of 0.56%.[36]

A larger trial of 50 subjects in Iran compared cysteamine 5% cream applied for 15 minutes to a modified Kligman formula (4% hydroquinone, 0.05% retinoic acid, and 0.1% betamethasone) applied once daily at night. The trial included 26 subjects with FST III and 24 subjects with FST IV. At month 4, the percentage reduction in mMASI score was approximately 9% greater in the cysteamine cream group compared to the modified Kligman group. These differences were statistically significant.[37] Cysteamine was better tolerated than the modified Kligman formula; however, some subjects complained of the strong odor of cysteamine in this study. This did not result in treatment discontinuation.

Cysteamine has become a frequently used therapy in the management of melasma. It is effective and well tolerated as a short contact therapy for melasma.

TRANEXAMIC ACID

Tranexamic acid (TXA) is another newer topical agent in the treatment of melasma. TXA may influence pigmentation through its anti-plasmin activity. Plasmin activity increases arachidonic acid and alpha-melanocyte-stimulating hormone, agents that can activate melanin synthesis.[38–40]

TXA has been studied as a topical, intradermal, and oral medication for melasma.[38,41,42] Although oral TXA has been demonstrated to be highly effective in melasma, there is an increased risk of thromboembolic events. For this reason, there is significant interest in the topical efficacy of TXA.

In a double-blind split-face 12-week trial including 50 Iranian women with melasma, tranexamic acid 3% solution daily was compared to hydroquinone 3%/dexamethasone 0.01% solution twice daily. At 12 weeks, there was no difference in the MASI reduction or in the investigators' and subjects' assessment of melasma improvement. Localized skin side effects were more frequent on the hydroquinone/dexamethasone-treated side.[38]

A randomized double-blinded clinical trial including 60 Iranian subjects with melasma compared TXA 5% twice daily to hydroquinone 2% twice daily. At week 12, the reduction in the mean MASI score was not significant between the two groups. The hydroquinone group had more side effects and patient satisfaction was greater in the TXA group.[43]

A 12-week split-face trial compared liposomal TXA 5% to HQ4% twice daily. Both formulations demonstrated a statistically significant reduction of mMASI at 12 weeks. A greater decrease of mMASI was observed with 5% liposomal TA, although this difference was not statistically significant. Local irritation was only observed in the hydroquinone group.[44]

TXA has emerged as another useful agent in the treatment of melasma. In clinical studies, TXA was reported to be well tolerated and offers similar efficacy to hydroquinone. Used alone or in combination formulas, TXA is a helpful addition to the melasma treatment armamentarium.

NIACINAMIDE

Niacinamide is a biologically active amide of vitamin B3. It inhibits melanosome transfer to keratinocytes and also has photoprotective effects. An 8 week split-face study of 27 subjects with melasma compared niacinamide 4% cream to hydroquinone 4% cream and showed no difference between the two treatments as measured by colorimetry. Good to excellent improvement was reported in 44% of subjects in the niacinamide group and 55% of subjects in the hydroquinone group. There were fewer side effects in the niacinamide-treated group.[45]

Niacinamide is an easily accessible ingredient and is often incorporated into cosmetic formulations including moisturizers and serums. In melasma, its use is most helpful as an adjunct in a comprehensive treatment regimen.

LICORICE EXTRACT

Licorice extract is a common ingredient in formulations to treat hyperpigmentation. There are three active components of licorice extract including glabridin, liquiritin, and licochalcone A. Glabridin and liquiritin inhibit tyrosinase while licochalcone A is an antiinflammatory. A study of 90 subjects with melasma in Pakistan compared liquirtin 2% and liquiritin 4% to hydroquinone 4% over 8 weeks. Improvement was seen in 96.7% of those in the 4% liquirtin group, 86.7% in the 2% liquirtin group, and 76.3% in the 4% hydroquinone group. The treatments were well tolerated with no adverse events reported.[46]

OTHER THERAPIES

Several other therapies have been reported to treat melasma. Kojic acid is often used alone or in combination formulas with beneficial results.[47,48] Other ingredients that have been studied for melasma in randomized controlled trials include methimazole,[49] silymarin,[50] undecylenoyl phenylalanine,[51] epidermal growth factor,[52] lignin peroxidase,[53] mulberry extract,[54] Rumex occidentalis,[55] 4-n-butylresorcinol,[56] glycolic acid,[57] aloe vera,[58] dioic acid,[59] ellagic acid and arbutin,[60] flutamide,[61] and parsley.[62,63]

SPECIAL CONSIDERATIONS

It is important to note that although published studies often focus on monotherapy with one ingredient compared to HQ or a modified Kligman-Willis formula, many commercially available products to treat melasma include a combination of ingredients.[64,65] Melanogenesis is a complex, multistage process so using topical agents that act on different stages of this process is thought to offer superior results.[66] In clinical practice, multimodal therapies are often required to approach the clinical efficacy of hydroquinone.

In addition, the importance of strict sun protection cannot be underestimated in the management of melasma. A comprehensive approach with an emphasis on sun protection and sun avoidance is critical. Broad-spectrum ultraviolet (UV) protection with mineral sunscreens is key for treatment success. In addition, sunscreens that offer visible light (VL) protection with the addition of iron oxides have been reported to be superior to UV-only coverage.[67] The limitation of tinted UV-VL sunscreen in darker skin types is matching the sunscreen to the wide range of hues represented by the skin of color population. Sunscreens with antioxidants and free radical quenchers also confer protection against VL and therefore may be an alternative to tinted sunscreens for some patients.[68]

Camouflage with makeup can also be helpful in melasma patients and has been reported to significantly improve the quality of life in patients with pigmentary disorders.[69] In patients who choose to wear makeup, foundations and coverage products can not only cover melasma patches but also help to improve cosmesis of mineral sunscreens that tend to have a greyish hue when applied on darker skin tones.

CONCLUSION

Melasma is one of the most challenging conditions to treat in a dermatology practice. It is important for patients to understand that melasma is a chronic condition that can be managed with multiple interventions. Topical therapy often involves initiation with a hydroquinone-based Kligman-Willis formula followed by hydroquinone-free maintenance therapy. Intermittent use of hydroquinone is often required; however, newer therapies and formulations have proven to be increasingly effective alternatives to treat melasma. Utilizing combination therapy with an emphasis on sun protection and sun avoidance offers patients a comprehensive and effective approach to the management of melasma.

REFERENCES

1. Hexsel D, Lacerda DA, Cavalcante AS, et al. Epidemiology of melasma in Brazilian patients: A multicenter study. *Int J Dermatol.* 2014;53(4):440-444.
2. KrupaShankar DSR, Somani VK, Kohli M, et al. A cross-sectional, multicentric clinico-epidemiological study of melasma in India. *Dermatol Ther.* 2014;4(1):71-81.
3. Moin A, Jabery Z, Fallah N. Prevalence and awareness of melasma during pregnancy. *Int J Dermatol.* 2006;45(3): 285-288.
4. Ogbechie-Godec OA, Elbuluk N. Melasma: An up-to-date comprehensive review. *Dermatol Ther (Heidelb).* 2017; 7(3):305-318.
5. Roberts WE. Pollution as a risk factor for the development of melasma and other skin disorders of facial hyperpigmentation is there a case to be made? *J Drugs Dermatol.* 2015:14:337-341.
6. Sanchez JL, Vazquez M. A hydroquinone solution in the treatment of melasma. *Int J Dermatol.* 1982;20:55-58.
7. Kligman AM, Willis I. A new formula for depigmenting human skin. *Arch Dermatol.* 1975;111(1):40-48.
8. Taylor SC, Torok H, Jones T, et al. Efficacy and safety of a new triple-combination agent for the treatment of facial melasma. *Cutis.* 2003;72(1):67-72.
9. Griffiths CEM, Finkel LJ, Ditre CM, et al. Topical tretinoin (retinoic acid) improves melasma. A vehicle-controlled, clinical trial. *Br J Dermatol.* 1993;129:415-421.
10. Neering H. Treatment of melasma (chloasma) by local application of a steroid cream. *Dermatologica.* 1975; 151(6):349-353.
11. Kligman LH, Schwartz E, Lesnik RH, et al. Topical tretinoin prevents corticosteroid-induced atrophy without lessening the anti-inflammatory effect. *Curr Probl Dermatol.* 1993;21:79-88.
12. Huang PY, Chu CY. Allergic contact dermatitis due to sodium metabisulfite in a bleaching cream. *Contact Dermatitis.* 2007;56:123-124.
13. Charlín R, Barcaui CB, Kac BK, et al. Hydroquinone-induced exogenous ochronosis: A report of four cases and usefulness of dermoscopy. *Int J Dermatol.* 2008; 47(1):19-23.
14. Bhawan J, Grimes P, Pandya AG, et al. A histological examination for skin atrophy after 6 months of treatment with fluocinolone acetonide 0.01%, hydroquinone 4%, and tretinoin 0.05% cream. *Am J Dermatopathol.* 2009; 31(8):794-798.

15. Grimes PE, Bhawan J, Guevara IL, at al. Continuous therapy followed by a maintenance therapy regimen with a triple combination cream for melasma. *J Am Acad Dermatol*. 2010;62(6): 962-967.

16. Pathak MA, Fitzpatrick TB, Kraus EW. Usefulness of retinoic acid in the treatment of melasma. *J Am Acad Dermatol*. 1986;15(4):894-899.

17. Griffiths CE, Finkel LJ, Ditre CM, Hamilton TA, Ellis CN, Voorhees JJ. Topical tretinoin (retinoic acid) improves melasma. A vehicle-controlled, clinical trial. *Br J Dermatol*. 1993;129(4):415-421.

18. Ortonne JP. Retinoid therapy of pigmentary disorders. *Dermatol Ther*. 2006;19(5):280-288.

19. Graupe K, Verallo-Rowell VM, Verallo V, Zaumseil RP. Combined use of 20% azelaic acid cream and 0.05% tretinoin cream in the topical treatment of melasma. *J Dermatolog Treat*. 1996;7(4):235-237.

20. Keeling J, Cardona L, Benitez A, Epstein R, Rendon M. Mequinol 2%/tretinoin 0.01% topical solution for the treatment of melasma in men: A case series and review of the literature. *Cutis*. 2008;81(2):179-183.

21. Halder R, Nordlund JJ. Topical treatment of pigmentary disorders. In: Nordlund JJ, Boissy RE, Hearing VJ, King RA, Ortonne JP, eds. *The Pigmentary System Physiology and Pathology*. New York: Oxford University Press; 1998: 969-975.

22. Neering H. Treatment of melasma (chloasma) by local application of a steroid cream. *Dermatology*. 1975;151(6): 349-353.

23. Kanwar AJ, Dhar S, Kaur S. Treatment of melasma with potent topical corticosteroids. *Dermatology*. 1994; 188(2):170.

24. Kirsch B, Hoesly PM, Jambusaria A, Heckman MG, Diehl NN, Sluzevich JC. Evaluating the efficacy, safety, and tolerability of the combination of tazarotene, azelaic acid, tacrolimus, and zinc oxide for the treatment of melasma: a pilot study. *J Clin Aesthet Dermatol*. 2019;12(5):40.

25. Farris PF. Topical vitamin C: A useful agent for treating photoaging and other dermatologic conditions. *Dermatol Surg*. 2005;31(7 Pt 2):814-817.

26. Espinal-Perez LE, Moncada B, Castanedo-Cazares JP. A double-blind randomized trial of 5% ascorbic acid vs. 4% hydroquinone in melasma. *Int J Dermatol*. 2004; 43(8):604-607.

27. Huh CH, Seo KI, Park JY, Lim JG, Eun HC, Park KC. A randomized, double-blind, placebo-controlled trial of vitamin C iontophoresis in melasma. *Dermatology*. 2003; 206(4):316-320.

28. Ismail ESA, Patsatsi A, Abd El-Maged WM, Nada EEAE. Efficacy of microneedling with topical vitamin C in the treatment of melasma. *J Cosmet Dermatol*. 2019;18(5):1342-1347.

29. Garcia-Lopez M. Double-blind comparison of azelaic acid and hydroquinone in the treatment of melasma. *Acta Derm Venereol (Stockh)*. 1989;143:58-61.

30. Baliña LM, Graupe K. The treatment of melasma 20% azelaic acid versus 4% hydroquinone cream. *Int J Dermatol*. 1991;30(12):893-895.

31. Kakita LS, Lowe NJ. Azelaic acid and glycolic acid combination therapy for facial hyperpigmentation in darker-skinned patients: A clinical comparison with hydroquinone. *Clin Ther*. 1998;20(5):960-970.

32. Kasraee B. Peroxidase-mediated mechanisms are involved in the melanocytotoxic and melanogenesis-inhibiting effects of chemical agents. *Dermatology*. 2002;205:329-339.

33. Mansouri P, Farshi S, Hashemi Z, Kasraee B. Evaluation of the efficacy of cysteamine 5% cream in the treatment of epidermal melasma: A randomized double-blind placebo-controlled trial. *Br J Dermatol*. 2015;173(1): 209-217.

34. Nguyen J, Remyn L, Chung IY, et al. Evaluation of the efficacy of cysteamine cream compared to hydroquinone in the treatment of melasma: A randomised, double-blinded trial. *Australas J Dermatol*. 2021;62(1):e41-e46.

35. Lima PB, Dias JAF, Cassiano D, et al. A comparative study of topical 5% cysteamine versus 4% hydroquinone in the treatment of facial melasma in women. *Int J Dermatol*. 2020;59(12):1531-1536.

36. Lee CM. A comparative study of topical 5% cysteamine versus 4% hydroquinone in the treatment of facial melasma in women: The devil is in the detail. *Int J Dermatol*. 2021;60(2):255.

37. Karrabi M, David J, Sahebkar M. Clinical evaluation of efficacy, safety and tolerability of cysteamine 5% cream in comparison with modified Kligman's formula in subjects with epidermal melasma: A randomized, double-blind clinical trial study. *Skin Res Technol*. 2021;27(1):24-31.

38. Ebrahimi B, Naeini FF. Topical tranexamic acid as a promising treatment for melasma. *J Res Med Sci*. 2014; 19(8):753.

39. Wang N, Zhang L, Miles L, Hoover-Plow J. Plasminogen regulates pro-opiomelanocortin processing. *J Thromb Haemost*. 2004;2:785-796.

40. Chang WC, Shi GY, Chow YH, et al. Human plasmin induces a receptor-mediated arachidonate release coupled with G proteins in endothelial cells. *Am J Physiol*. 1993; 264:C271-C281.

41. Lee JH, Park JG, Lim SH, et al. Localized intradermal microinjection of tranexamic acid for treatment of melasma in Asian patients: a preliminary clinical trial. *Dermatol Surg*. 2006;32:626-631.

42. Del Rosario E, Florez-Pollack S, Zapata Jr L, et al. Randomized, placebo-controlled, double-blind study of

oral tranexamic acid in the treatment of moderate-to-severe melasma. *J Am Acad Dermatol.* 2018;78(2):363-369.

43. Atefi N, Dalvand B, Ghassemi M, Mehran G, Heydarian A. Therapeutic effects of topical tranexamic acid in comparison with hydroquinone in treatment of women with melasma. *Dermatol Ther.* 2017;7(3):417-424.

44. Banihashemi M, Zabolinejad N, Jaafari MR, Salehi M, Jabari A. Comparison of therapeutic effects of liposomal tranexamic acid and conventional hydroquinone on melasma. *J Cosmet Dermatol.* 2015;14(3):174-177.

45. Navarrete-Solís J, Castanedo-Cázares JP, Torres-Álvarez B, et al. A double-blind, randomized clinical trial of niacinamide 4% versus hydroquinone 4% in the treatment of melasma. *Dermatol Res Pract.* 2011;2011:379173.

46. Zubair S, Mujtaba G. Comparison of efficacy of topical 2% liquiritin, topical 4% liquiritin and topical 4% hydroquinone in the management of melasma. *J Pak Assoc Dermatol.* 2009;19(3):158-163.

47. Monteiro RC, Kishore BN, Bhat RM, Sukumar D, Martis J, Ganesh HK. A comparative study of the efficacy of 4% hydroquinone vs 0.75% kojic acid cream in the treatment of facial melasma. *Indian J Dermatol.* 2013; 58(2):157.

48. Garcia A, Fulton Jr JE. The combination of glycolic acid and hydroquinone or kojic acid for the treatment of melasma and related conditions. *Dermatol Surg.* 1996;22(5): 443-447.

49. Gheisari M, Dadkhahfar S, Olamaei E, Moghimi HR, Niknejad N, Najar Nobari N. The efficacy and safety of topical 5% methimazole vs 4% hydroquinone in the treatment of melasma: A randomized controlled trial. *J Cosmet Dermatol.* 2020;19(1):167-172.

50. Nofal A, Ibrahim ASM, Nofal E, Gamal N, Osman S. Topical silymarin versus hydroquinone in the treatment of melasma: a comparative study. *J Cosmet Dermatol.* 2019;18(1):263-270.

51. Katoulis A, Alevizou A, Soura E, et al. A double-blind vehicle-controlled study of a preparation containing undecylenoyl phenylalanine 2% in the treatment of melasma in females. *J Cosmet Dermatol.* 2014;13(2):86-90.

52. Lyons A, Stoll J, Moy R. A randomized, double-blind, placebo-controlled, split-face study of the efficacy of topical epidermal growth factor for the treatment of melasma. *J Drugs Dermatol.* 2018;17(9):970-973.

53. Draelos ZD. A split-face evaluation of a novel pigment-lightening agent compared with no treatment and hydroquinone. *J Am Acad Dermatol.* 2015;72(1):105-107.

54. Alvin G, Catambay N, Vergara A, Jamora MJ. A comparative study of the safety and efficacy of 75% mulberry (Morus alba) extract oil versus placebo as a topical treatment for melasma: A randomized, single-blind, placebo-controlled trial. *J Drugs Dermatol.* 2011;10(9):1025-1031.

55. Mendoza CG, Singzon IA, Handog EB. A randomized, double-blind, placebo-controlled clinical trial on the efficacy and safety of 3% Rumex occidentalis cream versus 4% hydroquinone cream in the treatment of melasma among Filipinos. *Int J Dermatol.* 2014;53(11): 1412-1416.

56. Huh SY, Shin JW, NA JI, Huh CH, Youn SW, Park KC. Efficacy and safety of liposome-encapsulated 4-n-butyl-resorcinol 0.1% cream for the treatment of melasma: A randomized controlled split-face trial. *J Dermatol.* 2010; 37(4):311-315.

57. Ibrahim ZA, Gheida SF, El Maghraby GM, Farag ZE. Evaluation of the efficacy and safety of combinations of hydroquinone, glycolic acid, and hyaluronic acid in the treatment of melasma. *J Cosmet Dermatol.* 2015;14(2): 113-123.

58. Ghafarzadeh M, Eatemadi A. Clinical efficacy of liposome-encapsulated Aloe vera on melasma treatment during pregnancy. *J Cosmet Laser Ther.* 2017;19(3):181-187.

59. Tirado-Sánchez A, Santamaría-Román A, Ponce-Olivera RM. Efficacy of dioic acid compared with hydroquinone in the treatment of melasma. *Int J Dermatol.* 2009;48(8): 893-895.

60. Ertam I, Mutlu B, Unal I, Alper S, Kivcak B, Ozer O. Efficiency of ellagic acid and arbutin in melasma: A randomized, prospective, open-label study. *J Dermatol.* 2008; 35(9):570-574.

61. Adalatkhah H, Sadeghi-Bazargani H. The first clinical experience on efficacy of topical flutamide on melasma compared with topical hydroquinone: A randomized clinical trial. *Drug Des Devel Ther.* 2015;9:4219.

62. Khosravan S, Alami A, Mohammadzadeh-Moghadam H, Ramezani V. The effect of topical use of Petroselinum crispum (Parsley) versus that of hydroquinone cream on reduction of epidermal melasma: A randomized clinical trial. *Holist Nurs Pract.* 2017;31(1):16-20.

63. Austin E, Nguyen JK, Jagdeo J. Topical treatments for melasma: A systematic review of randomized controlled trials. *J Drugs Dermatol.* 2019;18(11):S1545 961619P1156X.

64. Seemal D, Ayres ME, Bak H, et al. Effect of a tranexamic acid, kojic acid, and niacinamide containing serum on facial dyschromia: A clinical evaluation. *J Drugs Dermatol.* 2019;18(5):454-459.

65. Makino ET, Mehta RC, Garruto J, Gotz V, Sigler ML, Herndon JH. Clinical efficacy and safety of a multimodality skin brightener composition compared with 4% hydroquinone. *J Drugs Dermatol.* 2013;12(3):s21-s26.

66. Bandyopadhyay D. Topical treatment of melasma. *Indian J Dermatol.* 2009;54(4):303.

67. Castanedo-Cazares JP, Hernandez-Blanco D, Carlos-Ortega B, Fuentes-Ahumada C, Torres-Álvarez B. Near-visible light

and UV photoprotection in the treatment of melasma: a double-blind randomized trial. *Photodermatol Photoimmunol Photomed*. 2014;30(1):35-42.

68. Lim HW, Kohli I, Ruvolo E, Kolbe L, Hamzavi IH. Impact of visible light on skin health: The role of antioxidants and free radical quenchers in skin protection. *J Am Acad Dermatol*. 2022;86(3):S27-S37.

69. Holme SA, Beattie PE, Fleming CJ. Cosmetic camouflage advice improves quality of life. *Br J Dermatol*. 2002; 147(5):946-949.

9

Procedural Therapies for Melasma

Mona Sadeghpour, Melissa Laughter, Chee Leok Goh

SUMMARY AND KEY FEATURES

- Sun protection and topical skin whiteners remain the first-line treatment for melasma.
- Lasers and EBD are not first-line treatment for melasma. They are used as adjunct treatment for melasma. Postinflammatory hyperpigmentation (PIH) is a common complication when treating melasma with lasers and EBD.

- Laser toning using low-fluence QS and picosecond pigment lasers has been reported to be effective for melasma but is not curative. Recurrence is the rule. Guttate hypomelanosis occurs when the procedure is carried out too frequently.
- Lasers and EBD should be used for treating melasma only if other treatment modalities fail.

INTRODUCTION

Melasma is a chronic and evolving hyperpigmentation disorder defined by increased activity of melanocytes resulting in pigment deposition within the dermis and/or epidermis. Melasma presents clinically as symmetric, hyperpigmented patches and macules most often involving the most photoexposed areas such as the forehead, malar cheeks, and perioral region. However, other skin areas may be affected including nonfacial skin, otherwise known as extrafacial melasma.[1] Melasma can significantly impact the patient's psychosocial wellbeing such as self-esteem, body image, anxiety, and depression.[2] Although the exact pathophysiology of melasma has not been established, there is increased risk with sun exposure, darker skin (Fitzpatrick skin types III–V), family history of melasma, pregnancy, and the use of oral contraceptives or hormone replacement therapy.[1,3–5]

Treatment of melasma centers around the prevention of additional melanin deposition as well as the removal of excess melanin within the skin. Successful treatment requires treatment of both of these aspects of the disease in order to prevent recurrence. The mainstay of treatment

focuses on the combination of vigilant photoprotection and topical therapy to block pigment production including hydroquinone 4% cream, tretinoin, or triple-combination therapy using hydroquinone, tretinoin, and a low-potency steroid.[6] Unfortunately, the treatment of melasma is challenging with high rates of unsatisfactory results and disease recurrence. Treatment efficacy can vary from patient to patient, and some patients may need to try multiple treatments to achieve satisfactory results. Given this clinical and therapeutic challenge, combinations of modalities, including resurfacing techniques and light or laser-based approaches, have been used as adjunctive to treat melasma. Table 9.1 lists the procedures that have been used as adjunctive treatment for melasma. It is important to understand that despite the variety of treatment modalities used for melasma, the gold standard and first-line treatment remains the combination of strict sun protection and topical lightening agents including hydroquinone, tretinoin, and triple-combination therapy. If a patient is not responding to topical therapy, the addition of laser treatments can be recommended as second- or third-line treatment modalities. Furthermore, it is imperative for providers to

---

TABLE 9.1 Procedures Used as Adjunctive Treatment for Melasma

1. Chemical peel
   - Glycolic acid, salicylic acid, trichloroacetic acid
2. Intense pulsed light
3. Pigment lasers: nanosecond and picosecond lasers
   - Nd:YAG, Alexandrite, Diode, Ruby
   - Laser toning (low-fluence large spot)
4. Vascular lasers
   - Pulsed dye laser
   - Copper bromide laser
   - IPL
5. Ablative and nonablative fractional lasers
6. Microneedling

---

better understand melasma treatment in patients with skin of color, as melasma has a higher prevalence in women of color and women with darker skin types (Fitzpatrick skin type IV–VI).[7] Patients with skin of color may have variable efficacy and risks associated with procedures aimed at treating melasma. In this chapter, we will review the various procedural-based treatments for melasma, with an additional focus on the efficacy and adverse risks within patients with skin of color.

1. CHEMICAL PEELS (LEVEL OF EVIDENCE C)

Chemical peels can be used in conjunction with other therapeutics for the treatment of melasma. Chemical peels are performed with various agents, most commonly glycolic acid (GA), salicylic acid (SA), and trichloroacetic acid (TCA). The peeling agent works by increasing epidermal remodeling and keratinocyte turnover, thereby removing epidermal melanin. The effects of chemical peels can be highly variable and are often dictated by the type of chemical peel, concentration of peeling agent, amount of chemical applied to the skin, and duration of application. Studies evaluating the efficacy of chemical peels for the treatment of melasma have shown inconsistent results. Furthermore, there is concern for dyspigmentation that can occur postprocedure. This is especially important when considering chemical peels as therapy in patients with skin of color. For example, stronger peeling agents such as TCA tends to cause more PIH in darker skin types.

The advantages of chemical peels is the ease of application, minimal downtime, and the ability of patients to return to work on the same day. Furthermore, unlike

laser devices, chemicawl peels do not require costly investments for practitioners. Their disadvantages include risk of PIH and unpredictability of treatment outcome. If chemical peel is considered, selection of low concentrations of glycolic acid is recommended. TCA should be avoided in patients with skin of color.

Glycolic Acid Peels

Among agents used for chemical peels, GA has been the most heavily investigated for its efficacy in treating melasma. The majority of studies evaluate serial GA peels with concentrations ranging from 10% to 70%. Glycolic acid peels should be used in combination with sun protection and other topical treatments. However, studies have shown inconsistent results. Sarkar et al., showed improved melasma clearance in the group with skin of color of 20 Indian patients who received a combination of serial GA peels and modified Kligman's formula topical therapy when compared to the 20 patients in the control group who received topical therapy alone.[8] However, the rate of postprocedure complication including postinflammatory hyperpigmentation and persistent erythema was higher in the GA peel treatment group. Other studies in contrast have not been able to demonstrate superior improvement in melasma using combination GA chemical peels and topical treatments when compared to topical monotherapy alone including 1% tretinoin[9] or 2% to 4% hydroquinone.[10,11] Furthermore, compared to topical therapy alone, glycolic acid was associated with lower tolerability as well as posttreatment burning and ensuing hyperpigmentation.[9,10] Thus, GA peels should only be used cautiously, judiciously, and under experienced supervision in darker-skinned patients, and risk and benefits of treatments must be weighed and thoroughly discussed with patients prior to treatment.

Salicylic Acid Peels

Salicylic acid (SA) is typically used at a concentration of 20% to 30% and works by removing excess epidermal pigment. However, similar to GA, SA has not been shown to be superior when used in conjunction to topical therapies compared to topical monotherapy of hydroquinone 4% used twice daily.[8] Within dark-skinned patients, studies have also shown variable results. Though one uncontrolled study that included six melasma patients with Fitzpatrick skin types V–VI showed that salicylic acid at concentrations of 20% to

30% at 2-week intervals had good improvement,[12] a prospective, randomized, split-face, controlled trial in 20 Latin American women did not show efficacy when a series of four 20% to 30% salicylic acid peels was added to twice-daily 4% hydroquinone cream.[12]

Lasers and Energy-Based Devices (EBD)

Lasers and EBD devices have become increasingly used in the treatment of melasma, particularly in patients with melasma that is refractory to standard topical therapies. Lasers and EBD are intended to assist in the removal of excess melanin deposition in melasma. Many studies have been conducted to assess the efficacy and adverse events with various lasers alone and as adjuvant therapies with mixed results. Generally, lasers and light devices can be divided by mechanism of action and their target chromophores (see Table 9.1) including intense pulsed light, pigment (nano and picosecond) lasers, vascular lasers, and ablative/nonablative/fractional lasers. The use of lasers and EBD for the treatment of melasma in patients with skin of color must be carried out with high caution due to the increased risk of postinflammatory hyperpigmentation. Melasma may in some cases darken following laser treatment, and patients at higher risk including those with higher Fitzpatrick skin types should be properly counseled prior to treatment. When treating patients with skin of color, it is almost always advised to prepare and pretreat the skin with a topical depigmenting agent such as hydroquinone 4%, tretinoin, or triple-combination therapy to lower the risk of postprocedure hyperpigmentation (though scientific evidence supporting efficacy of this technique is currently lacking).

2. INTENSE PULSED LIGHT (LEVEL OF EVIDENCE C)

Intense pulsed light (IPL) devices emit broadband light at a wavelength of 500 nm to 1200 nm. The energy from this broadband emission is absorbed by melanosomes and melanin in melanocytes and keratinocytes and thus can be used to treat pigmentation in melasma. Many studies have investigated the use of IPL as a monotherapy and as adjuvant with other topical therapies. In a study from Taiwan by Wang et al., 33 patients with mixed melasma and Fitzpatrick skin type III and IV received four monthly IPL sessions and topical hydroquinone compared to topical hydroquinone alone. In the

IPL and HQ group (17 females), 35% of patients had greater than 50% improvement of melanin index compared to the HQ alone group (16 control) where only 14% of patients experienced greater than 50% improvement. However, at the 24-week posttreatment follow up, the improvement on the IPL-treated side had decreased less to a mean of 24.2%, suggesting the need for maintenance treatments. Side effects seen in the IPL-treated group included crusting lasting for 1 to 2 weeks and transient PIH that was seen in 12% of patients and resolved with use of topical hydroquinone.[13] In another open-label study by Li et al., 89 Chinese females with predominantly mixed melasma unresponsive to topical therapy and chemical peels were treated with IPL every 3 weeks for four sessions. Patients were instructed to use broad-spectrum sunscreen and avoid bleaching creams. There was a statistically significant decrease in MASI score from 15.2 to 5.2 after four IPL sessions and to 4.5 at the 3-month follow-up visit. Additionally, there was a decrease in melanin index as measured by the Mexameter from a mean value of 140.8 to a value of 119. Of note, patients with epidermal melasma responded better than those with the mixed type. The most common side effects included temporary erythema, edema, microcrusting, and three patients experienced PIH.[14]

The advantage of IPL is its low complication rate and minimal downtime posttreatment. It also provides universal rejuvenation improving skin texture and superficial telangiectasia/erythema. The disadvantages of IPL include lack of predictable and sustained effectiveness and requirement for maintenance treatments.

3. PIGMENTARY LASERS (LEVEL OF EVIDENCE B)

Pigmentary lasers are groups of lasers with short-pulse duration that target melanin. Melanin has short thermal relaxation time and is best targeted using short-pulse duration. Such lasers have pulsed duration ranging from 50 nanoseconds to 5 nanoseconds. They are referred to as "quality-switched" (QS) lasers. Examples include QS Nd:YAG laser, QS Alexandrite laser, and QS Ruby laser.

Quality-Switched Lasers

Quality-switched lasers, including QS Ruby, QS Alexandrite, and QS Nd:YAG, have all been used in the treatment of melasma. However, given the high absorption of melanin by both QS Ruby and QS Alexandrite lasers, their use is generally not recommended for treatment of melasma in patients with skin of color. This is due to the shorter wavelengths of these lasers compared to the QS Nd:YAG lasers and hence their higher risk of postinflammatory hyperpigmentation and hypopigmentation. The QS lasers, if used with the conventional fluence to treat other pigmentation disorders, tends to cause severe PIH and are never recommended to be used to treat melasma. A "laser-toning" protocol using low fluence, large spot size, over multiple treatment sessions using the QS Nd:YAG lasers has been widely used in Asian patients.

Q-switched Neodymium:Yttrium-Aluminum-Garnet Laser (QS Nd:YAG) (Level of Evidence B)

Growing evidence around the globe has shown support for treatment of melasma using "laser-toning" procedure using low-fluence protocols with QS Nd:YAG lasers delivered over multiple passes (5–10) repeated every 2 to 4 weeks over 6 to 10 months. This laser treatment protocol can be safely used in all skin types including patients with skin of color. Using the principal of subcellular-selective photothermolysis, the laser can penetrate to the deep dermis and selectively target and suppress activity of melanocytes without causing melanocyte death.[15,16] Targeting melanosomes without causing collateral damage to surrounding tissue and melanocytes is important as it lowers the risk of postinflammatory pigmentary change, including both hypo- and hyperpigmentation, in patients with skin of color.

Numerous reports have investigated the efficacy of "laser toning" using QS Nd:YAG in patients with skin of color.[17–20] However, even despite evidence supporting efficacy of low-fluence QS Nd:YAG for treatment of melasma, "low-fluence" treatment protocols have not been standardized. Furthermore, many of the previously reported parameters, which initially appear effective, have been complicated by frequent and early melasma recurrence,[21–23] punctate leukoderma[22–24] (Figs. 9.1 and 9.2) and postinflammatory hyperpigmentation.[23,24] Conclusions from these studies have suggested that despite initial efficacy of QS-Nd:YAG laser treatment ("laser toning") for melasma in patients, including those with skin of color, improvements were only temporary and potential for side effects were common. The protocols in these earlier studies used higher fluences (>2 and up to 4 J/cm2), very frequent treatment sessions (weekly), and/or higher number of passes (up to 20). Lessons from these studies have highlighted the importance of protocols utilizing lower fluences (usually ≤ 2 J/cm2), lower number of passes (2 or 3 compared to 10 or 20 used in earlier studies), delivered with less frequency (monthly rather than weekly) to avoid treatment-related adverse events.

Taking these lessons into consideration, most recently Sadeghpour et al., sought to investigate the safety and efficacy of a combined treatment approach using low-fluence QS Nd:YAG laser, mechanical exfoliation, and 4% topical hydroquinone in treatment of melasma

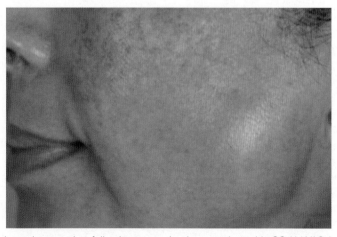

Fig. 9.1. Guttate hypopigmentation following excessive laser toning with QS Nd:YAG laser for melasma. Image courtesy of National Skin Centre, Singapore.

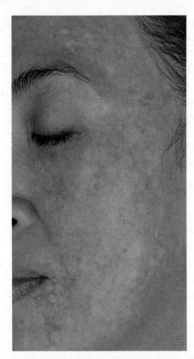

Fig. 9.2. Severe hypomelanotic macules on cheeks from excessive "laser toning" with QS Nd:YAG laser for facial melasma. Image courtesy of National Skin Centre, Singapore.

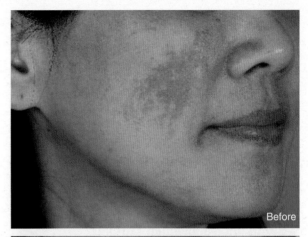

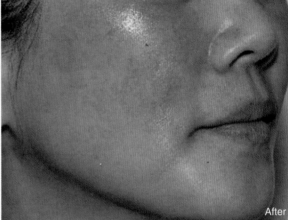

Fig. 9.3. Treatment outcome with "laser toning" using low fluence (1-2 J/cm2), 6 to 8 mm spot size using QS Nd:YAG laser, monthly treatment x 8 session for melasma. Images courtesy of National Skin Centre, Singapore.

through a prospective, split-face, placebo-controlled, randomized controlled study (Sadeghpour et al., unpublished data 2021). Eleven patients with FST III-IV were randomized to receive "treatment" versus "placebo" QS Nd: YAG laser treatment on either the right or left side of the face. "Treatment" laser was performed using two laser passes (treatment parameter: 1.6 J/cm^2, 6-mm spot-size, 5–7 nanoseconds pulse duration) (Rev-lite®, Cynosure, Westford, MA). "Placebo" treatment was delivered using a laser cap made of thick, opaque cardboard matching the size of the laser device tip that blocked all laser beams being emitted from the device. Study outcomes were measured using modified MASI (mMASI) scores and melanin index. At the 6-month follow up, the study found that reduction of mMASI and melanin index was similar in both laser-treated and placebo-treated sides, and the addition of QS Nd:YAG laser did not add significant benefit to baseline treatment. Importantly, there was no adverse events reported during 9-month study period.

Overall taken together, these studies suggest that even when delivered under safe dosing and frequency parameters, the improvement of melasma using QS Nd:YAG laser toning is modest (Fig. 9.3) at best and likely not superior to the improvement achievable by judicious use of topical therapy including broad-spectrum sunscreen and topical pigment blockers such as 4% HQ. Thus topical therapy should remain first line in treatment, including in patients of color.

Picosecond Lasers

Picosecond lasers have introduced a novel method for pigment fragmentation by delivering energy at a speed that is potentially three orders of magnitude faster than the nanosecond speed of Q-switched lasers. The fast delivery of energy from the picosecond lasers can target melanosomes through a photoacoustic mechanism, which minimizes the photothermal impact used in other lasers, decreasing the risk for thermally induced adverse events such as PIH. Therefore, in theory, with these lasers adjacent tissue suffers less thermal damage and melanosomes are shattered into smaller particles, which is then more efficiently cleared by macrophage system (Fig. 9.4). Picosecond lasers are currently available with laser outputs of 532 nm, 730 nm, 755 nm, 785 nm, and 1064 nm. A recent randomized split-face study of 39 Korean patients by Choi et al., utilizing a picosecond dual-wavelength 595-nm and 1064-nm laser in combination with 2% hydroquinone versus hydroquinone 2% alone showed superior improvement in relative lightness value

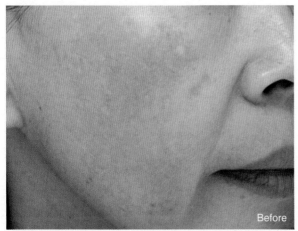

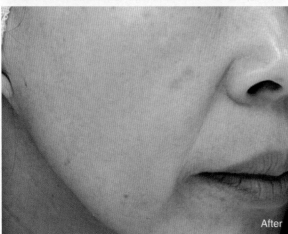

Fig. 9.4. Treatment outcome with "laser toning" using picosecond laser with *fluence 0.8 J/cm2, 8 mm* spot size, monthly treatment x 6 sessions. Images courtesy of National Skin Centre, Singapore.

at completion of trial and follow-up period for the laser-treated side, but no difference in modified melasma area and severity index (mMASI) scores or patient satisfaction for the laser-treated group during the follow-up period, indicating likelihood of melasma recurrence after treatment cessation.[25]

Newer generations of picosecond lasers employ diffractive lens array (DLA) technology, which enables the laser to fractionate the beam resulting in laser-induced optical breakdown (LIOB). LIOB in turn allows for higher levels of energy to be redistributed in a more widespread fashion in the skin. This decreased exposure of the skin to high fluences creates safer energy parameters, which then in turn decreases the overall risk for adverse events. This safety potential is especially important for treatment of pigment in patients with skin of color. In a recent prospective, a nonrandomized study by Wong et al., 20 patients of Asian descent received nine fractionated 1064-nm picosecond laser treatments using DLA technology. There was a statistically significant improvement in mMASI from 10.8 at baseline to 2.7 and 3.6 at 6 and 12 weeks posttreatment, respectively (both $P < 0.01$). However, there was no comparison to the nonfractionated picosecond laser, nor nanosecond devices. The only side effect reported was transient erythema and edema, which resolved spontaneously.[26]

Reports from studies comparing the safety and efficacy of picosecond laser treatments delivered by full beam (flat optic) versus fractionated beam (DLA) have been mixed. While one study reported higher safety and efficacy of treatments delivered with the fractionated beam,[27] another found no significant difference between the two and a higher incidence of adverse events with the fractionated beam treatments.[28] Further controlled studies are required to determine what treatment protocols, and which type of picosecond lasers are most effective for the treatment of melasma.

4. VASCULAR LASERS (PULSED DYE AND COPPER BROMIDE LASERS) (LEVEL OF EVIDENCE D)

Recent evidence suggests that altered vascularity may contribute to the pathogenesis of melasma, invoking the use of lasers that target the vasculature as a treatment modality for melasma. Kim et al., investigated the relationship between cutaneous vasculature and melanocyte by determining the expression of factor VIIIa-related antigen and vascular endothelial growth factor (VEGF) in lesional and nonlesional skin samples from 50 Korean women with melasma. In the melasma lesional skin samples, the study found a significant increase in both the number and the size of dermal blood vessels as well as increased expression of VEGF.[29] Hence vascular lasers and light devices are used for the treatment of melasma. They include the pulsed dye lasers, copper bromide lasers, and IPL. But there are relatively few reports on their effects on vascular component in melasma.

Pulsed Dye Laser

In a controlled, randomized, split-face, single blind trial Passeron et al., compared the efficacy of three sessions of weekly PDL combined with TCC (hydroquinone 4%, tretinoin 0.05%, and fluocinolone acetonide 0.01%) for the treatment of melasma. For each PDL treatment two passes were used: one with settings targeting hyperpigmentation followed immediately by a second pass with settings aimed at treatment of the vessels. Both groups used sunscreen with SPF of 50 or higher. At the 1-month time point, patients had greater improvement of melasma and higher patient satisfaction within the combination group of PDL and TCC; however, this improvement was only seen in patients with Fitzpatrick skin type of II and III. Within the 3-year follow-up period, only one patient presented with disease recurrence. However, half of the patients with darker skin types (Fitzpatrick IV) experience PIH with no improvement in their melasma or patient satisfaction following this combination treatment.[30] The authors of the study attributed the PIH to the PDL pass targeting melanin clearance and thus recommended avoidance of this specific passage in future studies and using only settings that target the vascular component.

Another retrospective study with 11 patients with an average age 38.7 years and Fitzpatrick skin type II (n = 4), III (n = 3), and IV (n = 4), whose melasma specifically showed telangiectatic erythema (identified through spectrocolorimetry analysis), were treated with PDL and 1927-nm fractional low-powered diode laser and subsequently showed more than 50% improvement in melasma in 54% of patients. Researchers specifically used settings targeting telangiectasias, suggesting that the treatment of the vascular component of melasma improvement treatment efficacy.[31] There were no adverse events reported.

Copper Bromide Lasers

The copper bromide laser (Dual Yellow; Norseld) have concomitant dual-wavelength light source output comprising 90% yellow light at 578 nm targeting vascular lesions, and 10% green light at 511 nm that targets pigmentary lesions, which can be emitted separately or simultaneously. Reports of the use of these lasers for treatment of melasma have been mixed.

In a study by Lee et al., 10 Korean women with mixed or epidermal melasma were treated with a copper bromide laser emitting both wavelengths simultaneously at 2-week intervals for a total of 8 weeks. MASI scores decreased modestly from an average of 12.3 pretreatment to 9.5 at 1-month posttreatment follow up, but the effects appeared to wane slightly at 1-month posttreatment follow up. Histologic examination from lesional skin of four patients also showed decreased levels of basal layer melanin (Melan-A), decreased CD34 staining for blood vessels, and decreased endothelin 1 and VEGF antigen posttreatment. However, clinical lightening appeared to wane slightly at the 1-month posttreatment follow up, and three patients were noted to have recurrence at the 6-month posttreatment follow up.[32] However, the study by Eimpunth et al., from Thailand with 20 melasma patients who were treated with the copper bromide laser did not show statistically significant improvement the in mean melanin index (MI) compared with baseline at any of the follow-up visits. The authors concluded that the copper bromide laser does not improve melasma in patients with skin phototypes III–V.[33] The randomized split-face study by Ghorbel et al., also failed to show any significant decrease in MASI score at the end of the study (6-month follow up) from baseline when the combination of copper bromide laser and triple-combination cream (hydroquinone, 5%, dexamethasone acetate, 0.1%, and retinoic acid, 0.1%) was compared to triple-combination cream alone.[34] Overall, these studies suggest that the use of copper bromide lasers is unlikely to be an effective treatment for melasma, including in patients with skin of color.

5. FRACTIONAL RESURFACING LASERS (LEVEL OF EVIDENCE D)

Developed in 2004, fractional resurfacing lasers work through creating microthermal damage targeting a fraction of the skin at a time. These lasers can be broadly split into ablative and nonablative fractional lasers (NAFL).

Nonablative Fractional Resurfacing Lasers

NAFL devices inducing microscopic areas of coagulative thermal injury termed microscopic treatment zones (MTZs). The injured skin clears damaged melanin through the skin's surface while the neighboring uninjured skin permits the migration of basal keratinocytes through the injured skin speeding up the healing process.[35] NAFL induces damage below the threshold of ablative fractional lasers and generally have a more rapid recovery and a lower risk of scarring or dyspigmentation.[36]

1927-nm Fractionated Nonablative Thulium Laser

The 1927-nm NAFL laser, introduced in 2009, has a higher absorption for water and ability to reduce hyperpigmentation when compared to other NAFLs. One nonrandomized pilot study with 14 melasma patients investigated the efficacy and safety of three to four treatments with 1927-nm NAFLs and topical 4% hydroquinone. Results showed a statistically significant reduction in MASI score by 51% at the 1-month time point and a 34% reduction at the 6-month time point. Although the study was not randomized or controlled, the treatment was safely used in patients with FST I-IV without any reports of postinflammatory hyperpigmentation or scarring following the treatment.[37] One prospective nonrandomized trial treated 23 patients with 1927-nm NAFLs and showed moderate improvement in standardized facial imaging photographs at 1-month and mild to moderate improvement at 3 months.[38]

Low-Energy, Low-Density 1927-nm Fractionated Nonablative Diode Laser

In contrast to the high-energy, high-density, 1927-nm nonablative fractionated thulium lasers, low-energy, low-density 1927-nm NAFLs deliver a low fluence and low-density energy with a broader safety profile in treatment of melasma. In one nonrandomized, single center study 23 female patients of FST I-VI (11 with diagnosis of photodamage, 10 with melasma, and 2 with PIH) were treated with Clear and Brilliant Permea ® fractional 1927 diode laser for 4 to 6 treatments. Blinded assessment showed that 55% of participants reported moderate to very significant improvement at both the 1-month and 3-month time points. Importantly, authors reported transient PIH in one Asian participant

with melasma, which subsequently resolved two months following completion of the study.[38]

Well-controlled, randomized studies comparing the efficacy of these lasers to standard topical therapies are currently lacking. The delivery of lower fluences and densities in these studies support the use of this laser as a treatment option for melasma in patients with skin of color especially when utilized with topical depigmenting agents, used either concomitantly or as pretreatment prior to laser therapy.

1550-nm Fractional Laser

A randomized, blinded control trial with 20 patients with moderate to severe melasma compared biweekly 1550-nm fractional laser for 8 weeks to triple-topical therapy with tretinoin 0.05%, hydroquinone 5%, and triamcinolone acetonide cream 0.1%. Results showed no difference in melasma improvement between the two groups. At the 6-week time point, both groups reported recurrence of disease, and patients tended to prefer the topical therapy to the laser treatments.[39] However, in a randomized controlled split-face study with 29 melasma patients comparing 1550 fractional laser therapy to triple-topical therapy for 15 weeks, patient global assessment and patient satisfaction were significantly lower on the laser-treated side of the face. Furthermore, physician's global assessment, melanin index, and lightness displayed a significant worsening of hyperpigmentation on the laser-treated side. However, a large proportion of patients (31%) reported postinflammatory hyperpigmentation and preferred the side treated with topical triple-combination therapy.[40]

6. MICRONEEDLING WITH TOPICAL DEPIGMENTING AGENTS (LEVEL OF EVIDENCE D)

Microneedling is a minimally invasive procedure in which sterilized microneedles create repetitive micropunctures within the skin. This controlled mechanical damage caused by the microneedles is aimed at inducing collagen regeneration and has been used to treat a wide variety of skin conditions, including melasma.[41] Unfortunately, there are limited well-controlled, rigorous studies investigating the efficacy and tolerability of microneedling for the treatment of melasma, particularly when used as a monotherapy. Microneedling used as an adjuvant therapy to topical monotherapies has also showed variable results. In a recent split-face trial, microneedling was combined with a depigmenting serum (containing two topicals, rucinol and sophora-alpha) for a 2-month treatment period. The 20 melasma patients showed a statistically significant improvement in both the Melasma Area Severity Index (MASI) Score and luminosity index (L) levels with the microneedling and topical depigmenting serum compared to depigmenting serum alone.[42] Another split-faced, investigator-blinded study investigated the combination of four monthly QS-Nd:YAG sessions followed by microneedling and topical vitamin C. Sixteen patients with recalcitrant dermal or mixed-type melasma showed significant improvement in their mean MASI score within the QS-Nd:YAG, microneedling, and topical therapy compared to QS-Nd:YAG alone.[43] There have also been multiple studies comparing topical tranexamic acid (TXA) combined with microneedling to either topical TXA[44] or intradermal injections of TXA.[45,46]

It is thought that the adjuvant potential of microneedling likely stems from its ability to improve penetration of depigmenting agents within the skin rather than the induction of pigment turnover caused from the micro punctures themselves.[42] Although there have been many studies incorporating microneedling in some form, there are no prospective, well-controlled randomized trials comparing microneedling to first-line topical therapy including hydroquinone and triple-combination topical creams. Thus, though microneedling may provide some benefit to patients as an adjuvant therapy, it should not take the place of well-established topical therapies and strict photoprotection.

SUMMARY AND FUTURE DIRECTIONS

Melasma has a complex pathogenesis and is more prevalent amongst patients of color. To this day, data from well-designed, randomized, controlled trials still support topical therapy along with diligent photoprotection as first line of treatment. Though many procedural treatments have been tried and reported in the literature for melasma, no one procedural modality is consistently successful long term, and procedure-related adverse events are common. Patients with skin of color are especially at risk for developing complications following procedural treatments for melasma given the higher content of melanin in their skin. Extreme caution must be exercised when selecting procedures for these groups

of patients in order to prevent excessive injury or heating of skin. Furthermore, no one laser has proven to be consistently effective for melasma treatment, and selection of lasers as a treatment modality should be second or third line in treatment. When lasers or other procedures are selected, it is highly recommended to use topical therapy (such as hydroquinone, tretinoin, or TCC) as well as strict photoprotection for 2 to 4 weeks prior to the procedure in order to suppress melanocyte activity and to decrease the risk of postinflammatory hypo- or hyperpigmentation in the skin for patients.

The advent of picosecond lasers with both flat optic and DLA technology has provided promising potential for removing pigmentation in melasma through photoacoustic mechanisms that are less disruptive and damaging to the surrounding skin. However, long-term benefits remain to be confirmed by additional randomized, controlled trials in the future.

REFERENCES

1. Sanchez NP, Pathak MA, Sato S, Fitzpatrick TB, Sanchez JL, Mihm MC. Melasma: A clinical, light microscopic, ultrastructural, and immunofluorescence study. *J Am Acad Dermatol*. 1981;4(6):698-710. doi:10.1016/S0190-9622(81)70071-9.
2. Fatma F, Baati I, Mseddi M, Sallemi R, Turki H, Masmoudi J. The psychological impact of melasma. A report of 30 Tunisian women. *Eur Psychiatry*. 2016;33:S327. doi:10.1016/j.eurpsy.2016.01.1130.
3. Guinot C, Cheffai S, Latreille J, et al. Aggravating factors for melasma: A prospective study in 197 Tunisian patients. *J Eur Acad Dermatol Venereol*. 2010;24(9):1060-1069. doi:10.1111/j.1468-3083.2010.03592.x.
4. Tamega ADA, Miot LDB, Bonfietti C, Gige TC, Marques MEA, Miot HA. Clinical patterns and epidemiological characteristics of facial melasma in Brazilian women. *J Eur Acad Dermatol Venereol*. 2013;27(2):151-156. doi:10.1111/j.1468-3083.2011.04430.x.
5. Achar A, Rathi SK. Melasma: A clinico-epidemiological study of 312 cases. *Indian J Dermatol*. 2011;56(4):380-382. doi:10.4103/0019-5154.84722.
6. Lakhdar H, Zouhair K, Khadir K, et al. Evaluation of the effectiveness of a broad-spectrum sunscreen in the prevention of chloasma in pregnant women. *J Eur Acad Dermatol Venereol*. 2007;21(6):738-742. doi:10.1111/j.1468-3083.2007.02185.x.
7. Grimes PE. Melasma: Etiologic and therapeutic considerations. *Arch Dermatol*. 1995;131(12):1453-1457. doi:10.1001/archderm.131.12.1453.

8. Kodali S, Guevara IL, Carrigan CR, et al. A prospective, randomized, split-face, controlled trial of salicylic acid peels in the treatment of melasma in Latin American women. *J Am Acad Dermatol.* 2010;63(6):1030-1035. doi:10.1016/j.jaad.2009.12.027.

9. Faghihi G, Shahingohar A, Siadat AH. Comparison between 1% tretinoin peeling versus 70% glycolic acid peeling in the treatment of female patients with melasma. *J Drugs Dermatol.* 2011;10(12):1439-1442.

10. Lim JTE, Tham SN. Glycolic acid peels in the treatment of melasma among Asian women. *Dermatol Surg.* 1997;23(3):177-179. doi:10.1111/j.1524-4725.1997.tb00016.x.

11. Hurley ME, Guevara IL, Gonzales RM, Pandya AG. Efficacy of glycolic acid peels in the treatment of Melasma. *Arch Dermatol.* 2002;138(12):1578-1582. doi:10.1001/archderm.138.12.1578.

12. Grimes PE. The safety and efficacy of salicylic acid chemical peels in darker racial-ethnic groups. *Dermatol Surg.* 1999;25(1):18-22. doi:10.1046/j.1524-4725.1999.08145.x.

13. Wang CC, Hui CY, Sue YM, Wong WR, Hong HS. Intense pulsed light for the treatment of refractory melasma in Asian persons. *Dermatol Surg.* 2004;30(9):1196-1200. doi:10.1111/j.1524-4725.2004.30371.x.

14. Li YH, Chen JZS, Wei HC, et al. Efficacy and safety of intense pulsed light in treatment of melasma in Chinese patients. *Dermatol Surg.* 2008;34(5):693-701. doi:10.1111/j.1524-4725.2008.34130.x.

15. Kim JH, Kim H, Park HC, Kim IH. Subcellular selective photothermolysis of melanosomes in adult zebrafish skin following 1064-nm Q-switched Nd:YAG laser irradiation. *J Invest Dermatol.* 2010;130(9):2333-2335. doi:10.1038/jid.2010.129.

16. Mun JY, Jeong SY, Kim JH, Han SS, Kim IH. A low fluence Q-switched Nd:YAG laser modifies the 3D structure of melanocyte and ultrastructure of melanosome by subcellular-selective photothermolysis. *J Electron Microsc (Tokyo).* 2011;59(2):103-112. doi:10.1093/jmicro/dfq068.

17. Polnikorn N. Treatment of refractory dermal melasma with the MedLite C6 Q-switched Nd:YAG laser: Two case reports. *J Cosmet Laser Ther.* 2008;10(3):167-173. doi:10.1080/14764170802179687.

18. Kim MJ, Cho SB, Kim JS. Melasma treatment in Korean women using a 1064-nm Q-switched Nd:YAG laser with low pulse energy. *Clin Exp Dermatol.* 2009;34(8):e847-e850. doi:10.1111/j.1365-2230.2009.03599.x.

19. Jeong SY, Shin J Bin, Yeo UC, Kim WS, Kim IH. Low-fluence Q-switched neodymium-doped yttrium aluminum garnet laser for melasma with pre- or post-treatment triple combination cream. *Dermatol Surg.* 2010;36(6):909-918. doi:10.1111/j.1524-4725.2010.01523.x.

20. Choi M, Choi JW, Lee SY, et al. Low-dose 1064-nm Q-switched Nd:YAG laser for the treatment of melasma. *J Dermatol Treat.* 2010;21(4):224-228. doi:10.3109/09546630903401462.

21. Parra CAH, Careta MF, Valente NYS, De Sanches Osório NEG, Torezan LAR. Clinical and histopathologic assessment of facial melasma after low-fluence q-switched neodymium-doped yttrium aluminium garnet laser. *Dermatol Surg.* 2016;42(4):507-512. doi:10.1097/DSS.0000000000000653.

22. Polnikorn N. Treatment of refractory melasma with the MedLite C6 Q-switched Nd:YAG laser and alpha arbutin: A prospective study. *J Cosmet Laser Ther.* 2010;12(3):126-131. doi:10.3109/14764172.2010.487910.

23. Wattanakrai P, Mornchan R, Eimpunth S. Low-fluence q-switched neodymium-doped yttrium aluminum garnet (1,064 nm) laser for the treatment of facial melasma in Asians. *Dermatol Surg.* 2010;36(1):76-87. doi:10.1111/j.1524-4725.2009.01383.x.

24. Suh KS, Sung JY, Roh HJ, Jeon YS, Kim YC, Kim ST. Efficacy of the 1064-nm Q-switched Nd:YAG laser in melasma. *J Dermatol Treat.* 2011;22(4):233-238. doi:10.3109/09546631003686051.

25. Choi YJ, Nam JH, Kim JY, et al. Efficacy and safety of a novel picosecond laser using combination of 1 064 and 595 nm on patients with melasma: A prospective, randomized, multicenter, split-face, 2% hydroquinone cream-controlled clinical trial. *Lasers Surg Med.* 2017. doi:10.1002/lsm.22735.

26. Wong CSM, Chan MWM, Shek SYN, Yeung CK, Chan HHL. Fractional 1064 nm picosecond laser in treatment of melasma and skin rejuvenation in Asians, a prospective study. *Lasers Surg Med.* 2021;53(8):1032-1042. doi:10.1002/lsm.23382.

27. Polnikorn N, Tanghetti E. Treatment of refractory melasma in Asians with the picosecond Alexandrite laser. *Dermatol Surg.* 2020;46(12):1651-1656. doi:10.1097/DSS.0000000000002612.

28. Manuskiatti W, Yan C, Tantrapornpong P, Cembrano KAG, Techapichetvanich T, Wanitphakdeedecha R. A prospective, split-face, randomized study comparing a 755-nm picosecond laser with and without diffractive lens array in the treatment of melasma in Asians. *Lasers Surg Med.* 2021;53(1):95-103. doi:10.1002/lsm.23312.

29. Kim EH, Kim YC, Lee ES, Kang HY. The vascular characteristics of melasma. *J Dermatol Sci.* 2007;46(2):111-116. doi:10.1016/j.jdermsci.2007.01.009.

30. Passeron T, Fontas E, Kang HY, Bahadoran P, Lacour JP, Ortonne JP. Melasma treatment with pulsed-dye laser and triple combination cream: A prospective, randomized, single-blind, split-face study. *Arch Dermatol.* 2011;147(9):1106-1108.doi:10.1001/archdermatol.2011.255.

31. Geddes ERC, Stout AB, Friedman PM. Retrospective analysis of the treatment of melasma lesions exhibiting

increased vascularity with the 595-nm pulsed dye laser combined with the 1927-nm fractional low-powered diode laser. *Lasers Surg Med.* 2017;49(1):20-26. doi:10.1002/lsm.22518.

32. Lee HI, Lim YY, Kim BJ, et al. Clinicopathologic efficacy of copper bromide plus/yellow laser (578 nm with 511 nm) for treatment of melasma in Asian patients. *Dermatol Surg.* 2010;36(6):885-893. doi:10.1111/j.1524-4725.2010.01564.x.

33. Eimpunth S, Wanitphakdeedecha R, Triwongwaranat D, Varothai S, Manuskiatti W. Therapeutic outcome of melasma treatment by dual-wavelength (511 and 578 nm) laser in patients with skin phototypes III-V. *Clin Exp Dermatol.* 2014;39(3):292-297. doi:10.1111/ced.12267.

34. Ghorbel HH, Boukari F, Fontas E, et al. Copper bromide laser vs triple-combination cream for the treatment of melasma: a randomized clinical trial. *JAMA Dermatol.* 2015;151(7):791-792. doi:10.1001/jamadermatol.2014.5580.

35. Hantash BM, Bedi VP, Sudireddy V, Struck SK, Herron GS, Chan KF. Laser-induced transepidermal elimination of dermal content by fractional photothermolysis. *J Biomed Opt.* 2006;11(4):041115. doi:10.1117/1.2241745.

36. Manstein D, Herron GS, Sink RK, Tanner H, Anderson RR. Fractional photothermolysis: A new concept for cutaneous remodeling using microscopic patterns of thermal injury. *Lasers Surg Med.* 2004;34(5):426-438. doi:10.1002/lsm.20048.

37. Polder KD, Bruce S. Treatment of melasma using a novel 1,927-nm fractional thulium fiber laser: A pilot study. *Dermatol Surg.* 2012;38(2):199-206. doi:10.1111/j.1524-4725.2011.02178.x.

38. Brauer JA, Alabdulrazzaq H, Cindy Bae YS, Geronemus RG. Evaluation of a low energy, low density, non-ablative fractional 1927nm wavelength laser for facial skin resurfacing. *J Drugs Dermatol.* 2015;14(11):1262-1267.

39. Kroon MW, Wind BS, Beek JF, et al. Nonablative 1550-nm fractional laser therapy versus triple topical therapy for the treatment of melasma: A randomized controlled pilot study. *J Am Acad Dermatol.* 2011;64(3):516-523. doi:10.1016/j.jaad.2010.01.048.

40. Wind BS, Kroon MW, Meesters AA, et al. Non-ablative 1,550nm fractional laser therapy versus triple topical therapy for the treatment of melasma: A randomized controlled split-face study. *Lasers Surg Med.* 2010;42(7):607-612. doi:10.1002/lsm.20937.

41. Iriarte C, Awosika O, Rengifo-Pardo M, Ehrlich A. Review of applications of microneedling in dermatology. *Clin Cosmet Investig Dermatol.* 2017;10:289-298. doi:10.2147/CCID.S142450.

42. Fabbrocini G, De Vita V, Fardella N, et al. Skin needling to enhance depigmenting serum penetration in the treatment of melasma. *Plast Surg Int.* 2011;2011:158241. doi:10.1155/2011/158241.

43. Ustuner P, Balevi A, Ozdemir M. A split-face, investigator-blinded comparative study on the efficacy and safety of Q-switched Nd:YAG laser plus microneedling with vitamin C versus Q-switched Nd:YAG laser for the treatment of recalcitrant melasma. *J Cosmet Laser Ther.* 2017;19(7):383-390. doi:10.1080/14764172.2017.1342036.

44. Xu Y, Ma R, Juliandri J, et al. Efficacy of functional microarray of microneedles combined with topical tranexamic acid for melasma. *Med (United States).* 2017;96(19):e6897. doi:10.1097/MD.0000000000006897.

45. Budamakuntla L, Loganathan E, Suresh D, et al. A randomised, open-label, comparative study of tranexamic acid microinjections and tranexamic acid with microneedling in patients with melasma. *J Cutan Aesthet Surg.* 2013;6(3):139-143. doi:10.4103/0974-2077.118403.

46. Ebrahim HM, Said Abdelshafy A, Khattab F, Gharib K. Tranexamic acid for melasma treatment: A split-face study. *Dermatol Surg.* 2020;46(11):e102-e107. doi:10.1097/DSS.0000000000002449.

10

Postinflammatory Hyperpigmentation: Treatment and Prevention

Oma N. Agbai, Rebecca L. Quiñonez, Susan C. Taylor

SUMMARY AND KEY FEATURES

- Postinflammatory hyperpigmentation (PIH) is one of the most common chief complaints in people of color and has a profound impact on quality of life.
- Although PIH can be treated with a variety of cosmetic procedures, these procedures often pose a risk for stimulating a hypermelanotic state and subsequent postprocedural hyperpigmentation.
- Strict photoprotection following cosmetic procedures is paramount to the prevention of postprocedural hyperpigmentation.

- Combining topical melanogenesis inhibitors and procedures may improve cosmetic outcomes and mitigate postprocedural hyperpigmentation when topicals are used several weeks prior to and following procedures.
- For treatment of PIH, topical melanogenesis inhibitor use should be optimized prior to adding procedures such as chemexfoliants and laser procedures.

INTRODUCTION

Postinflammatory hyperpigmentation (PIH) is one of the most common chief complaints in people of color (POC) and has a profound impact on quality of life.[1] PIH is an acquired reactive hypermelanosis caused by inflammatory skin conditions such as acne, contact dermatitis, psoriasis, seborrheic dermatitis, or atopic dermatitis. Additionally, PIH can be caused by external factors such as superficial skin trauma, cosmetic procedures, or radiation therapy. While there are several therapeutic modalities discussed in the literature for hypermelanoses such as melasma, there remains a paucity of data on treatments for PIH. Although PIH can be treated with a variety of cosmetic procedures, these procedures often pose a risk for stimulating a hypermelanotic state and subsequent postprocedural hyperpigmentation. Therefore, careful

preprocedural management is required for PIH prevention. Herein we discuss current knowledge on cosmetic procedures for management of PIH, in addition to a detailed discussion on topical therapeutic options for PIH, as well as preprocedural risk assessment and prevention of PIH.

PRE- AND POSTPROCEDURAL MANAGEMENT FOR PREVENTION OF POSTPROCEDURAL PIH

Risk Stratification for Postinflammatory Hyperpigmentation Based on Skin Type

The FST scale is the most widely used method to classify skin phenotype. The ability to tan or burn after exposure to UV radiation is the basis on which type I–VI skin types are classified.[2] While it remains the gold standard of classification for skin type in the setting of phototherapy, it must be remembered that this classification only measures the skin's immediate response to UV exposure and does not necessarily predict the skin's response to manipulation from cosmetic procedures. Traditionally, individuals with FST IV–VI may be considered high risk for development of postprocedural PIH, requiring optimized procedure selection and preprocedural management, as will be discussed later in this chapter. The FST scale is commonly used to assess the suitability of laser treatments and the selection of optical settings in POC.

The Roberts Skin Type Classification System (RSTCS) is a four-part scale that assesses and assigns a numerical value to the patient's phototype, hyperpigmentation, photoaging, and scarring capability.[3] It was constructed to allow dermatologists to anticipate short- and long-term effects of cosmetic procedures and individualize procedure recommendations in the full spectrum of POC. The RSTCS assesses the patient's past medical history, ancestral background, history of scarring, and pigmentary changes and includes a full skin evaluation and, potentially, a skin-site reaction test.[4,5] From the assessment, the propensity for pigmentation, for example, is determined and graded on a 0–VI scale (H0 = hypopigmentation to HVI = severe and permanent hyperpigmentation for greater than 1 year). The RSTCS may be used to evaluate all skin types. The RSTCS offers a more individualized and complete assessment approach for optimizing cosmetic treatments particularly for increasing numbers of POC.

Hector Leal Silva, MD, of Monterrey, Mexico, uses a simple method for evaluating the risk or degree of postprocedure PIH according to the color of the patient's palmar creases.[6,7] The scale classifies individuals into four groups (0–3 scale) where the darker the palmar creases, the greater the incidence of PIH after cosmetic procedures.

Medical Considerations

Particular attention should be given to photosensitizing and phototoxic medications including thiazide diuretics, calcium channel blockers, anticoagulation therapy, tetracyclines, oral retinoids, and oral contraceptives or hormonal agents.[8] These medications may increase the risk of procedural bleeding, delayed wound healing, postprocedure hyperpigmentation, or cutaneous eruptions.[9]

Photoprotection

The importance of photoprotection cannot be underestimated for both the treatment of cosmetic concerns in POC and as postprocedure prevention of hyperpigmentation.[10–13] Given reduced rates of regular sunscreen use in the Black population, education on the benefits of routine sunscreen application is paramount in reducing the risk for UV-related dyschromias, skin cancer, and photoaging in this population.[14–18] In addition to UV radiation, visible light (VL) has been shown to increase melanogenesis, thus impacting prevention, development, and treatment of pigmentary disorders such as melasma and PIH.[18] Tinted sunscreens containing iron oxide and pigmentary titanium dioxide provide protection against VL, in addition to UV radiation. Use of tinted sunscreens containing these ingredients has been shown to be more effective in prevention of hyperpigmentation disorders when compared to nontinted broad-spectrum sunscreen without these filters and should be strongly recommended for cosmetic patients of color.[15,17] It is important to note that mineral sunscreens containing inorganic filters such as zinc oxide and titanium dioxide leave a white, gray, or violaceous cast in dark skin, causing an unwanted chalky film. Micronized sunscreen formulations using nanoparticles of zinc oxide and titanium dioxide reduce the appearance of a chalky film on dark skin and may be viewed as cosmetically favorable, but they do not protect against visible light. Given these considerations, tinted broad-spectrum sunscreens, which are now available in a variety of hues to match most skin colors, are favored.

Topical Melanogenesis Inhibitors

There is an array of topical melanogenesis inhibitors that may be utilized for preprocedure management and address the cosmetic concerns of POC (Table 10.1). Additionally, these agents may be used to treat PIH caused by cosmetic procedures. For cosmetic procedures in POC that have melanocyte stimulatory potential including laser treatments, microneedling, and chemexfoliation, pretreatment use of inhibitors of melanogenesis may be considered. Hydroquinone in a 4% concentration applied once daily for up to 6 weeks preprocedure is commonly selected to decrease the potential for postprocedure hyperpigmentation and as concurrent treatment of

TABLE 10.1	Studies of Topical Therapy for PIH				
Author, Year	**Study Design**	**Patients (Condition)**	**Intervention/ Treatment**	**Outcome Measures**	**Results**
Bulengo-Ransby[35] (1993) PMID: 8479462	Randomized, controlled	68, Black subjects (PIH)	Tretinoin 0.1% Once daily 40 weeks	Clinical Evaluation Colorimetric and Biopsy Analysis	Lightening of PIH lesions with tretinoin after 40 weeks ($P < 0.001$). Colorimetry demonstrates an increase of 2.6 +/– 0.7 units in value for lesions in tretinoin group, compared with an increase of 1.2 +/– 0.4 units for control ($P = 0.05$).
Grimes[34] (2006) PMID: 16475496	Randomized, controlled	74, FST III-VI (acne)	Tazarotene 0.1% cream Once daily 18 weeks	Clinical Evaluation Medication tolerability	Tazarotene-associated decrease in overall severity of PIH by a mean of 1.2 compared with 0.2 ($P < 0.01$). Pigmentary mean reduction in tazarotene group by 1.1 vs. 0.5 grades ($P = 0.22$).
Jacyk[36] (2001) PMID: 11843232	Open-label, prospective	65, Black South African patients (PIH and acne)	0.1% Adapalene gel Once daily 12 weeks	Number and density of hyperpigmentation	Decline in mean number of lesions ranged from 46% to 72% from baseline to week 12 ($P < 0.01$). Decrease in severity of PIH after 12 weeks ($P < 0.01$).
Callender[37] (2012) PMID: 22798973	Randomized, double-blind, placebo-controlled	33, FST IV-VI (acne, PIH)	Topical clindamycin phosphate 1.2% and tretinoin 0.025% gel or placebo Once daily 12 weeks	Evaluators Global Acne Severity Scale • Lesion counts • PIH Severity Scale • Patient's Global Assessment scale	Clindamycin/tretinoin patients had a decrease lesion count of 11.9 to 5.5 from baseline to week 12 vs. 13.6 to 11.35 in placebo group ($P = 0.05$). Clindamycin/tretinoin topical had superior efficacy.
DuBois[38] (2019) PMID: 31251543	Open-label, prospective	50, FST IV–VI (acne, PIH)	0.3 % adapalene gel/ 2.5% benzoyl peroxide gel Once daily 16 weeks	• IGA • QoL and subject questionnaire • GAI • Presence of PIH	77% subjects were satisfied/ very satisfied. 56% subjects had clear/almost clear results per IGA. 87% good to excellent improvement in GAI 75% had no or mild PIH by week 16.
Yoshimura[28] (1999) PMID: 10441721	Open-label, prospective	61, oriental patients (Senile lentigines, melasma, PIH)	5% hydroquinone, 7% lactic acid ointment + 0.1% all trans retinoic acid ointment or 0.1% all trans retinoic acid aqueous gel Twice daily	• Clinical Evaluation • Colorimetry	Improvement of hyperpigmentation in 18 cases (82% patients) in hydroquinone group, and in 100% cases in the gel group. Treatment time required was 62 days for hydroquinone group and 20 days for gel group.

Continued

TABLE 10.1		Studies of Topical Therapy for PIH—cont'd			
Author, Year	**Study Design**	**Patients (Condition)**	**Intervention/ Treatment**	**Outcome Measures**	**Results**
Cook-Bolden FE[29] (2008) PMID: 18491487	Open-label, prospective	21, FST II–VI (17 with PIH)	Microencapsulated hydroquinone 4% and retinol 0.15% with antioxidants (not specified) Twice daily in face and body 12 weeks	• Lesion number, size, darkness, and disease severity upon clinical evaluation • Reflectance spectrophotometer • Global improvement assessment • Participant satisfaction questionnaire	Reduction in lesion size, darkness, and severity reduced throughout the 12 weeks ($P < .032$). 63% of patients had marked improvement or complete clearing of hyperpigmentation.
Grimes PE[30] (2004) PMID: 15663072	Open-label study	28, FST I–IV (12 PIH, 16 melasma)	Microentrapped hydroquinone 4% with retinol 0.15% Twice daily 12 weeks	• Evaluation of disease severity, pigmentation intensity, lesion area, colorimetry measurements. • Global evaluation • Spectrophotometer	Mean disease severity decreased from 4.6 at baseline to 2.7 by week 12 ($P < .001$). Pigmentation intensity decreased from 3.2 at baseline to 1.8 by week 12 ($P < .001$). Lesion area decreased from 2.8 to 1.8 from baseline to week 12 ($P < .001$). Colorimetry measurements showed improvements from baseline 23% to 39.7% by week 12.
Lowe NJ[33] (1998) PMID: 9829446	Randomized, double-masked, Parallel	52, FST IV–VI (melasma, PIH, idiopathic melanosis, drug-induced hyperpigmentation)	20% azelaic acid cream or placebo Twice daily 24 week	• Global Physician assessment • Lesion size, pigmentary intensity (chromometer) • Clinical photography • Patient questionnaire	Decreases in pigment intensity in both investigator subjective scale ($P = 0.032$) and chromometer analysis ($P = 0.039$). Global improvement noted with azelaic acid at end of study ($P = 0.008$). Patients reported smoother skin and very satisfied with treatment.
Kircik LH[32] (2011) PMID: 21637899	Open-label, prospective	20, FST IV–VI (hyperpigmentation, acne)	15% azelaic acid gel Twice daily 16 weeks	• Investigator Global Assessment of acne and PIH	92% of patients had at least 1-point improvement in IGA for acne. 85% of total patients had at least 2-point improvement of IGA. At week 16, 69% of all subjects were rated as clear based on IGA ($P = .0005$).

TABLE 10.1	Studies of Topical Therapy for PIH—cont'd				
Author, Year	Study Design	Patients (Condition)	Intervention/ Treatment	Outcome Measures	Results
Castanedo-Cazares JP[43] (2013) PMID: 23355788	Randomized, double-blind, placebo-controlled	24, FST III-V (axillary hyperpig-mentation)	Niacinamide 4%, desonide 0.05%, or placebo	• Colorimetry • Quantitative evaluation of melanin, inflammatory infiltrates, NKI/Beteb, CD1a, CD68, and Collagen type IV via histo-chemistry, immunohisto-chemistry	24% of cases had excellent response with niacinamide, 30% for desonide, and 6% for placebo.
Kurokawa I[41] (2017) PMID: 31149741	Split-face, open-label, prospective	10 (PIH, PIE, AS in acne vulgaris)	Combination of glycerol-octyl-ascorbic acid/ascorbyl 2-phos-phate 6 palmi-tate and DL-al-pha-tocopherol phosphate lotion	• IGA • Clinical observation • Photography	Greater improvement in PIH, PIE, and AS observed on the combination treated side vs. control.
Boissy RE[40] (2005) PMID: 16026582	Paired comparison, vehicle-controlled, double-blind study	50, 35 Caucasian light skin, 16 non-Caucasian darker skin (solar lentigines)	3% Arbutin (de-oxyArbutin) Daily treatment (does not state the daily regimen) 12 weeks	• Skin lightness with Chro-mameter • Digital image evaluation for solar lentigi-nes by three independent clinicians	Expert blinded visual assess-ment noted statistically signif-icant improvement in solar lentigines of Caucasian group ($P = 0.05$) but not darker skinned group ($P = 0.08$).
Taylor MB[42] (2013) PMID: 23377327	Open-label, prospective	35, 32/35 FST III-V (melasma, PIH)	Vitamin C with full-face ionto-phoresis mask and mandelic/malic acid skin care regimen One in office treat-ment and 12 to 24 at-home treatments (1-hour applica-tion 3x each week) over 1 to 2 months treatment	• Clinical pho-tos evaluated by four independent observers • MASI score	Greater than 25% improvement observed in 32/35 patients, and >50% improvement in 22/35 patients. MASI scores demonstrated improvement from baseline for all patients.

AS, atrophic scars; *FST*, Fitzpatrick skin type; *GAI*, Global assessment of improvement; *IGA*, Investigator Global Assessment; *MASI*, Melasma Area and Severity Index; *PIE*, postinflammatory erythema; *PIH*, postinflammatory hyperpigmentation; *QoL*, quality of life.

dyschromias.[9,11,19–21] Topical retinoids may be used as either adjunctive or preprocedure therapy for inhibition or treatment of dyschromias as well as for facial rejuvenation (Fig. 10.1). Topicals containing ingredients including azelaic acid, ascorbic acid, or niacinamide may be used in combination to decrease the activity of melanocytes and mitigate the effects of pigment production and/or transfer and thus lessen the risk of postprocedural hyperpigmentation while treating any underlying pigmentary disorders.[12,22–24] Of note, topical retinoids are often discontinued 1 week prior to resurfacing of the skin with chemexfoliation or laser procedures to minimize the penetration of the peeling agent with resulting irritation, desquamation, or ulceration.[3,9,11,12,25] Dermatologists should encourage cosmetic patients to communicate openly about the use of any cosmeceuticals and monitor the ingredients for their safety profile. Of note, it has been documented that some patients use skin-bleaching agents that contain high-potency corticosteroids that may adversely affect postprocedure wound healing.[26]

Hydroquinone and Hydroquinone Combinations

While the adaptations of the Kligman-Willis formula (comprised of 0.1% tretinon, 5.0% hydroquinone, 0.1% dexamethasone)[27] have been used for decades for treatment of PIH and other disorders of hyperpigmentation, newer

studies have emerged demonstrating additional options for combination therapy of hydroquinone and topical retinoids. In this study of 792 patients (the largest study to date), the safety and efficacy of triple combination therapy (fluocinolone acetonide 0.01%/hydroquinone 4%/tretinoin 0.05.%) in the treatment of acne-induced PIH was investigated. 40% of patients treated with the triple-combination cream were clear or almost clear at 8 weeks. The triple-combination cream demonstrated numerical but not statistical superiority when compared to each of its dyads.[27a] Multiple studies have demonstrated efficacy of topical hydroquinone use in combination with retinoids and chemexfoliants. For example, in a study performed in eight Asian subjects with PIH, combination treatment of 5% hydroquinone, 7% lactic acid ointment, and topical 0.1% all trans retinoic acid applied twice daily, 50% of these demonstrated a "good" response, as defined by final relative melanin value (RMV) reduction to less than 20% of the RMV before treatment through Mexameter assessment.[28] Hydroquinone 4% cream has also been assessed in combination with retinol 0.15% twice daily for 12 weeks, with one study showing either marked improvement or complete clearing in 12 of 19 PIH subjects, as assessed with reflectance spectrophotometry.[29] Similarly, an open-label study of 28 FST I–IV subjects with PIH evaluated the application of microentrapped hydroquinone 4% with retinol 0.15% twice daily for 12 weeks and noted significant

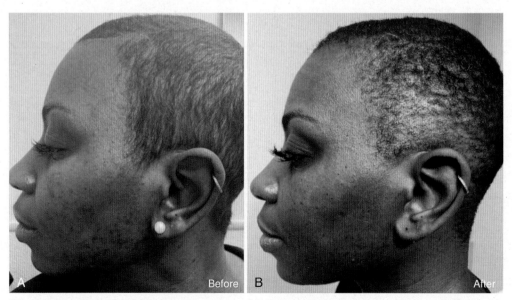

Fig. 10.1 (A and B) Black/African-American women with PIH and acne prior to (A) and following (B) treatment with hydroquinone 4% cream BID daily and tretinoin 0.05% nightly cream for 3 months. (*Image courtesy of Oma N. Agbai, MD*).

improvement of disease severity and pigmentation intensity from baseline as assessed by global evaluation, colorimetry, and spectrophotometry.[30]

Given the rare risk of exogenous ochronosis with hydroquinone use, strict photoprotective measures and pulse application are often used and encouraged to reduce the risk of this adverse effect. For example, in a pulse application regimen, consistent use 1 to 2 times daily for 3 to 6 months would typically be followed by an in-office skin examination to assess for efficacy and monitor for adverse effects prior to resuming, as clinically indicated. Patients with sensitive skin may need to apply a combination treatment containing a topical retinoid 3 to 4 times weekly during the initial treatment period to optimize tolerance prior to advancing to daily application.

Azelaic Acid (AzA)

Azelaic acid is a naturally occurring dicarboxylic acid with antityrosinase activity, as well as antiinflammatory, antikeratinizing, antimicrobial, and antioxidant effects, making it a management option for both acne and PIH.[31] One study treated 20 Fitzpatrick skin type (FST) IV–VI subjects with acne and associated PIH with topical 15% AzA gel twice daily for 16 weeks.[32] At the conclusion of the treatment period, 100% of subjects had at least a 2-point improvement on investigator global assessment scores for PIH (ranging from 0-clear, to 6-very severe) and reported a significant decrease of hyperpigmentation assessed by colorimetry after 16 weeks of treatment. Possible adverse effects included irritation, erythema, and stinging. One author has observed that initiating therapy every other day for 2 weeks before advancing to daily or twice-daily application may reduce the stinging sensation that some patients may experience at the onset of treatment. In another multicenter, randomized, double-blind, placebo-controlled study, 52 FST IV–VI subjects with facial hyperpigmentation were treated with 20% azelaic acid gel twice daily for a period of 24 weeks.[33] At the conclusion of this study, azelaic acid gel produced a significant reduction in pigment intensity, as assessed by both investigator's subjective scale and chromometer analysis.

Topical Retinoids

Although evidence suggests that a combination of topical retinoids with other depigmenting agents such as hydroquinone is more effective than with retinoids alone (see previous section on hydroquinone combination therapy), topical retinoids have been studied as monotherapy for PIH. Statistically significant improvement in clinical PIH assessment compared to placebo has been reported in randomized controlled trials utilizing topical retinoids. For example, in one study of 74 FST III–VI subjects with PIH applying topical tazarotene 0.1% cream nightly for 18 weeks, the pigmentary severity of hyperpigmented lesions was decreased by an average of 1.1 (treatment) versus 0.5 (placebo) grades, a difference that was found to be statistically significant.[34] There was no significant difference in mild erythema, burning, and peeling between the treatment and placebo groups and no reports of tazarotene-induced hyperpigmentation. Similarly, in a study of 68 Black subjects with PIH, in which topical tretinoin 0.1% was applied daily for 40 weeks, the hyperpigmentation of 58% of subjects was classified as "much lighter" and 38% classified as "lighter."[35] These findings were statistically significant when compared to placebo and were assessed through colorimetry. No significant adverse effects or   were reported. An open-label prospective study of 65 Black South African subjects with PIH and acne-evaluated application of 0.1% Adapalene gel once daily for 12 weeks noted two-thirds of subjects experienced a reduction of the number and density of hyperpigmented macules at the conclusion of the treatment period.[36]

Combined therapies for acne including topical retinoids have also been assessed in their efficacy at reducing acne-related PIH. For example, in a double-blind, placebo-controlled study, 33 FST IV–VI subjects with acne and PIH were treated with topical tretinoin 0.025% gel and topical clindamycin phosphate 1.2% versus placebo once daily for 12 weeks.[37] The reduction in mean PIH score signifying improvement from baseline to week 12 was higher for the clindamycin/tretinoin gel group versus placebo group (−1.2 vs. −0.9). Similarly, in an open-label, prospective study of 50 FST IV–VI subjects with acne and PIH, 0.3% adapalene gel/2.5% benzoyl peroxide gel was applied once daily for 16 weeks.[38] At the conclusion of the treatment period, 77% of subjects were satisfied/very satisfied, 56% subjects had clear/almost clear results per investigator's global assessment, 87% reported good to excellent improvement in global assessment of improvement, and 75% had no or mild PIH by week 16.

Arbutin

Arbutin has been employed for treatment of disorders of hyperpigmentation due to its tyrosinase inhibition in vitro.[39] Despite this function, arbutin was shown to be ineffective in reduction of skin pigmentation,[39] potentially due to poor skin penetration through topical application in vivo. Conversely, a modified form of arbutin, deoxyarbutin, has been shown to reduce skin pigmentation in animal studies, more so than 3% hydroquinone after 9 weeks of use.[40] Topical arbutin has not been extensively studied specifically for PIH management in human studies, though it has been studied in POC for management of unspecified hyperpigmentation and solar lentigines. One paired comparison, vehicle-controlled, double-blind study of 50 postmenopausal women using 3% deoxyarbutin topical versus vehicle to the dorsal surface of each forearm showed a significant reduction in pigmentation compared to placebo in the total population, which included 16 POC, after 12 weeks of daily use as assessed by colorimetry.[40] Of note, the reduction in pigmentation in the POC group was not shown to be statistically significant. More studies at varying concentrations and longer duration of treatment are needed to determine the efficacy of topical arbutin and its derivatives in POC.

Vitamin C (Ascorbic Acid)

Topical ascorbic acid has gained interest as a management option for hyperpigmentation disorders, though its instability and suboptimal cutaneous penetration pose challenges to its efficacy as a management option for PIH. In a split-face trial of 10 Asian patients with acne and PIH, in which topical glyceryl-octyl–ascorbic acid (GOVC), ascorbyl 2-phosphate 6-palmitate (APP), and DL-α- tocopherol phosphate (TP) was applied twice daily for 3 months, there was a greater improvement in PIH on the side with GOVC/APP/TP compared to the side without as assessed by clinical evaluation and photography.[41] In a study of 35 melasma and PIH patients, including 21 patients with FST IV–VI, a proprietary ascorbyl glucoside preparation was delivered via iontophoresis to improve absorption. Additionally, a 6% mandelic/malic acid skin care regimen was used.[42] After one in-office treatment and 12 to 24 home treatments, the authors noted a rapid improvement in the appearance of melasma and PIH within 1 to 2 months in all skin types included, and these improvements were sustained for up to 54 months.[42] Specific data for the PIH subset were not discussed.

Niacinamide (B3)

Topical niacinamide (B3) has been shown to reduce melanogenesis in vitro, as well as facial hyperpigmentation in vivo in Japanese women. In a vehicle-controlled study, 18 Japanese subjects with hyperpigmentation applied a 5% niacinamide moisturizer and a vehicle moisturizer in a paired design.[23] Through assessments with computer analysis and visual grading of high-resolution digital facial images, niacinamide showed a 10% decrease in total hyperpigmented area after 4 weeks of use and a 25% decrease after 8 weeks of use, a statistically significant reduction when compared to the vehicle-treated side.[23] A randomized study of 24 subjects with axillary PIH using niacinamide 4% and desonide 0.05% versus placebo showed a significantly greater reduction in hyperpigmentation when compared to placebo after 9 weeks of therapy, as assessed through NC2 melanin concentration maps and colorimetry L-values.[43] Furthermore, there was a greater reduction in hyperpigmentation with desonide use when compared to niacinamide.[43] A randomized double-blind trial of 207 adult Indian women age 30 to 60 years evaluated daily use of a facial lotion containing vitamins B and E and provitamin B5 for treatment of epidermal hyperpigmentation.[44] The test lotion included 4% niacinamide (vitamin B3) 0.5% panthenol, 0.5% tocopheryl acetate (vitamin E), sunscreen, and glycerol in addition to other cosmetic ingredients that made up the control lotion. Evaluation of L values on a chromameter and clinical photography indicated significant reduction in facial hyperpigmentation when compared with baseline and the control lotion after 10 weeks of daily use.

Lignin Peroxidase

Lignin peroxidase is a naturally occurring enzyme derived from the tree fungus *Phanerochaete chrysosporium* that has been observed to induce depigmentation in plants. One study compared twice-daily lignin peroxidase (LIP) cream with twice daily 2% hydroquinone cream and placebo in Asian women for mottled hyperpigmentation.[45] In this randomized, double-blind split-face study of 51 patients, LIP-treated subjects showed a 7.6% reduction in pigmentation after 31 days of treatment, as shown through Mexameter measurement of pigmentation. Contrarily, there was no statistically significant pigmentation reduction in the hydroquinone-treated group. While more studies are needed for treatment of postinflammatory hyperpigmentation specifically, topical lignin peroxidase may be an alternative to 2% hydroquinone.

CHEMEXFOLIATION

Chemexfoliation is an emerging cosmetic intervention for management of dyschromias (Table 10.2). The superficial chemexfoliants, glycolic acid (GA) 35%–70%, salicylic acid (SA) 20%–30%, mandelic acid (MA) 40%, Jessner's solution (JS), lactic acid (LA) 88%, phytic acid, and trichloroacetic acid (TCA) <15% remove the stratum corneum and penetrate to various lengths of the epidermis, resulting in an improvement in pigmentation and textural roughness.[46] Medium or deeper chemexfoliants, specifically including TCA peels with a concentration greater than 15%, penetrate the dermal layer, improving scarring but with the potential adverse effects of dyspigmentation and enhanced scarring. Therefore, TCA-containing medium-depth or deep peels should be avoided in FST IV–VI patients. Additionally, chemical peels considered safe in POC, such as the 20% salicylic acid peel, must be performed at intervals greater than 2 weeks apart to avoid extensive desquamation, subsequent burns, and PIH (seen in Fig. 10.2).

TABLE 10.2 Studies of Chemexfoliation for PIH

Author, Year	Study Design	Patients (Condition)	Intervention/ Treatment	Outcomes	Results
Joshi SS[85] (2009) PMID: 19400885	Split-face, randomized, controlled, open	11, FST IV–VI (PIH)	5 SA peels at 20% to 30%	• Blinded, independent photographic assessment • Treatment versus control ratings by dermatologists • Subjects DLQI • Subjects visual analog scale and treatment quality questionnaire	Improvement of PIH on treatment side was noted, but not significant ($P = .11$) according to the raters. Patient's reported significant improvement of PIH on treatment side ($P = .004$). No statistical significance in QoL ($P = .13$)
Grimes PE[18] (1999) PMID: 9935087	Open-label, prospective	25, FST V–VI (20) Black/ African-American (5) Hispanic (acne vulgaris, PIH, melasma, textured skin)	Pretreated with hydroquinone 4% for 2 weeks prior to 5 SA peels at 20% to 30% + hydroquinone 4% for 2 days after Peels were performed at 2-week intervals 12 weeks	• Clinical photography evaluated by independent investigator	Moderate to significant improvement in 5/5 patients with PIH. 88% improvement was noted on 22/25 patients.
Mohamed Ali BM[48] (2017) PMID: 27976510	Open-label, prospective	45, FST II–VI (PIH lesions)	SA 20% to 30% for up to 10 sessions at weekly intervals; or topical tretinoin 0.1% every other night; or the combination of the two 12 weeks	• Clinical photography • Physician evaluation • Patient evaluation • Dermoscopy for recurrent lesions or lesions with poor improvement	> number of patients with "good" (n = 5) and "very good" (5) results with combination of tretinoin 0.1% with SA peels compared to SA or topical tretinoin alone.

Continued

TABLE 10.2 Studies of Chemexfoliation for PIH—cont'd

Author, Year	Study Design	Patients (Condition)	Intervention/ Treatment	Outcomes	Results
Burns RL[47] (1997) PMID: 9145958	Randomized, controlled	19, FST IV–VI (PIH)	Tretinoin 0.05% once nightly and hydroquinone 2% GA 10% gel twice daily; or same treatment + 6 GA peels at 50% to 68% concentration at 3-week intervals 22 weeks	• Clinical photography • Colorimetry • Subjective evaluation	50% decrease in HASI scores in peel group by week 22. No significant difference with control. Colorimetric analysis in peel group showed greater improvement of PIH via lightening of pigmentation (47.1 l at baseline to 51.4 at week 22 ($P = 0.001$) compared to control group.
Sarkar R[86] (2017) PMID: 28114204	Randomized controlled	30, FST III–V Indian patients (facial PIH)	GA peels at 30% to 50% + (MKF = hydroquinone 2%, tretinoin 0.05%, hydrocortisone 1%), or the MKF alone 12 weeks	• Photographic evaluation • Scoring of HASI • Patient subjective assessment	HASI score of the peels group was 1.56 vs. MKF group was 5.13 at week 21, statistically significant ($P < .001$).
Sharad J[82] (2011) PMID: 22151943	Nonrandomized controlled	30, FST III–V (acne scars)	Group 1: 5 microneedling treatments Once every 6 weeks or Group 2: Microneedling treatments once every 6 weeks + 5 GA peels at 35% at same intervals	• Clinical Photographs • Scar assessment and objective grading	Mean improvement in scars was 31.33% in Group A and 62% in group B. PIH was observed in three patients in Group A that resolved with bleaching cream.
Kurokawa I[87] (2017) PMID: 27743393	Open-label, prospective	31 Japanese patients, FST not mentioned (PIH, atrophic acne scars)	20% GA peels + iontophoresis 3 to 4 times at 1- to 2-month intervals	• Clinical Photographs • Investigators Global Improvement rating • Acne severity grading	PIH improved in 26/31 patients (excellent), 3/31 (good), 2/31 (fair).

DLQI, Dermatology Life Quality Index; *FST*, Fitzpatrick skin type; *GA*, glycolic acid; *HASI*, Hyperpigmentation Area and Severity Index; *MASI*, Melasma Area and Severity Index; *MKF*, Modified Kligman Formula; *PIH*, postinflammatory hyperpigmentation; *QoL*, quality of life; *SA*, salicylic acid.

The safety and efficacy of chemexfoliation for the treatment of PIH was demonstrated in one study of POC with PIH, who underwent six total glycolic acid (GA) 50% to 68% peels at 3-week intervals.[47] GA peels were combined with once-daily topical treatment (2% hydroquinone/10% GA/0.05% tretinoin). Combined therapy led to a more rapid reduction of PIH than topical therapy alone. An open-label, prospective study of 31 Japanese patients with PIH and atrophic acne scars assessed 20% GA peels combined with iontophoresis 3 to 4 times at 1- to 2-month intervals. Patient scores for PIH after treatment were as follows: 4 (excellent, n = 26), 3

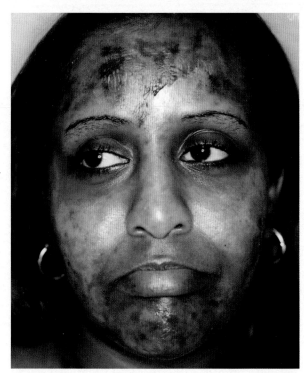

Fig. 10.2 Chemical peel burn on the face of a Black/African-American woman from 20% salicylic acid peel in a hydroethanolic vehicle, performed approximately 10 days after a previous SA 20% peel. Caution must be taken to avoid performing chemical peels at intervals less than 2 weeks apart. (*Image Courtesy of Cheryl Burgess, MD. Cosmetic Dermatology* [Cheryl Burgess, Editor] Springer-Verlag 2005).

(good, n = 3), 2 (fair, n = 1), 0 (none, n = 1). The mean score value was 3.7, indicating clinically apparent improvement of PIH and acne scars.

In addition to glycolic acid peels, salicylic acid (SA) peels have been studied for management of PIH. For example, five POC with PIH underwent five sessions of SA 20% to 30% peels performed at 2-week intervals with over 50% improvement demonstrated through serial photography in 100% of subjects.[18] Similarly, an open-label prospective study of 45 FST II–VI subjects with PIH evaluated use of salicylic acid 20% to 30% for up to 10 sessions at weekly intervals, compared to topical tretinoin 0.1% every other night, compared to a combination of the two for a duration of 12 weeks.[48] A significantly greater improvement with combination of tretinoin 0.1% with SA peels was noted when compared to the use of either individually. Interestingly, whereas some dermatologists recommend holding topical retinoids for 1 week

prior to chemical peels, this combination therapy was tolerated with minimum adverse effects.

Due to its lipophilic properties, SA peels are beneficial for the treatment of acne, as well as acne-induced PIH. In this study, nine acne patients underwent the forementioned regimen with over 50% improvement in 89% of subjects.[18] The Vitalize peel (SkinMedica, Carlsbad, CA) is a superficial chemexfoliant similar to the Jessner's peel that has been anecdotally reported to significantly reduce facial hyperpigmentation and photoaging in Asians.[49] One author reports that the Vi peel (Vitality Institute, Los Angeles, CA), a superficial to medium-depth peel, has been used extensively with excellent results in POC.

Procedure Counseling and Technique

Patients should be advised that the procedure involves application of a chemexfoliant that will cause mild to moderate pain, burning, or stinging sensations. To alleviate this discomfort, a fan blowing cool air to the treated area may be utilized during the peel procedure. Additionally, oral pain medications may be used pre- and postprocedure as indicated. Normal postprocedural reactions include mild to moderate skin peeling, sensitivity, and erythema, which typically resolve within 7 days. Patients with a history of herpes simplex virus infection may be pretreated with valacyclovir 500 mg to 1000 mg BID to TID for 14 days, starting one day prior to procedure. Preprocedural clinical photos are advisable. After obtaining written consent, the patient should be positioned with the head elevated at approximately 30% with the eyelids closed. To remove oil and debris, facial skin is cleansed thoroughly with isopropyl alcohol or acetone. This process may be repeated as indicated to remove excess amounts of soil and debris. Petrolatum may be applied to the bilateral lateral canthi, alar grooves, and oral commissures to protect these sensitive areas from excessive peeling and cracking. A 2x2-cm gauze folded twice can be used as an applicator for the chemical peel solution. One must ensure that the gauze is not excessively saturated to cause dripping of the peel solution when applied to the skin. With regards to endpoints of the chemical peel procedure, one must consider the peel solution used. For glycolic acid peels, the peel is neutralized with 10% to 15% sodium bicarbonate solution after approximately 3 to 4 minutes of peel application. However, if erythema or signs of epidermolysis occur, manifesting as grayish-white discoloration of the epidermis or vesicle formation, the peel must be immediately neutralized, regardless of the duration of peel application. For salicylic acid peels, the endpoint is the pseudofrost formed when the salicylic acid crystallizes. One to four coats may be applied to attain an even pseudofrost, after which the precipitated salicylate is removed with water after 3 to 5 minutes. Jessner's solution is applied in one to three coats until even frosting is achieved or erythema is visible. Peels may be repeated weekly, biweekly, or monthly, depending on the type and depth of the peel.[50]

Postchemexfoliation recommendations include ultraviolet avoidance and sun protection as well as prohibition of any procedures, scrubs, waxing, or manipulation of the skin.[51,52] Moisturization with moisturizing creams or petrolatum-based emollients should be performed 2 to 3 times daily, as well as strict photoprotection with a broad-spectrum sunscreen. Hydroquinone 4% to 8% cream 2 to 4 weeks pre- and posttreatment may been utilized to decrease the risk of chemexfoliant-induced PIH and for continued treatment of the underlying disorder.[8,18,24] Topical tretinoin 0.05% when used as adjunctive therapy for melasma, PIH, and facial rejuvenation may be discontinued 1 week prior to chemexfoliation to minimize irritation and unintended increased depth of the peel.[10,24,25] Topical corticosteroids may also be added if significant erythema, eczematoid reaction and/or PIH are present.[8,52]

LASER TREATMENTS (TABLE 10.3)

Despite their potential for induction of PIH, laser devices have been successfully utilized for the cosmetic treatment thereof (Fig. 10.3). A retrospective evaluation of 61 FST IV–VI patients with PIH treated with 1927-nm nonablative fractional laser showed a mean percent improvement of 43.24%, as assessed by two dermatologists.[53] One retrospective study of 25 patients employed laser-assisted drug delivery using the low-density 1927-nm fractional thulium fiber laser, followed by topical tranexamic acid for PIH. After an average of 3.3 treatments per patient, 16.0% had complete clearance (100% improvement), 68.0% had excellent clearance (76%–99% improvement), and 16.0% had good clearance (51%–75% improvement), as assessed by clinical photography.[54] Additionally, the Nd:YAG 1064-nm 650-microsecond pulse duration laser is an emerging treatment that delivers high and low fluences between 4 J/cm2 and 255 J/cm2 within a single 650-microsecond pulse duration.[55,56] The short-pulse duration avoids overheating the skin, mitigating procedural

discomfort and the risk of adverse effects commonly seen with the previous generation of long-pulsed lasers. In addition to PIH, this laser has been successfully used to treat melasma and pseudofolliculitis barbae in POC. In an observational study, the Q-switched Nd:YAG was used to treat 17 FST IV–V subjects with axillary PIH and found the mean improvement to be "good" after a minimum of three sessions, an improvement that lasted 6 months.[57] A systematic review assessed the efficacy data from 20 original studies[35,58–78] on laser therapeutics for PIH including 224 subjects.[79] Lasers such as the copper bromide laser and light-emitting diodes, intense pulsed light, QS Ruby, QS Nd:YAG 1064-nm, fractional laser were included. Most of the studies were not methodologically rigorous. Outcome measures varied from study to study and included concentration of melanin and hemoglobin, patient satisfaction questionnaires, clinical photography, subjective clinical improvement, light microscopy, melanin index, reflectance spectroscopy, and/or skin biopsy evaluated by a blinded dermatopathologist. Some studies showed no improvement or worsening of PIH after laser treatment.[62–64,68,71] The most extensively studied device was the Q-switched Nd: YAG laser, which has shown promising results based on multiple outcome measures as listed above.

Pre- and Posttreatment Considerations for Laser Therapy in POC

To avoid adverse pigmentation in POC, strict photoprotection to the treated areas should be advised. Proper cooling of the area during laser treatment is required to minimize PIH as it decreases tissue damage and excessive thermal injury. Test spots should be considered prior to initiation of the full laser treatment.[80] Hydroquinone in a 4% concentration applied once daily for 2 to 6 weeks preprocedure is commonly employed to decrease the risk for postprocedural hyperpigmentation.

MICRONEEDLING

In recent years, microneedling has expanded to include additional indications for acne-induced scarring, melasma, and hyperpigmentation. Studies have reported that microneedling combined with other therapies resulted in better outcomes and are safe and effective for patients with darker skin types.[81] For example, in one study of 30 Indian FST III–IV subjects with acne scars and acne-related postinflammatory hyperpigmentation,

TABLE 10.3   Studies of Laser Therapy for PIH

Author, Year	Study Design	Patients (Condition)	Intervention/ Treatment	Laser Settings	Outcomes	Results
Agbai O (2017)[78] PMID: 27973642	Systematic review	224	20 studies: copper bromide laser and light-emitting diodes, intense pulsed light, QS Ruby, QS Nd:YAG 1064 nm, fractional laser	Various	• Laser most used for PIH • Effectiveness of laser treatment	QS Nd:YAG laser therapy had promising results
Ghannam S[56] (2017) PMID: 29141060	Observational	17, FST IV–V Axillary PIH	QS Nd:YAG 1064 nm	Width: 5 ns +/– 2 ns 3 to 12 sessions One session every 2 weeks	• Clinical photographs • Practitioner, patient evaluation, and independent non-medical observer using standardized grading scale	One participant presented with hypopigmentation after sixth session. All other patients were treated successfully without any major adverse events. Minimum number of sessions for results was 3. Results lasted for 6 months.
West TB[88] (1999) PMID: 9935086	Randomized, controlled	100, FST I–III	CO_2 laser resurfacing alone or CO_2 laser + preoperative 10% GA cream twice daily or CO_2 laser + hydroquinone 4% cream qHS and tretinoin 0.025% cream twice daily (n = 25) 12 weeks	Laser settings not described	• Clinical and photographic assessments	No difference in incidence of post-CO_2 laser resurfacing PIH between pretreatment groups and no pretreatment group.
Techapichet- vanich[89] (2018) PMID: 29956440	Split-face, randomized, controlled	19, FST III–V (acne scars, enlarged pores)	CO_2 laser on both cheeks topical application of EGF (1 ug/g) ointment to half of face and petrolatum to other half of face Twice a day until crusting healed	Single pass of 10,600-nm CO_2 laser Energy: 10 mJ Density: 10%	• Wound healing (duration of scab shedding, post-laser erythema, erythema index, TEWL) • PIH evaluation with clinical photographs and Melanin Index	Incidence of PIH was not statistically different on either side of face ($P = .56$). Similar findings with melanin index ($P = .96$).

Continued

TABLE 10.3   Studies of Laser Therapy for PIH—cont'd

Author, Year	Study Design	Patients (Condition)	Intervention/ Treatment	Laser Settings	Outcomes	Results
Cheyasak N[90] (2015) PMID: 24854088	Split-face, randomized	40, FST IV (atrophic acne scars)	Fractional CO_2 laser on both sides of face and postoperative clobetasol propionate 0.05% ointment for 2 days on half face, and petrolatum on other half face for 7 days	Single-pass fractional CO_2 laser Pulse: 950 us Energy: 12.75 mJ (range 10–15 mJ) Coverage: 5% skin No use of cooling device	• Clinical evaluation • Photographic assessment • Scar volume evaluation • Colorimetry for degree of skin pigmentation and erythema	Petrolatum-treated side had higher incidence of PIH ($P < 0.001$) compared to topical corticosteroid and petrolatum-treated side.
Lueangarun S[91] (2018) PMID: 29431228	Split-face, randomized, controlled	16, FST III–IV (moderate -severe atrophic scar)	AFCO2 laser + Multicomponent nonsteroidal antiinflammatory moisturizer (MAS063DP) or AFCO2 + 0.02% triamcinolone acetonide (TA) Twice daily 7 days	Single pass of 10,600-nm eCO2 laser Energy: 30 mJ Density: 100 spots/cm2 Coverage: 7.7% area No use of cooling device	• Digital photography • Hemoglobin and melanin Index • Erythema, edema, PIH evaluation	Melanin index was less than baseline in both groups ($P < 0.001$). Improvement of edema, erythema, crusting and hyperpigmentation in all patients after 1 month ($P < 0.001$). No statistical difference in hemoglobin, melanin index, and texture between groups.
Waniphakdeedecha R[92] (2014) PMID: 24320057	Split-faced, randomized, controlled	30, Asian (PIH)	AFCO2 laser + petrolatum for 1 week vs. AFCO2 laser + petrolatum + broad-spectrum sunscreen with antinflammatory agents 1-session	AF CO2 resurfacing laser Both sides of face Energy: 10 mJ Density: 10% No use of cooling device	• TEWL • Melanin and erythema index	After 1 week, melanin index was less in sunscreen group vs. control group (197.98 vs. 230.77, $P < 0.001$).
Manuskiatti W[93] (2007) PMID: 17875874	Split-faced, randomized, controlled	23, Thai women (bilateral nevus of Ota-like macules, PIH)	Nd: YAG 1064-nm	1064-nm Nd: YAG Fluence: 7 J/cm2 Spot size: 3-mm Cold air-cooling device during and 30 seconds before and after laser on 1/2 face	• Clinical evaluation • Digital photography • Spectrometry	Cooled side had higher rate of PIH after laser (RR:2.6; 95% CI, 1.13–6.00; $P = .03$) 13/21 patients on cooled side developed PIH. 5/21 patients on uncooled side developed PIH.

Study	Study design	Patients/skin type	Intervention	Laser parameters	Outcome measures	Results
Chan HH[94] (2007) PMID: 17518354	Retrospective and Prospective study	Retrospective: 37, Chinese (acne scarring, skin rejuvenation, pigmentation). Prospective: 18	Retrospective: 119 treatment sessions. 1540-nm Erbium glass laser 68 sessions: high energy, low density 51 sessions: low energy, high density. Prospective:	Retrospective High energy, low density Energy: 7–20 mK average energy 16.3 mJ 1000 MTZ Time not mentioned Low energy, high density Energy: 6–12 mJ average energy 8.2 mJ 2000 MTZ Time not mentioned Prospective: 6,12, and 24 mJ, and 250 MTZ versus 6–12 mJ, and 1000–4000 MTZ) 1–16 passes Time not mentioned	• Clinical photography pre- and post-treatment for evidence of PIH	Retrospective: No statistical significance in PIH occurrence between groups. Localized peri-oral PIH occurred in patients without air cooling. Prospective: Low densities of total 250 MTZ had lower rate of PIH (<0–2 instances per site) compared to those receiving a total of 1000–4000 MTZ (9 instances per site).
Rutnin D[95] (2019) PMID: 31302943	Blinded, randomized, controlled	40, Asian Solar lentigines	QS 532-nm Nd:YAG laser with oral TA 1500 mg daily or placebo 6 weeks	Single session QS: Nd:YAG laser Spot size: 2-mm Energy: 1.8–2.3 J/cm at 2Hz	• Digital photographs • Dermoscopy • Colorimetry • Physician grading scores • Patient satisfaction scores	No statistical significance of incidence of PIH, melanin value, lightness index, and clinical improvement scores between the two groups. TA group demonstrated lower number of pigmented granules on dermoscopy at 6th ($P = 0.038$) and 12th weeks ($P = 0.013$).

AF, ablative fractional; *FST*, Fitzpatrick skin type; *MASI*, Melasma Area and Severity Index; *MTZ*, microthermal zone; *PIH*, postinflammatory hyperpigmentation; *TA*, tranexamic acid; *TEWL*, transepidermal water loss.

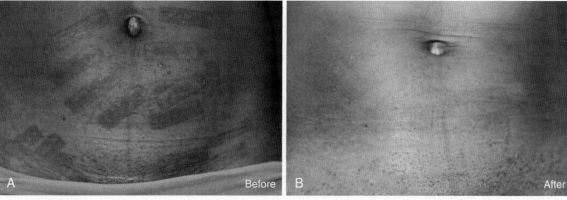

Fig. 10.3 (A and B) IPL burns on the abdomen before (A) and after (B) treatment with HQ 6% cream, Jessner's Peel, and Aerolase 650-microsec 1064-nm Nd:YAG at 18 J/cm2. (*Image courtesy of Cheryl Burgess, MD. Dermatology Times October 2020*).

subjects were divided into two groups: Group A was treated with microneedling (Derrmaroller MF8) every 6 weeks for a total of five treatments, and Group B was treated with a combination of alternating microneedling treatments and 35% GA peels every 3 weeks, with a total of five treatments for each.[81] There was an excellent improvement of PIH in Group B compared to Group A, as demonstrated through clinical photography. No permanent sequelae were noted in either group. Similarly, another study of 39 FST III-VI subjects with acne scarring and PIH were treated with an electric microneedling device (e Dermastamp, Dermaroller) for one session.[83] At 2 and 4 weeks following treatment, a 22% improvement in the postacne hyperpigmentation index (PAHPI) was noted.[76] This statistically significant improvement in mean PAHPI scores was also reflected in clinical photography. No significant adverse effects were reported. In addition to PIH, microneedling has been reported as a management option for periorbital hypermelanosis. A case report of a 48-year-old man (FST V) with idiopathic periorbital melanosis documented his treatment with the DermaFrac device, which employs microneedling in addition to infusion of a serum containing antiaging and lightening agents.[84] Physician global assessment demonstrated 50% to 75% and 75% to 90% improvement after 4 and 12 sessions, respectively, and no adverse effects were noted. The proposed mechanism of action may be related to optimized skin hydration and induction of collagen and elastin synthesis, which may diminish the visibility of dermal pigment.

In POC it is especially important to avoid the scrubbing technique of the microneedles along the skin, which may increase the risk of PIH. Repeatedly pressing and lifting the pen in a "jackhammer" technique to avoid harmful abrasion is the preferred technique when performing microneedling in POC.

CONCLUSION

Herein we discussed topical and procedural modalities for PIH. It is the author's opinion that topical melanogenesis inhibitor use should be optimized prior to adding procedures such as chemexfoliants and laser procedures. Combining topicals and procedures may improve cosmetic outcomes and mitigate postprocedural hyperpigmentation when topicals are used several weeks prior to and following procedures. With further research in this area, cosmetic therapeutic options may become more readily available to individuals of all ethnic skin types.

REFERENCES

1. Darji K, Varade R, West D, Armbrecht ES, Guo MA. Psychosocial impact of postinflammatory hyperpigmentation in patients with acne vulgaris. *J Clin Aesthet Dermatol.* 2017;10:18-23.
2. Fitzpatrick TB. The validity and practicality of sun-reactive skin types I through VI. *Arch Dermatol.* 1988;124:869-871.
3. Taylor SC, Burgess CM, Callender VD, et al. Postinflammatory hyperpigmentation: Evolving combination treatment strategies. *Cutis.* 2006;78:6-19.

4. Roberts WE. The Roberts skin type classification system. *J Drugs Dermatol.* 2008;7:452-456.

5. Roberts WE. Skin type classification systems old and new. *Dermatol Clin.* 2009;27:529-533, viii.

6. Jalalat S, Weiss E. Cosmetic laser procedures in Latin skin. *J Drugs Dermatol.* 2019;18:s127-s131.

7. Rossi AM, Perez MI. Laser therapy in Latino skin. *Facial Plast Surg Clin North Am.* 2011;19:389-403.

8. Deere BP, Ferdinand KC. Hypertension and race/ethnicity. *Curr Opin Cardiol.* 2020;35:342-350.

9. Roberts WE. Chemical peeling in ethnic/dark skin. *Dermatol Ther.* 2004;17:196-205.

10. Cole PD, Hatef DA, Taylor S, Bullocks JM. Skin care in ethnic populations. *Semin Plast Surg.* 2009;23:168-172.

11. Callender VD. Acne in ethnic skin: Special considerations for therapy. *Dermatol Ther.* 2004;17:184-195.

12. Sarkar R, Arsiwala S, Dubey N, et al. Chemical peels in melasma: A review with consensus recommendations by Indian Pigmentary Expert Group. *Indian J Dermatol.* 2017;62:578-584.

13. Schalka S. New data on hyperpigmentation disorders. *J Eur Acad Dermatol Venereol.* 2017;31 suppl 5:18-21.

14. Kaidbey KH, Agin PP, Sayre RM, Kligman AM. Photo-protection by melanin—a comparison of black and Caucasian skin. *J Am Acad Dermatol.* 1979;1:249-260.

15. Boukari F, Jourdan E, Fontas E, et al. Prevention of melasma relapses with sunscreen combining protection against UV and short wavelengths of visible light: A prospective randomized comparative trial. *J Am Acad Dermatol.* 2015;72:189-190.e1.

16. Agbai ON, Buster K, Sanchez M, et al. Skin cancer and photoprotection in people of color: A review and recommendations for physicians and the public. *J Am Acad Dermatol.* 2014;70:748-762.

17. Castanedo-Cazares JP, Hernandez-Blanco D, Carlos-Ortega B, Fuentes-Ahumada C, Torres-Alvarez B. Near-visible light and UV photoprotection in the treatment of melasma: A double-blind randomized trial. *Photodermatol Photoimmunol Photomed.* 2014;30:35-42.

18. Randhawa M, Seo I, Liebel F, Southall MD, Kollias N, Ruvolo E. Visible light induces melanogenesis in human skin through a photoadaptive response. *PLoS One.* 2015; 10:e0130949.

19. Grimes PE. The safety and efficacy of salicylic acid chemical peels in darker racial-ethnic groups. *Dermatol Surg.* 1999;25:18-22.

20. Kaushik SB, Alexis AF. Nonablative fractional laser resurfacing in skin of color: Evidence-based review. *J Clin Aesthet Dermatol.* 2017;10:51-67.

21. Javaheri SM, Handa S, Kaur I, Kumar B. Safety and efficacy of glycolic acid facial peel in Indian women with melasma. *Int J Dermatol.* 2001;40:354-357.

22. Chaowattanapanit S, Silpa-Archa N, Kohli I, Lim HW, Hamzavi I. Postinflammatory hyperpigmentation: A comprehensive overview: Treatment options and prevention. *J Am Acad Dermatol.* 2017;77:607-621.

23. Davis EC, Callender VD. Postinflammatory hyperpigmentation: A review of the epidemiology, clinical features, and treatment options in skin of color. *J Clin Aesthet Dermatol.* 2010;3:20-31.

24. Hakozaki T, Minwalla L, Zhuang J, et al. The effect of niacinamide on reducing cutaneous pigmentation and suppression of melanosome transfer. *Br J Dermatol.* 2002;147:20-31.

25. Callender VD, St Surin-Lord S, Davis EC, Maclin M. Postinflammatory hyperpigmentation: Etiologic and therapeutic considerations. *Am J Clin Dermatol.* 2011;12:87-99.

26. Dey VK. Misuse of topical corticosteroids: A clinical study of adverse effects. *Indian Dermatol Online J.* 2014; 5:436-440.

27. Bulengo-Ransby SM, Griffiths CE, Kimbrough-Green CK, et al. Topical tretinoin (retinoic acid) therapy for hyperpigmented lesions caused by inflammation of the skin in Black patients. *N Engl J Med.* 1993;328:1438-1443.

27a. Taylor S, Grimes P, Lim J, Im S, Kui H. Postinflammatory hyperpigmentation. *J Cutan Med Surg.* 2009;13(4): 183-191.

28. Grimes P, Callender V. Tazarotene cream for postinflammatory hyperpigmentation and acne vulgaris in darker skin: A double-blind, randomized, vehicle-controlled study. *Cutis.* 2006;77:45-50.

29. Jacyk WK. Adapalene in the treatment of African patients. *J Eur Acad Dermatol Venereol.* 2001;15 suppl 3:37-42.

30. Callender VD, Young CM, Kindred C, Taylor SC. Efficacy and safety of clindamycin phosphate 1.2% and tretinoin 0.025% gel for the treatment of acne and acne-induced post-inflammatory hyperpigmentation in patients with skin of color. *J Clin Aesthet Dermatol.* 2012;5:25-32.

31. DuBois J, Ong GCW, Petkar G, et al. Patient-reported outcomes in acne patients with skin of color using adapalene 0.3%-benzoyl peroxide 2.5%: a prospective real-world study. *J Drugs Dermatol.* 2019;18:514.

32. Yoshimura K, Harii K, Aoyama T, Shibuya F, Iga T. A new bleaching protocol for hyperpigmented skin lesions with a high concentration of all-trans retinoic acid aqueous gel. *Aesthetic Plast Surg.* 1999;23:285-291.

33. Cook-Bolden FE, Hamilton SF. An open-label study of the efficacy and tolerability of microencapsulated hydroquinone 4% and retinol 0.15% with antioxidants for the treatment of hyperpigmentation. *Cutis.* 2008;81:365-371.

34. Grimes PE. A microsponge formulation of hydroquinone 4% and retinol 0.15% in the treatment of melasma and postinflammatory hyperpigmentation. *Cutis.* 2004;74: 362-368.

35. Lowe NJ, Rizk D, Grimes P, Billips M, Pincus S. Azelaic acid 20% cream in the treatment of facial hyperpigmentation in darker-skinned patients. *Clin Ther.* 1998;20:945-959.

36. Kircik LH. Efficacy and safety of azelaic acid (AzA) gel 15% in the treatment of post-inflammatory hyperpigmentation and acne: A 16-week, baseline-controlled study. *J Drugs Dermatol.* 2011;10:586-590.

37. Castanedo-Cazares JP, Larraga-Pinones G, Ehnis-Perez A, et al. Topical niacinamide 4% and desonide 0.05% for treatment of axillary hyperpigmentation: A randomized, double-blind, placebo-controlled study. *Clin Cosmet Investig Dermatol.* 2013;6:29-36.

38. Kurokawa I, Yoshioka M, Ito S. Split-face comparative clinical trial using glyceryl-octyl-ascorbic acid/ascorbyl 2-phosphate 6-palmitate/DL-alpha-tocopherol phosphate complex treatment for postinflammatory hyperpigmentation, postinflammatory erythema and atrophic scar in acne vulgaris. *J Dermatol.* 2019;46:e347-e348.

39. Boissy RE, Visscher M, DeLong MA. DeoxyArbutin: A novel reversible tyrosinase inhibitor with effective in vivo skin lightening potency. *Exp Dermatol.* 2005;14:601-608.

40. Taylor MB, Yanaki JS, Draper DO, Shurtz JC, Coglianese M. Successful short-term and long-term treatment of melasma and postinflammatory hyperpigmentation using vitamin C with a full-face iontophoresis mask and a mandelic/malic acid skin care regimen. *J Drugs Dermatol.* 2013;12:45-50.

41. Kligman AM, Willis I. A new formula for depigmenting human skin. *Arch Dermatol.* 1975;111:40-48.

42. Draelos ZDKAL. Implication of azelaic acid's multiple mechanisms of action: Therapeutic versatility. American Academy of Dermatology 66th Annual Meeting. San Antonio, TX.

43. Chakraborty AK, Funasaka Y, Komoto M, Ichihashi M. Effect of arbutin on melanogenic proteins in human melanocytes. *Pigment Cell Res.* 1998;11:206-212.

44. Jerajani HR, Mizoguchi H, Li J, Whittenbarger DJ, Marmor MJ. The effects of a daily facial lotion containing vitamins B3 and E and provitamin B5 on the facial skin of Indian women: A randomized, double-blind trial. *Indian J Dermatol Venereol Leprol.* 2010;76:20-26.

45. Mauricio T, Karmon Y, Khaiat A. A randomized and placebo-controlled study to compare the skin-lightening efficacy and safety of lignin peroxidase cream vs. 2% hydroquinone cream. *J Cosmet Dermatol.* 2011;10:253-259.

46. Joshi SS, Boone SL, Alam M, et al. Effectiveness, safety, and effect on quality of life of topical salicylic acid peels for treatment of postinflammatory hyperpigmentation in dark skin. *Dermatol Surg.* 2009;35:638-644; discussion 644.

47. Mohamed Ali BM, Gheida SF, El Mahdy NA, Sadek SN. Evaluation of salicylic acid peeling in comparison with topical tretinoin in the treatment of postinflammatory hyperpigmentation. *J Cosmet Dermatol.* 2017;16:52-60.

48. Burns RL, Prevost-Blank PL, Lawry MA, Lawry TB, Faria DT, Fivenson DP. Glycolic acid peels for postinflammatory hyperpigmentation in Black patients. A comparative study. *Dermatol Surg.* 1997;23:171-174; discussion 175.

49. Sarkar R, Parmar NV, Kapoor S. Treatment of postinflammatory hyperpigmentation with a combination of glycolic acid peels and a topical regimen in dark-skinned patients: A comparative study. *Dermatol Surg.* 2017;43:566-573.

50. Sharad J. Combination of microneedling and glycolic acid peels for the treatment of acne scars in dark skin. *J Cosmet Dermatol.* 2011;10:317-323.

51. Kurokawa I, Oiso N, Kawada A. Adjuvant alternative treatment with chemical peeling and subsequent iontophoresis for postinflammatory hyperpigmentation, erosion with inflamed red papules and non-inflamed atrophic scars in acne vulgaris. *J Dermatol.* 2017;44:401-405.

52. Vemula S, Maymone MBC, Secemsky EA, et al. Assessing the safety of superficial chemical peels in darker skin: a retrospective study. *J Am Acad Dermatol.* 2018;79:508-513.e2.

53. Kim MM, Byrne PJ. Facial skin rejuvenation in the Asian patient. *Facial Plast Surg Clin North Am.* 2007;15:381-386, vii.

54. Wang JV, Lopez A, Geronemus RG. Safety and Effectiveness of Low-Energy, Low-Density 1927-nm Fractional Thulium Fiber Laser With Tranexamic Acid for Postinflammatory Hyperpigmentation. *Dermatol Surg.* 2022;48(10):1131-1133.

54a. Bae YC, Rettig S, Weiss E, Bernstein L, Geronemus R. *Lasers Surg Med.* 2020;52(1):7-12.

55. Khunger N, Force IT. Standard guidelines of care for chemical peels. *Indian J Dermatol Venereol Leprol.* 2008; 74 suppl:S5-S12.

56. Sharad J. Glycolic acid peel therapy—a current review. *Clin Cosmet Investig Dermatol.* 2013;6:281-288.

57. Rullan P, Karam AM. Chemical peels for darker skin types. *Facial Plast Surg Clin North Am.* 2010;18:111-131.

58. Ghannam S, Al Otabi FK, Frank K, Cotofana S. Efficacy of low-fluence Nd:YAG 1064-nm laser for the treatment of post-inflammatory hyperpigmentation in the axillary area. *J Drugs Dermatol.* 2017;16:1118-1123.

59. West TB, Alster TS. Effect of pretreatment on the incidence of hyperpigmentation following cutaneous CO2 laser resurfacing. *Dermatol Surg.* 1999;25:15-17.

60. Techapichetvanich T, Wanitphakdeedecha R, Iamphonrat T, et al. The effects of recombinant human epidermal growth factor containing ointment on wound healing and post inflammatory hyperpigmentation prevention after fractional ablative skin resurfacing: A split-face randomized controlled study. *J Cosmet Dermatol.* 2018;17:756-761.

61. Cheyasak N, Manuskiatti W, Maneeprasopchoke P, Wanitphakdeedecha R. Topical corticosteroids minimise the risk of postinflammatory hyper-pigmentation after

ablative fractional CO2 laser resurfacing in Asians. *Acta Derm Venereol.* 2015;95:201-205.

62. Lueangarun S, Tempark T. Efficacy of MAS063DP lotion vs 0.02% triamcinolone acetonide lotion in improving post-ablative fractional CO2 laser resurfacing wound healing: a split-face, triple-blinded, randomized, controlled trial. *Int J Dermatol.* 2018;57:480-487.

63. Wanitphakdeedecha R, Phuardchantuk R, Manuskiatti W. The use of sunscreen starting on the first day after ablative fractional skin resurfacing. *J Eur Acad Dermatol Venereol.* 2014;28:1522-1528.

64. Manuskiatti W, Eimpunth S, Wanitphakdeedecha R. Effect of cold air cooling on the incidence of postinflammatory hyperpigmentation after Q-switched Nd:YAG laser treatment of acquired bilateral nevus of Ota like macules. *Arch Dermatol.* 2007;143:1139-1143.

65. Chan HH, Manstein D, Yu CS, Shek S, Kono T, Wei WI. The prevalence and risk factors of post-inflammatory hyperpigmentation after fractional resurfacing in Asians. *Lasers Surg Med.* 2007;39:381-385.

66. Rutnin S, Pruettivorawongse D, Thadanipon K, Vachiramon V. A prospective randomized controlled study of oral tranexamic acid for the prevention of postinflammatory hyperpigmentation after Q-switched 532-nm Nd:YAG laser for solar lentigines. *Lasers Surg Med.* 2019;51:850-858.

67. Bae YC, Rettig S, Weiss E, Bernstein L, Geronemus R. Treatment of post-inflammatory hyperpigmentation in patients with darker skin types using a low energy 1,927 nm non-ablative fractional laser: a retrospective photographic review analysis. *Lasers Surg Med.* 2020;52:7-12.

68. Burgess C, Chilukuri S, Campbell-Chambers DA, Henry M, Saedi N, Roberts WE. Practical applications for medical and aesthetic treatment of skin of color with a new 650-microsecond laser. *J Drugs Dermatol.* 2019;18:s138-s143.

69. Roberts WE, Henry M, Burgess C, Saedi N, Chilukuri S, Campbell-Chambers DA. Laser treatment of skin of color for medical and aesthetic uses with a new 650-microsecond Nd:YAG 1064nm laser. *J Drugs Dermatol.* 2019;18:s135-s137.

70. Park KY, Choi SY, Mun SK, Kim BJ, Kim MN. Combined treatment with 578-/511-nm copper bromide laser and light-emitting diodes for post-laser pigmentation: A report of two cases. *Dermatol Ther.* 2014;27:121-125.

71. Ho WS, Chan HH, Ying SY, Chan PC, Burd A, King WW. Prospective study on the treatment of postburn hyperpigmentation by intense pulsed light. *Lasers Surg Med.* 2003;32:42-45.

72. Augustyniak A, Erkiert-Polguj A, Rotsztejn H. Variable pulsed light treatment of melasma and post-inflammatory hyperpigmentation—a pilot study. *J Cosmet Laser Ther.* 2015;17:15-19.

73. Park JH, Kim JI, Kim WS. Treatment of persistent facial postinflammatory hyperpigmentation with novel pulse-in-pulse mode intense pulsed light. *Dermatol Surg.* 2016;42:218-224.

74. Kopera D, Hohenleutner U. Ruby laser treatment of melasma and postinflammatory hyperpigmentation. *Dermatol Surg.* 1995;21:994.

75. Taylor CR, Anderson RR. Ineffective treatment of refractory melasma and postinflammatory hyperpigmentation by Q-switched ruby laser. *J Dermatol Surg Oncol.* 1994;20:592-597.

76. Mitra A, Yeung R, Sheehan-Dare R, Wilson CL. Lentiginous hyperpigmentation confined to resolved psoriatic plaques and treated with a Q-switched ruby laser. *Clin Exp Dermatol.* 2006;31:298-299.

77. Cho SB, Park SJ, Kim JS, Kim MJ, Bu TS. Treatment of post-inflammatory hyperpigmentation using 1064-nm Q-switched Nd:YAG laser with low fluence: Report of three cases. *J Eur Acad Dermatol Venereol.* 2009;23:1206-1207.

78. Kim S, Cho KH. Treatment of procedure-related postinflammatory hyperpigmentation using 1064-nm Q-switched Nd:YAG laser with low fluence in Asian patients: Report of five cases. *J Cosmet Dermatol.* 2010;9:302-306.

79. Kim S, Cho KH. Treatment of facial postinflammatory hyperpigmentation with facial acne in Asian patients using a Q-switched neodymium-doped yttrium aluminum garnet laser. *Dermatol Surg.* 2010;36:1374-1380.

80. Ho SG, Yeung CK, Chan NP, Shek SY, Kono T, Chan HH. A retrospective analysis of the management of acne postinflammatory hyperpigmentation using topical treatment, laser treatment, or combination topical and laser treatments in oriental patients. *Lasers Surg Med.* 2011;43:1-7.

81. Cho SB, Lee SJ, Kang JM, Kim YK, Oh SH. Treatment of refractory arcuate hyperpigmentation using a fractional photothermolysis system. *J Dermatol Treat.* 2010;21:107-108.

82. Katz TM, Goldberg LH, Firoz BF, Friedman PM. Fractional photothermolysis for the treatment of postinflammatory hyperpigmentation. *Dermatol Surg.* 2009;35:1844-1848.

83. Kroon MW, Wind BS, Meesters AA, et al. Non-ablative 1550 nm fractional laser therapy not effective for erythema dyschromicum perstans and postinflammatory hyperpigmentation: A pilot study. *J Dermatol Treat.* 2012;23:339-344.

84. Lee SJ, Chung WS, Lee JD, Kim HS. A patient with cupping-related post-inflammatory hyperpigmentation successfully treated with a 1,927 nm thulium fiber fractional laser. *J Cosmet Laser Ther.* 2014;16:66-68.

85. Lee YB, Park SM, Kim JW, Yu DS. Combination treatment of low-fluence Q-switched Nd:YAG laser and oral tranexamic acid for post-inflammatory hyperpigmentation due to allergic contact dermatitis to henna hair dye. *J Cosmet Laser Ther.* 2016;18:95-97.

86. Oram Y, Akkaya AD. Refractory postinflammatory hyperpigmentation treated fractional CO2 laser. *J Clin Aesthet Dermatol.* 2014;7:42-44.

87. Rokhsar CK, Ciocon DH. Fractional photothermolysis for the treatment of postinflammatory hyperpigmentation after carbon dioxide laser resurfacing. *Dermatol Surg.* 2009;35:535-537.

88. Savory SA, Agim NG, Mao R, et al. Reliability assessment and validation of the postacne hyperpigmentation index (PAHPI), a new instrument to measure postinflammatory hyperpigmentation from acne vulgaris. *J Am Acad Dermatol.* 2014;70:108-114.

89. Zawar VP, Agarwal M, Vasudevan B. Treatment of postinflammatory pigmentation due to acne with Q-switched

90. neodymium-doped yttrium aluminum garnet In 78 Indian cases. *J Cutan Aesthet Surg.* 2015;8:222-226.

90. Abstracts of the American Society for Laser Medicine and Surgery. March 30–April 3, 2011. Grapevine, Texas, USA. *Lasers Surg Med Suppl.* 2011;23:907-1018.

91. Agbai O, Hamzavi I, Jagdeo J. Laser treatments for postinflammatory hyperpigmentation: A systematic review. *JAMA Dermatol.* 2017;153:199-206.

92. Woolery-Lloyd H, Viera MH, Valins W. Laser therapy in black skin. *Facial Plast Surg Clin North Am.* 2011;19:405-416.

93. Singh A, Yadav S. Microneedling: Advances and widening horizons. *Indian Dermatol Online J.* 2016;7:244-254.

94. Al Qarqaz F, Al-Yousef A. Skin microneedling for acne scars associated with pigmentation in patients with dark skin. *J Cosmet Dermatol.* 2018;17:390-395.

95. Sahni K, Kassir M. Dermafrac: An innovative new treatment for periorbital melanosis in a dark-skinned male patient. *J Cutan Aesthet Surg.* 2013;6:158-160.

11

Prevention and Treatment of Keloids and Hypertrophic Scars

Alana Kurtti, Jared Jagdeo

SUMMARY & KEY FEATURES

- Keloids and hypertrophic scars represent fibrotic skin conditions with high resistance to therapy.
- Key strategies for prevention of keloid and hypertrophic scarring include avoiding unnecessary skin injury, rapid primary closure of wounds, precise wound edge approximation, and minimizing tension on the wound.
- Commonly used therapies include occlusive dressings, pressure therapy, intralesional corticosteroids, cryotherapy, and excisions.
- Newer therapies include radiotherapy, bleomycin, 5-fluorouracil, botulinum toxin type A, pulsed dye lasers, ablative lasers, nonablative fractional lasers, laser-assisted drug delivery, and light-emitting diode phototherapy.

- Although a variety of medical and surgical therapies are available, most treatments have not been adequately evaluated in high-quality studies and there is no universally accepted approach.
- Before selecting a treatment modality, it is important to discuss desired treatment outcomes (e.g., symptom relief, scar volume reduction, functional improvement, and aesthetic improvement) with the patient. It is also essential to review common side effects as several therapies cause dyspigmentation, a major concern for patients with skin of color. The patient's treatment goals should help guide the provider's choice of therapy.

CLINICOHISTOPATHOLOGIC FEATURES

Keloids and hypertrophic scars are pathologic scars characterized by excessive tissue response to dermal injury (i.e., surgery, burns, trauma).[1] The two scars share several features but have aesthetic, pathogenic, and histopathologic distinctions (Table 11.1).[1] The hypertrophic scar is typically firm, raised within the boundaries of the wound, and occasionally symptomatic, causing pruritus or pain. This type of scar typically develops within 4 to 8 weeks of injury, commonly forming over extensor joints and areas of high mechanical tension.[2] While it may take years, hypertrophic scars can regress spontaneously over time.[3]

Contrarily, keloids are raised scars that extend beyond the original site of injury.[2] They can appear months to many years after injury and do not regress spontaneously over time. The most common sites of occurrence include the upper chest, shoulders, upper back, neck, and head, especially the ear.[4] Compared to hypertrophic scars, keloids are typically more clinically severe, causing pruritus and pain more frequently in patients.[1]

From a histopathologic perspective, both keloids and hypertrophic scars result from excess collagen deposition. Keloids display a random organization of Type I and Type III collagen fibers, while hypertrophic scars primarily have an organized, parallel pattern of Type III collagen.[2,5]

TABLE 11.1   Comparison of Keloids and Hypertrophic Scars

	Keloid	Hypertrophic Scar
Incidence	Rare	Frequent
Associated skin type	Higher prevalence in darker-skinned individuals	None
Predilection site	Upper chest, shoulders, upper back, neck, head, especially earlobes	Shoulders, neck, pre-sternum, knees and ankles
Time course	Proliferation months to years after injury or spontaneous formation, no regressive phase	Emergence within 4–8 weeks of injury, rapid growth for several months then regression
Spontaneous regression	No	Yes, possible
Extension	Extends beyond original borders of wound	Confined to original borders of wound
Contracture	Rare	Often
Recurrence rate after surgical excision	High	Low
Histological characteristics	Random orientation of Type I and III collagen	Organized, parallel pattern of primarily Type III collagen

EPIDEMIOLOGY

There is strong evidence for a genetic component of keloid development, given the familial predisposition, varied incidence in different ethnic populations, and presence in twins.[6] Racial/ethnic variations in keloid prevalence have been reported, with most of the published literature describing an increased prevalence among Black populations. However, the strength of the association of keloids with socially determined race has been recently called into question.[7] Keloids affect men and women equally, with the highest incidence between age 11 to 30 years.[8,9] There is a familial tendency to develop keloids, with familial studies suggesting an autosomal dominant pattern of inheritance with incomplete penetrance.[6,10] Contrarily, there is no strong evidence of a genetic susceptibility to hypertrophic scar development.

PREVENTION

Prevention of keloid and hypertrophic scarring is more successful than treatment. It is thus essential that patients avoid unnecessary skin injury, including nonessential and cosmetic surgeries, regardless of whether the patient is prone to pathologic scarring.[8,11] Since delayed epithelialization beyond 10 to 14 days substantially increases the rate of hypertrophic scarring, prompt epithelialization is crucial for preventing aberrant scar development.[8,12] Additionally, wounds subject to tension due to movement, anatomic location, or loss of tissue have a greater risk of hypertrophy and expansion.[8,13] Thus, rapid primary closure of wounds under minimal tension with precise wound edge approximation is of the utmost importance.[8]

MANAGEMENT

Keloids and hypertrophic scars represent fibrotic skin conditions with high resistance to therapy.[14,15] The two types of scars may be accompanied by pain, pruritus, functional impairment, aesthetic deformity, and low self-reported quality of life.[2,15] Although a variety of medical and surgical therapies have been used for the treatment of keloids and hypertrophic scars, most of these treatments have not been adequately evaluated in high-quality studies and there is no universally accepted treatment approach. In this section, we explore both common and emerging therapies for keloids and hypertrophic scars in patients with skin of color.

A. Standard Therapies
1. Occlusive Dressings

Occlusive dressings are routinely used for the treatment and prevention of keloids and hypertrophic scars. Silicone gel sheeting (SGS) is a commonly used occlusive dressing composed of a semiocclusive silicone gel sheet combined with a durable silicone membrane.[1,16] The antiscarring effects of occlusive dressings are believed to result from a combination of occlusion and hydration of the wound bed.[17] The SGS creates a moisture-rich environment, preventing dehydration of the stratum corneum and ultimately reducing activation of fibroblasts and thus collagen synthesis.[17]

Silicone gel sheeting is easily accessible over the counter and by prescription. The clear, sticky sheeting is sized to the scar and fixed with tape. SGS requires tremendous patient compliance, often requiring patients to wear the SGS at least 12 hours per day for 12 months or more.[1,18,19]

Efficacy of SGS has primarily been demonstrated when the dressing is used as a prophylactic measure rather than a treatment.[1] A systematic review including 20 trials totaling 873 patients compared adhesive silicone gel sheeting with various treatments and no therapy.[20] In the prevention studies, SGS reduced the incidence of hypertrophic scarring in people prone to scarring (risk ratio 0.46 compared with no treatment). In the treatment studies, SGS statistically significantly reduced scar thickness and improved scar color. However, because the prevention and treatment studies were highly susceptible to bias, the reviewers concluded that there is weak evidence for SGS as an effective preventative and therapeutic method for hypertrophic scars and keloids.[20] Side effects associated with SGS include skin breakdown, skin rash, skin maceration, and foul smell from the gel.[21]

2. Pressure Therapy

Pressure therapy (PT) is regularly used for the prevention and treatment of pathologic scars, especially hypertrophic scars from burns. Compression treatments include button compression, pressure earrings, ACE bandages, elastic adhesive bandages, spandex or elastane bandages, and support bandages.[1] PT is believed to trigger apoptosis of cells in the extracellular matrix via activation of mechanoreceptors and reduce oxygen tension in the wound through occlusion of blood vessels, ultimately reducing fibroblast proliferation and collagen deposition.[1,2,22]

Regarding usage protocol, there are no comparative analyses of pressure amount.[23] Thus, the pressure used clinically typically relies on empirical reports.[23] Most articles indicate a pressure of 25 mm Hg or greater.[24] It

has been recommended that pressure garments be worn at least 23 hours daily starting immediately after wound reepithelialization, for 6 to 24 months.[25,26]

Evidence in support of PT is limited. When used as a prevention technique, a 2009 metaanalysis of six RCTs including 316 patients demonstrated no difference in global scar assessment between patients treated with pressure garments and controls.[27] However, a 2017 metaanalysis of 12 RCTs involving 710 patients with hypertrophic scars from burn injuries showed that patients managed with PT (15–25 mm Hg) showed significant improvements in Vancouver Scar Scale (VSS) score, pigmentation, redness, and brightness.[28] Observational studies of patients with keloids, especially of the earlobe, have shown that custom-made pressure devices may reduce the risk of recurrence after surgical excision.[29,30] In a study including 1436 ear keloids in 883 patients treated with surgical excision followed by pressure magnet use for 12 hours daily for 6 months, 89.4% did not have recurrence at 18 months.[29] A study of 88 subjects postexcision of earlobe keloids treated with custom-made pressure clips for 12 hours a day for 6 to 18 months had a recurrence rate of only 29.5% at a mean follow up of 6.5 years.[30]

PT is typically well tolerated. However, if excessive pressure is used, the compression may cause tissue necrosis or parasthesias.[29,31] In addition, higher pressures may cause discomfort and thus increase the rate of noncompliance.[28]

3. Intralesional Corticosteroids

Intralesional triamcinolone acetonide (TAC) is a mainstay treatment for hypertrophic scars and keloids. Corticosteroids improve scar pliability and decrease scar volume by reducing the synthesis of collagen and glycosaminoglycans.[32,33] The decrease in collagen synthesis is believed to be due to fibroblast hypoactivity, reduction in fibroblast density, or modification of the maturation of fibroblasts.[32] Intralesional corticosteroids also confer antiinflammatory and vasoconstrictive effects, which are believed to reduce pain and pruritus.[2,25]

Intralesional TAC is typically administered at a concentration of 10 to 40 mg/mL every 4 to 6 weeks.[2] The injections are given for several months or until the scar has flattened.[2] Keloids and hypertrophic scars are typically directly injected with corticosteroids. However, thick and longstanding keloids are often so firm that they must be softened with cryotherapy pretreatment for 5 to 20 seconds.[13]

The rates of response to intralesional corticosteroid injections vary from 50% to 100%, with a recurrence rate of 9% to 50%.[25,34] Results from a metaanalysis showed that TAC treatment results in marked reduction in keloid size in comparison with the untreated control.[35] Further, TAC was found to be more effective in improving scars than SGS, verapamil, and cryotherapy.[35] Outcomes may be improved when corticosteroids are given in combination with other therapies. For example, randomized trials and observational studies have reported that combination TAC and 5-fluorouracil (5-FU) is more effective than intralesional corticosteroids alone in reducing keloid size, induration, and erythema.[36–38]

Side effects of treatment with intralesional steroids include telangiectasia, atrophy, and dyspigmentation.[2] The risk of local complications is higher when adjacent healthy tissue is inadvertently injected.[39]

4. Cryotherapy

Cryotherapy has been used as both monotherapy and adjunct therapy for pathologic scars.[34] This modality is believed to induce ischemic damage, leading to necrosis and reduction of tumor bulk.[1] Cryotherapy can be administered as a contact or spray session, or intralesionally. Typically, a freeze–thaw cycle up to 30 seconds is used and repeated up to three times in a single treatment visit. Treatments are given every 4 to 6 weeks or until response occurs. Intralesional cryotherapy can be performed through single or multiple needles of varying gauges or an intralesional cryoprobe.[2] The CryoShape (Etgar Group International Ltd, Kfar Saba, Israel), an FDA-approved intralesional cryotherapy device consisting of a 14-gauge double-lumen cryoneedle, is commercially available in the United States.[40,41] Alternatively, intralesional cryotherapy can be performed using disposable needles by connecting the needle hub to a cryotherapy gun nozzle.[42] The connection should be secured in place with tape, also preventing leakage. This technique offers the provider the advantage of using different size needles.

Remission rates between 68% and 81% and low recurrence rates have been reported for spray and contact sessions, respectively.[40] However, this may require numerous treatment sessions.[43] Compared to spray or contact cryotherapy, intralesional cryotherapy freezes the scar from the core outwards, achieving deeper, more complete freezing of the scar and often requires fewer treatment sessions for sufficient scar outcomes.[1,40,44,45] Studies using the CryoShape have reported that intralesional cryotherapy reduces keloid volume by an average of 51.4% to 67.4% after a single treatment.[40,41] Improvements in hardness, elevation, and redness as well as itching and tenderness were also reported, with none of the subjects experiencing permanent hypopigmentation or recurrence.[40,41] Evidence suggests intralesional cryotherapy is more efficacious in small scars and ear keloids.[44,46]

Side effects include permanent hypo- and hyperpigmentation, skin atrophy, and blistering.[47,48] Because melanocytes are more sensitive to cold temperatures, contact or spray sessions often result in significant hypopigmentation, limiting its use in darker skin types.[2] Contrarily, intralesional cryotherapy localizes freezing within the lesion, averting damage to the surface skin better than contact or spray therapy.[2] For this reason, intralesional therapy may be a more suitable option than contact or spray therapy for patients with skin of color as it less frequently results in hypopigmentation.

5. Excision

Excision may be used as monotherapy to treat hypertrophic scars and keloids but is often used in combination with other therapies. Surgical treatment may include full excision with primary closure or shave excision left to heal by secondary intention.[2] Optimal techniques for primary wound closure after complete excision include gentle handling of tissue, avoidance of wound bed tension, closure within relaxed skin tension lines, eversion of wound edges, precise approximation of wound edges, and careful control of infection and inflammation.[1,2,49,50]

For hypertrophic scars, the timing of surgical treatment is a crucial consideration as hypertrophic scars may regress naturally without any physical manipulation.[8] Surgery may not be necessary, although postexcisional recurrence rates of hypertrophic scars are usually small.[8,51,52] For keloids, full or shave excision is rarely used as monotherapy as recurrence rates range from 45% to 100%.[53] In a study of 43 subjects that underwent surgical excision of ear keloids, the recurrence rate was 51.2%.[54] Decreased recurrence rates have been reported with adjuvant therapies. For example, in a retrospective analysis of 80 patients with keloid scars managed with excision and immediate postoperative radiotherapy, the recurrence rate was 9% at one year and 16% at 5 years.[55]

A major risk of excision is creating a longer scar than the original, and recurrence may lead to an even larger keloid.[8] For this reason, surgical excision for keloids and hypertrophic scars should be used with extreme caution.

Emerging Therapies

6. Radiotherapy

There is a consensus that radiation is an effective therapy for keloids and hypertrophic scars.[56] While the exact mechanism is unknown, radiotherapy is believed to inhibit fibroblast proliferation, thereby decreasing collagen production. In vitro, radiotherapy has been shown to inhibit proliferation and induce senescence of keloidal fibroblasts by promoting cell cycle arrest.[57]

Brachytherapy and external beam therapy (EBT) have been used for the treatment of keloids and hypertrophic scars. Brachytherapy delivers targeted radiation through a hollow catheter incorporated into the lesion and can be administered as a low-dose rate (LDR) or high-dose rate (HDR).[1,58] LDR typically requires longer treatment periods, inpatient hospitalization, and therefore is not as practical for treatment of pathologic scars.[2] In contrast, HDR typically requires just 5 to 10 minutes of treatment.[59]

EBT involves delivery of targeted radiation beams from outside the body.[58] Numerous techniques and modalities, including megavoltage electrons and low-energy kilovoltage, have been used for EBT.[60] Compared to brachytherapy, traditional electron EBT has been said to require higher radiation doses due to the larger distance between the radiation source and scar and inadvertently expose adjacent healthy skin to radiation.[2,58] However, superficial X-ray radiation therapy (SRT) is a low-energy EBT that delivers energy to a depth of 5 mm. SRT targets the skin while avoiding damage to deeper tissues.[61] SRT is believed to be simpler, less costly, and convenient as it can be performed in office.

A 2017 systematic review and metaanalysis including 72 studies and 9048 keloids demonstrated that surgery combined with postoperative radiotherapy yields a lower recurrence rate than radiotherapy alone (22% and 37%, respectively).[62] Postoperative brachytherapy was associated with a lower recurrence rate than postoperative EBT with electron beam and X-ray therapy

(15% and 23%, respectively).[62] Among the two EBT modalities, similar control of keloid recurrence was noted.[62] Compared with LDR, HDR has been shown to provide better relief of keloid symptoms, including pain and pruritus and has the advantage of shorter treatment times and no inpatient hospitalization requirement.[63]

A variety of radiation modalities, doses, and schedules have been shown to effectively treat pathologic scars. Numerous groups have sought to determine the biologically effective dose (BED) necessary for successfully treating keloids. A BED of ≥ 30 Gy has been suggested as it is associated with <10% recurrence.[64,65] This can be attained with a single dose of 13 to 15 Gy, two fractions of 8.5 to 10 Gy, or three fractions of 6 to 7.5 Gy, administered within 2 days postoperatively.[65] In 2019, consensus guidelines asserted that postsurgical SRT significantly reduces keloid recurrence rates and that fractionation of the SRT dose reduces the risk of hyperpigmentation and other adverse events.[66] The optimal treatment protocol was said to be a biologically effective dose of 3000 cGy with three fractions of 600 cGy on postoperative days 1, 2, and 3.[66] Consideration of equipment accessibility, cost, and provider experience are essential when selecting a radiation modality and technique.

A major concern for radiotherapy is the possibility of radiation-induced malignancy years after treatment. While causation cannot be confirmed, several cases of malignancy that may have been associated with radiation therapy for keloids have been reported.[55,67] Patients may also experience several skin-related side effects. In the short term, erythema, desquamation, and pigmentary changes may occur.[62,67] In the long term, patients may experience permanent pigmentary changes, atrophy, telangiectasias, and subcutaneous fibrosis.[67,68] Radiation therapy is not suggested for pregnant patients, patients less than 12 years old, or radiosensitive anatomic locations, such as the thyroid.[2]

7. Bleomycin

Bleomycin is a cytotoxic, antineoplastic, antiviral, and antibacterial agent derived from *Streptomyces verticillus*.[2] It is thought to inhibit collagen synthesis via decreased stimulation by TGF-β1.[69] There are multiple methods by which bleomycin is administered for the treatment of pathologic scars, including tattooing, dermojet intralesional injection, and intralesional injection with or without electroporation therapy.[1]

Several studies have demonstrated significant improvement in hypertrophic scar and keloid height and pliability as well as reduction in erythema, pruritus, and pain after bleomycin treatment.[69–71] In a study by Saray et al., involving 15 keloids and hypertrophic scars treated with multiple jet injections of bleomycin (1.5 IU/mL) repeated monthly, for an average of two to six sessions, 73.3% of lesions showed complete flattening and there were no recurrences during a mean 19-month follow up.[71] While studies have shown favorable results, bleomycin use is still uncommon.

Regardless of the method of bleomycin delivery, common side effects include hyperpigmentation, pain on injection, ulceration and crusting at injection sites, and dermal atrophy.[69-73] Although systemic administration of bleomycin can cause pulmonary, renal, cutaneous, hepatic, and myelogenous toxicity, systemic effects appear to be rare when low doses are used.[52]

8. 5-Fluorouracil

5-FU is a medication primarily used for oncologic purposes but has also been used for pathologic scars.[8] In vitro and in vivo, 5-FU has been shown to inhibit fibroblast proliferation and TGF-β–induced expression of type I collagen.[23,37,74] This therapy can be used as monotherapy or in combination with other treatments, with intralesional injection being the preferred delivery technique.[23]

As a monotherapy, 5-FU tattooing every 4 weeks for a total of three treatments has been reported to significantly reduce keloid surface, height, induration, erythema, and pruritus.[75] In a systematic review of 18 small trials and 482 patients, intralesional 5-FU alone resulted in good or excellent outcomes in 45% to 78% of patients, while a combination of 5-FU and TAC injections increased good or excellent outcomes to 50% to 96%.[76]

A combination of 5-FU and TAC in a ratio of 9:1 can be used for intralesional injections of keloids and hypertrophic scars.[37] A mixture of 45 mg of 5-FU (0.9 ml of 250 mg/5 ml) with 4 mg TAC (0.1 ml of 40 mg/1 ml) has been shown to be effective, with few side effects.[37,77] A systematic review including six studies revealed that intralesional combination of TAC and 5-FU is more effective than TAC alone in the treatment of keloids and hypertrophic scars, as shown by greater improvements in scar height, erythema, observer assessment, and patient self-assessment.[77]

Wound ulceration, hyperpigmentation, and pain on injection are common side effects of treatment.[8,47] Systemic side effects of 5-FU include anemia, leukopenia, and thrombocytopenia but have not been observed to date after intralesional injection.[1,19]

9. Botulinum toxin type A

Botulinum toxin type A (BTXA) is a potent neurotoxin that produces a temporary flaccid paralysis of striated muscle for a period of 2 to 6 months.[25] Tension is believed to facilitate the development of pathologic scars. By inhibiting underlying muscle contraction during wound healing, BTXA is thought to minimize tension on the wound edges.[2] Studies also have shown that BTXA influences fibroblast proliferation.[78]

BTXA is administered by intralesional injection and while the optimal regimen has not been determined, studies have reported success injecting 70 to 140 U of BTXA at 1- to 3-month intervals for 3 to 9 months.[78–81]

Elhefnawy et al., demonstrated that intralesional injection of BTXA given once a month for 3 months in 20 patients with hypertrophic scars resulted in statistically significant improvements in erythema, pliability, and itching scores, with high patient satisfaction.[80] Favorable outcomes have also been observed in studies of BTXA for keloids.[82] A systematic review and meta-analysis of 14 clinical trials showed that injection of intralesional BTXA was more effective in the treatment of hypertrophic scars and keloids than injection of intralesional corticosteroid or placebo and was also associated with reduced pain following injection.[83] BTXA treatment is typically well tolerated with few side effects, which may make it a more preferrable treatment than intralesional TAC.

10. Pulsed dye laser

Pulsed dye laser (PDL) is a form of nonablative laser therapy initially engineered to treat vascular lesions.[1] The PDL at 585-nm and 595 nm wavelengths has been extensively investigated for scar therapy.[84] PDL is believed to induce microvascular damage leading to local hypoxia and decreased nutrient supply, ultimately altering collagen metabolism and inducing expression of matrix metalloproteinases (MMPs) and collagenase.[1,19]

Based on current recommendations, nonoverlapping laser pulses at fluences ranging from 6.0 to 7.5 J/cm^2 (7-mm spot) or from 4.5 to 5.5 J/cm^2 (10-mm spot) should be applied over the entire surface of the scar.[85]

Two to six treatments at 4 to 8 week intervals may be necessary to achieve scar resolution.[25]

The main clinical effects of PDL therapy include reductions of scar erythema and pruritus.[86,87] Additional benefits include improvements in scar height, volume, texture, and pliability.[88] A systematic review including 10 studies assessing PDL therapy for hypertrophic scars demonstrated low or moderate improvements in erythema, scar volume, and pliability with PDL 585-nm and 595-nm treatment, respectively.[89]

The most common adverse effect of 585-nm PDL treatment is postoperative purpura, which can persist for 7 to 14 days.[8] Other adverse effects include hyperpigmentation, especially in darker skin tones, hypopigmentation, and blistering.[86,90]

11. Ablative Lasers

Ablative resurfacing lasers, the 10,600-nm carbon dioxide (CO_2) and 2940-nm erbium doped yttrium aluminium garnet (Er:YAG) lasers, are used for scar revision by means of superficial ablation or excision. Ablative lasers vaporize superficial tissue and stimulate contraction and remodeling of the dermis.[91] At the molecular level, the lasers target water molecules to cause local tissue changes, including alteration of collagen deposition, upregulation of MMPs, and downregulation of TGF-β.[92] Ablative fractional lasers (AFL) use thermal damage to create numerous vertical microcolumns, with the tissue spared around each column stimulating remodeling.[93]

Laser settings depend on several factors including scar thickness, scar location, and Fitzpatrick skin type. Penetration depth correlates with pulse energy level and should be adjusted for scar thickness.[94] High-energy levels are typically used for thick scars on the extremities and torso while lower-energy levels are used for thin scars, facial scars, and young patients.[94] Several treatment sessions at monthly intervals are often needed to achieve notable scar improvements.[95,96]

CO_2 laser treatments have been reported to improve keloid texture, pigmentation, and overall appearance.[96] When compared to surgical removal of keloids, CO_2 laser excision has similar, high rates of recurrence, ranging from 74% to 100% at 1 year, but is associated with less blood loss and postoperative pain.[1,97,98] In a pilot study including 21 patients with keloids or hypertrophic scars, Er:YAG laser therapy significantly reduced scar redness, hardness, and elevation.[99] In a study comparing the efficacy of CO_2 and Er:YAG AFL in 23 patients with hypertrophic scars, remarkable improvements in pliability were noted with both AFL, but the CO_2 laser appeared to yield superior results.[100] Repeated ablative fractional CO_2 laser treatments have been reported to mainly improve hypertrophic and keloid scar pliability.[101]

Side effects of laser therapy for pathologic scars include erythema, edema, and hyperpigmentation.[96]

12. Nonablative Fractional Lasers

A variety of nonablative fractional lasers (NAFL) have been investigated for the treatment of pathologic scars.[102] Similar to AFL, NAFL create numerous microscopic heat columns with intervening spared skin stimulating tissue remodeling.[103] Unlike with AFL, NAFL leave the epidermis relatively spared.

While NAFL have shown great promise in the treatment of lacerations and surgical scars, robust studies evaluating NAFL for the management of keloids and hypertrophic scars are lacking.[104,105] In a split-lesion RCT involving 18 patients with hypertrophic scars, there was no statistically significant difference in visual and palpable scoring of the side treated with 1540-nm NAFL compared with the untreated side as determined by physician assessment.[102] In a study of 38 patients with hypertrophic and keloid scars, combination treatment with 1550-nm erbium glass NAFL and steroid injections was compared to steroid injections alone.[106] There was no significant difference in observer ratings or recurrence rate. However, the combination treatment group required fewer treatment sessions and showed greater improvements in patient ratings.[106] High-quality studies investigating the efficacy of NAFL for keloid and hypertrophic scar treatment are needed.

Side effects of NAFL for pathologic scars include erythema, edema, hyperpigmentation.[102]

13. Laser-Assisted Drug Delivery

Laser-assisted drug delivery (LADD) is an evolving treatment modality. AFL have been used to facilitate topical drug delivery past the epidermal barrier, thereby increasing bioavailability and efficacy.[107] CO_2 and Er:YAG AFL create microscopic vertical channels in the skin that allow for deep delivery of topical agents, such as corticosteroids and 5-FU.[108]

There is limited high-quality evidence comparing LADD techniques in the treatment of keloids and hypertrophic scars. In a recent case report, combination CO_2 laser with TAC resulted in significant reduction in thickness, improvement in texture, and overall aesthetic appearance of a keloid in a patient with skin of color. This improvement was maintained at 22 months post-initial treatment, without complications or adverse events.[109] In a prospective case series including 15 subjects with hypertrophic scars, combination same session laser therapy and immediate postoperative corticosteroid delivery resulted in overall improvement scores of greater than 50% on average as determined by blinded evaluators.[107] Initial reports have been promising, but additional studies are necessary to explore the effectiveness of different topical therapies with LADD for pathologic scar treatment.

14. Light-Emitting Diode

Light-emitting diode (LED) phototherapy, also known as low-level light therapy (LLLT), is an emerging treatment modality for keloids and hypertrophic scars. In vitro studies have shown that LED phototherapy yields antifibrotic effects by decreasing fibroblast proliferation.[110–112]

Studies investigating the efficacy of LLLT for pathologic scars are lacking. A case series involving three patients with keloids or hypertrophic scars demonstrated that near-infrared LED phototherapy (805 nm at 30 mW/cm²) postexcision or CO_2 laser ablation markedly improved VSS score, scar height as measured by quantitative skin topography, and blinded clinical assessment of photographs compared with control scars, with no significant side effects.[113]

Potential side effects include posttreatment erythema, hypo- or hyperpigmentation, and blistering.[114] LED phototherapy may be a simple, convenient adjunct therapy for at-home management of pathologic scars.[115] However, future studies are needed to determine its clinical efficacy.

15. MicroRNA

The dysregulation of microRNAs (miRNAs) have been implicated in the pathogenesis of keloids and hypertrophic scars.[116] miRNAs are short noncoding RNA molecules approximately 22 nucleotides in length that modify gene expression at the posttranscriptional level by targeting complimentary mRNA sequences.[117]

By performing miRNA expression microarrays in keloids, hypertrophic scars, and normal tissues, researchers have identified numerous upregulated and downregulated miRNAs in pathologic scars compared to normal tissue.[23,116] miR-196a was reported to be significantly underexpressed in keloid fibroblasts compared with normal fibroblasts, resulting in increased expression of type I and III collagens.[118] In a separate study, miR-130a was found to be increased in hypertrophic scar tissues and derived primary fibroblasts and positively correlated with expression of type I and III collagen and α-smooth muscle actin, indicating that miR-130a has significant profibrotic potential.[119]

Using miRNA mimics that enhance antifibrotic activity, miRNA-based therapy represents a promising new therapeutic approach for the treatment of keloids and hypertrophic scars. However, this modality remains in the infancy stage of development.

CONCLUSION

The abundance of therapies available for the prevention and treatment of hypertrophic scars and keloids continues to expand, but no standardized guidelines for the management of pathologic scars exist. The lack of high-quality studies evaluating scar therapies combined with the plethora of available treatments can make selecting a treatment an overwhelming task. Before devising a management plan, it is important to discuss goals of therapy with the individual patient. Desired treatment outcomes may include symptom relief, scar volume reduction, functional improvement, and aesthetic improvement. It is also important to review common side effects, as several modalities cause dyspigmentation, a major concern for patients with skin of color. The individual patient's treatment goals should help guide the provider's choice of therapy.

REFERENCES

1. Betarbet U, Blalock TW. Keloids: A review of etiology, prevention, and treatment. *J Clin Aesthet Dermatol.* 2020;13(2):33-43.
2. Berman B, Maderal A, Raphael B. Keloids and hypertrophic scars: Pathophysiology, classification, and treatment. *Dermatol Surg.* 2017;43(suppl 1):S3-S18.
3. Mahdavian Delavary B, Van der Veer WM, Ferreira JA, Niessen FB. Formation of hypertrophic scars: Evolution and susceptibility. *J Plast Surg Hand Surg.* 2012;46(2):95-101.
4. Robles DT, Berg D. Abnormal wound healing: Keloids. *Clin Dermatol.* 2007;25(1):26-32.

5. Leong M, Murphy K, Phillips L. Wound healing. In: Townsend CJ, Beauchamp R, Evers B, Mattox K, eds. *Sabiston Textbook of Surgery.* vol. 6. Philadelphia, PA: Elsevier; 2012:130-162.

6. Brown JJ, Bayat A. Genetic susceptibility to raised dermal scarring. *Br J Dermatol.* 2009;161(1):8-18.

7. Deyrup A, Graves Jr JL. Racial biology and medical misconceptions. *N Engl J Med.* 2022;386(6):501-503.

8. Gauglitz GG, Korting HC, Pavicic T, Ruzicka T, Jeschke MG. Hypertrophic scarring and keloids: Pathomechanisms and current and emerging treatment strategies. *Mol Med.* 2011;17(1-2):113-125.

9. Ramakrishnan KM, Thomas KP, Sundararajan CR. Study of 1,000 patients with keloids in South India. *Plast econstr Surg.* 1974;53(3):276-280.

10. Marneros AG, Norris JE, Olsen BR, Reichenberger E. Clinical genetics of familial keloids. *Arch Dermatol.* 2001; 137(11):1429-1434.

11. Slemp AE, Kirschner RE. Keloids and scars: A review of keloids and scars, their pathogenesis, risk factors, and management. *Curr Opin Pediatr.* 2006;18(4): 396-402.

12. Mustoe TA, Cooter RD, Gold MH, et al. International clinical recommendations on scar management. *Plast Reconstr Surg.* 2002;110(2):560-571.

13. Mutalik S. Treatment of keloids and hypertrophic scars. *Indian J Dermatol Venereol Leprol.* 2005;71(1):3-8.

14. Bran GM, Goessler UR, Hormann K, Riedel F, Sadick H. Keloids: Current concepts of pathogenesis (review). *Int J Mol Med.* 2009;24(3):283-293.

15. Bock O, Schmid-Ott G, Malewski P, Mrowietz U. Quality of life of patients with keloid and hypertrophic scarring. *Arch Dermatol Res.* 2006;297(10):433-438.

16. Monstrey S, Middelkoop E, Vranckx JJ, et al. Updated scar management practical guidelines: Non-invasive and invasive measures. *J Plast Reconstr Aesthet Surg.* 2014; 67(8):1017-1025.

17. Tandara AA, Mustoe TA. The role of the epidermis in the control of scarring: Evidence for mechanism of action for silicone gel. *J Plast Reconstr Aesthet Surg.* 2008;61(10): 1219-1225.

18. Gold MH, Berman B, Clementoni MT, Gauglitz GG, Nahai F, Murcia C. Updated international clinical recommendations on scar management: part 1—evaluating the evidence. *Dermatol Surg.* 2014;40(8):817-824.

19. Heppt MV, Breuninger H, Reinholz M, Feller-Heppt G, Ruzicka T, Gauglitz GG. Current strategies in the treatment of scars and keloids. *Facial Plast Surg.* 2015;31(4): 386-395.

20. O'Brien L, Jones DJ. Silicone gel sheeting for preventing and treating hypertrophic and keloid scars. *Cochrane Database Syst Rev.* 2013;(9):CD003826.

21. Nikkonen MM, Pitkanen JM, Al-Qattan MM. Problems associated with the use of silicone gel sheeting for hypertrophic scars in the hot climate of Saudi Arabia. *Burns.* 2001;27(5):498-501.

22. Reno F, Grazianetti P, Cannas M. Effects of mechanical compression on hypertrophic scars: Prostaglandin E2 release. *Burns.* 2001;27(3):215-218.

23. Lee HJ, Jang YJ. Recent understandings of biology, prophylaxis and treatment strategies for hypertrophic scars and keloids. *Int J Mol Sci.* 2018;19(3):711.

24. Anderson JB, Foglio A, Harrant AB, et al. Scoping review of therapeutic strategies for keloids and hypertrophic scars. *Plast Reconstr Surg Glob Open.* 2021;9(3):e3469.

25. Arno AI, Gauglitz GG, Barret JP, Jeschke MG. Up-to-date approach to manage keloids and hypertrophic scars: A useful guide. *Burns.* 2014;40(7):1255-1266.

26. Macintyre L, Baird M. Pressure garments for use in the treatment of hypertrophic scars—a review of the problems associated with their use. *Burns.* 2006;32(1):10-15.

27. Anzarut A, Olson J, Singh P, Rowe BH, Tredget EE. The effectiveness of pressure garment therapy for the prevention of abnormal scarring after burn injury: A meta-analysis. *J Plast Reconstr Aesthet Surg.* 2009;62(1):77-84.

28. Ai JW, Liu JT, Pei SD, et al. The effectiveness of pressure therapy (15-25 mmHg) for hypertrophic burn scars: A systematic review and meta-analysis. *Sci Rep.* 2017;7: 40185.

29. Park TH, Seo SW, Kim JK, Chang CH. Outcomes of surgical excision with pressure therapy using magnets and identification of risk factors for recurrent keloids. *Plast Reconstr Surg.* 2011;128(2):431-439.

30. Tanaydin V, Beugels J, Piatkowski A, et al. Efficacy of custom-made pressure clips for ear keloid treatment after surgical excision. *J Plast Reconstr Aesthet Surg.* 2016;69(1): 115-121.

31. Niessen FB, Spauwen PH, Schalkwijk J, Kon M. On the nature of hypertrophic scars and keloids: A review. *Plast Reconstr Surg.* 1999;104(5):1435-1458.

32. Hochman B, Locali R, Matsuoka P, Ferreira L. Intralesional triamcinolone acetonide for keloid treatment: A systematic review. *Aesthetic Plast Surg.* 2008;32(4): 705-709.

33. Saki N, Mokhtari R, Nozari F. Comparing the efficacy of intralesional triamcinolone acetonide with verapamil in treatment of keloids: A randomized controlled trial. *Dermatol Pract Concept.* 2019;9(1):4-9.

34. Shaffer JJ, Taylor SC, Cook-Bolden F. Keloidal scars: A review with a critical look at therapeutic options. *J Am Acad Dermatol.* 2002;46(2 Suppl Understanding): S63-S97.

35. Wong TS, Li JZH, Chen S, Chan JYW, Gao W. The efficacy of triamcinolone acetonide in keloid treatment:

A systematic review and meta-analysis. *Front Med (Lausanne)*. 2016;3:71.

36. Davison SP, Dayan JH, Clemens MW, Sonni S, Wang A, Crane A. Efficacy of intralesional 5-fluorouracil and triamcinolone in the treatment of keloids. *Aesthet Surg J*. 2009;29(1):40-46.

37. Darougheh A, Asilian A, Shariati F. Intralesional triamcinolone alone or in combination with 5-fluorouracil for the treatment of keloid and hypertrophic scars. *Clin Exp Dermatol*. 2009;34(2):219-223.

38. Asilian A, Darougheh A, Shariati F. New combination of triamcinolone, 5-Fluorouracil, and pulsed-dye laser for treatment of keloid and hypertrophic scars. *Dermatol Surg*. 2006;32(7):907-915.

39. Roques C, Téot L. The use of corticosteroids to treat keloids: a review. *Int J Low Extrem Wounds*. 2008;7(3):137-145.

40. Har-Shai Y, Amar M, Sabo E. Intralesional cryotherapy for enhancing the involution of hypertrophic scars and keloids. *Plast Reconstr Surg*. 2003;111(6):1841-1852.

41. Har-Shai Y, Sabo E, Rohde E, Hyams M, Assaf C, Zouboulis CC. Intralesional cryosurgery enhances the involution of recalcitrant auricular keloids: A new clinical approach supported by experimental studies. *Wound Repair Regen*. 2006;14(1):18-27.

42. Altalhab S, AlJasser MI. Intralesional cryotherapy using disposable needles. *Dermatol Surg*. 2021;47(5):727-728.

43. Shepherd J, Dawber R. The historical and scientific basis of cryosurgery. *Clin Exp Dermatol*. 1982;7(3):321-328.

44. Abdel-Meguid AM, Weshahy AH, Sayed DS, Refaiy AE, Awad SM. Intralesional vs. contact cryosurgery in treatment of keloids: A clinical and immunohistochemical study. *Int J Dermatol*. 2015;54(4):468-475.

45. Gupta S, Kumar B. Intralesional cryosurgery using lumbar puncture and/or hypodermic needles for large, bulky, recalcitrant keloids. *Int J Dermatol*. 2001;40(5):349-353.

46. Chopinaud M, Pham AD, Labbé D, et al. Intralesional cryosurgery to treat keloid scars: Results from a retrospective study. *Dermatology*. 2014;229(3):263-270.

47. Atiyeh BS. Nonsurgical management of hypertrophic scars: evidence-based therapies, standard practices, and emerging methods. *Aesthetic Plast Surg*. 2007;31(5):468-492.

48. Zouboulis CC, Blume U, Büttner P, Orfanos CE. Outcomes of cryosurgery in keloids and hypertrophic scars: A prospective consecutive trial of case series. *Arch Dermatol*. 1993;129(9):1146-1151.

49. Kim DY, Kim ES, Eo SR, Kim KS, Lee SY, Cho BH. A surgical approach for earlobe keloid: Keloid fillet flap. *Plast Reconstr Surg*. 2004;113(6):1668-1674.

50. Balaraman B, Geddes ER, Friedman PM. Best reconstructive techniques: improving the final scar. *Dermatol Surg*. 2015;41:S265-S275.

51. Muir I. On the nature of keloid and hypertrophic scars. *Br J Plast Surg*. 1990;43(1):61-69.

52. Leventhal D, Furr M, Reiter D. Treatment of keloids and hypertrophic scars: A meta-analysis and review of the literature. *Arch Facial Plast Surg*. 2006;8(6):362-368.

53. Berman B, Bieley HC. Adjunct therapies to surgical management of keloids. *Dermatol Surg*. 1996;22(2):126-130.

54. Berman B, Flores F. Recurrence rates of excised keloids treated with postoperative triamcinolone acetonide injections or interferon alfa-2b injections. *J Am Acad Dermatol*. 1997;37(5):755-757.

55. Ragoowansi R, Cornes PG, Moss AL, Glees JP. Treatment of keloids by surgical excision and immediate postoperative single-fraction radiotherapy. *Plast Reconstr Surg*. 2003;111(6):1853-1859.

56. Ogawa R, Mitsuhashi K, Hyakusoku H, Miyashita T. Postoperative electron-beam irradiation therapy for keloids and hypertrophic scars: Retrospective study of 147 cases followed for more than 18 months. *Plast Reconstr Surg*. 2003;111(2):547-555.

57. Ji J, Tian Y, Zhu YQ, et al. Ionizing irradiation inhibits keloid fibroblast cell proliferation and induces premature cellular senescence. *J Dermatol*. 2015;42(1):56-63.

58. Van Leeuwen MC, Stokmans SC, Bulstra AEJ, et al. Surgical excision with adjuvant irradiation for treatment of keloid scars: A systematic review. *Plast ic Reconstr Surg Glob Open*. 2015;3(7):e440.

59. van Leeuwen MCE, Stokmans SC, Bulstra AJ, Meijer OWM, van Leeuwen PAM, Niessen FB. High-dose-rate brachytherapy for the treatment of recalcitrant keloids: A unique, effective treatment protocol. *Plast Reconstr Surg*. 2014;134(3):527-534.

60. Hoang D, Reznik R, Orgel M, Li Q, Mirhadi A, Kulber DA. Surgical excision and adjuvant brachytherapy vs external beam radiation for the effective treatment of keloids: 10-year institutional retrospective analysis. *Aesthet Surg J*. 2017;37(2):212-225.

61. Cheraghi N, Cognetta Jr A, Goldberg D. Radiation therapy for the adjunctive treatment of surgically excised keloids: a review. *J Clin Aesthet Dermatol*. 2017;10(8):12-15.

62. Mankowski P, Kanevsky J, Tomlinson J, Dyachenko A, Luc M. Optimizing radiotherapy for keloids: A meta-analysis systematic review comparing recurrence rates between different radiation modalities. *Ann Plast Surg*. 2017;78(4):403-411.

63. De Cicco L, Vischioni B, Vavassori A, et al. Postoperative management of keloids: Low-dose-rate and high-dose-rate brachytherapy. *Brachytherapy*. 2014;13(5):508-513.

64. Duan Q, Liu J, Luo Z, Hu C. Postoperative brachytherapy and electron beam irradiation for keloids: A single institution retrospective analysis. *Mol Clin Oncol*. 2015;3(3):550-554.

65. Kal HB, Veen RE, Jürgenliemk-Schulz IM. Dose–effect relationships for recurrence of keloid and pterygium after surgery and radiotherapy. *Int J Radiat Oncol Biol Phys.* 2009;74(1):245-251.

66. Nestor MS, Berman B, Goldberg D, et al. ConSENSUS Guidelines on the use of superficial radiation therapy for treating nonmelanoma skin cancers and keloids. *J Clin Aesthet Dermatol.* 2019;12(2):12-18.

67. Ogawa R, Yoshitatsu S, Yoshida K, Miyashita T. Is radiation therapy for keloids acceptable? The risk of radiation-induced carcinogenesis. *Plast Reconstr Surg.* 2009; 124(4):1196-1201.

68. Bijlard E, Verduijn GM, Harmeling J, et al. Optimal high-dose-rate brachytherapy fractionation scheme after keloid excision: A retrospective multicenter comparison of recurrence rates and complications. *Int J Radiat Oncol Biol Phys.* 2018;100(3):679-686.

69. España A, Solano T, Quintanilla E. Bleomycin in the treatment of keloids and hypertrophic scars by multiple needle punctures. *Dermatol Surg.* 2001;27(1):23-27.

70. Naeini FF, Najafian J, Ahmadpour K. Bleomycin tattooing as a promising therapeutic modality in large keloids and hypertrophic scars. *Dermatol Surg.* 2006;32(8): 1023-1030.

71. Saray Y, Güleç AT. Treatment of keloids and hypertrophic scars with dermojet injections of bleomycin: A preliminary study. *Int J Dermatol.* 2005;44(9):777-784.

72. Manca G, Pandolfi P, Gregorelli C, Cadossi M, De Terlizzi F. Treatment of keloids and hypertrophic scars with bleomycin and electroporation. *Plast Reconstr Surg.* 2013;132(4): 621e-630e.

73. Aggarwal H, Saxena A, Lubana PS, Mathur R, Jain D. Treatment of keloids and hypertrophic scars using bleomycin. *J Cosmet Dermatol.* 2008;7(1):43-49.

74. Nanda S, Reddy BSN. Intralesional 5-fluorouracil as a treatment modality of keloids. *Dermatol Surg.* 2004;30(1): 54-57.

75. Sadeghinia A, Sadeghinia S. Comparison of the efficacy of intralesional triamcinolone acetonide and 5-fluorouracil tattooing for the treatment of keloids. *Dermatol Surg.* 2012;38(1):104-109.

76. Bijlard E, Steltenpool S, Niessen FB. Intralesional 5-fluorouracil in keloid treatment: A systematic review. *Acta Derm Venereol.* 2015;95(7):778-782.

77. Jiang ZY, Liao XC, Liu MZ, et al. Efficacy and safety of intralesional triamcinolone versus combination of triamcinolone with 5-fluorouracil in the treatment of keloids and hypertrophic scars: A systematic review and meta-analysis. *Aesthet Plast Surg.* 2020;44(5):1859-1868.

78. Zhibo X, Miaobo Z. Botulinum toxin type A affects cell cycle distribution of fibroblasts derived from hypertrophic scar. *J Plast Reconstr Aesthet Surg.* 2008;61(9):1128-1129.

79. Xiao Z, Zhang F, Cui Z. Treatment of hypertrophic scars with intralesional botulinum toxin type A injections: A preliminary report. *Aesthet Plast Surg.* 2009;33(3):409-412.

80. Elhefnawy AM. Assessment of intralesional injection of botulinum toxin type A injection for hypertrophic scars. *Indian J Dermatol Venereol Leprol.* 2016;82(3):279-283.

81. Shaarawy E, Hegazy RA, Abdel Hay RM. Intralesional botulinum toxin type A equally effective and better tolerated than intralesional steroid in the treatment of keloids: A randomized controlled trial. *J Cosmet Dermatol.* 2015;14(2):161-166.

82. Zhibo X, Miaobo Z. Intralesional botulinum toxin type A injection as a new treatment measure for keloids. *Plast Reconstr Surg.* 2009;124(5):275e-277e.

83. Bi M, Sun P, Li D, Dong Z, Chen Z. Intralesional injection of botulinum toxin type A compared with intralesional injection of corticosteroid for the treatment of hypertrophic scar and keloid: A systematic review and meta-analysis. *Med Sci Monit.* 2019;25:2950-2958.

84. Alster TS. Improvement of erythematous and hypertrophic scars by the 585-nm flashlamp-pumped pulsed dye laser. *Ann Plast Surg.* 1994;32(2):186-190.

85. Tanzi EL, Alster TS. Laser treatment of scars. *Skin Therapy Lett.* 2004;9(1):4-7.

86. Chan HH, Wong DS, Ho WS, Lam LK, Wei W. The use of pulsed dye laser for the prevention and treatment of hypertrophic scars in chinese persons. *Dermatol Surg.* 2004;30(7):987-994; discussion 994.

87. Reish RG, Eriksson E. Scars: A review of emerging and currently available therapies. *Plast Reconstr Surg.* 2008; 122(4):1068-1078.

88. Parrett BM, Donelan MB. Pulsed dye laser in burn scars: Current concepts and future directions. *Burns.* 2010;36(4): 443-449.

89. Vrijman C, van Drooge AM, Limpens J, et al. Laser and intense pulsed light therapy for the treatment of hypertrophic scars: A systematic review. *Br J Dermatol.* 2011;165(5):934-942.

90. Alster T. Laser scar revision: comparison study of 585-nm pulsed dye laser with and without intralesional corticosteroids. *Dermatol Surg.* 2003;29(1):25-29.

91. Preissig J, Hamilton K, Markus R. Current laser resurfacing technologies: A review that delves beneath the surface. *Semin Plast Surg.* 2012;26(3):109-116.

92. Qu L, Liu A, Zhou L, et al. Clinical and molecular effects on mature burn scars after treatment with a fractional CO_2 laser. *Lasers Surg Med.* 2012;44(7):517-524.

93. Bogdan Allemann I, Kaufman J. Fractional photothermolysis—an update. *Lasers Med Sci.* 2010;25(1):137-144.

94. McGoldrick RB, Sawyer A, Davis CR, Theodorakopoulou E, Murison M. Lasers and ancillary treatments for scar management: Personal experience over two decades and contextual review of the literature. Part I: Burn scars. *Scars Burn Heal.* 2016;2:2059513116642090.

95. Akaishi S, Koike S, Dohi T, Kobe K, Hyakusoku H, Ogawa R. Nd:YAG laser treatment of keloids and hypertrophic scars. *Eplasty.* 2012;12:e1.

96. Nicoletti G, De Francesco F, Mele CM, et al. Clinical and histologic effects from CO2 laser treatment of keloids. *Lasers Med Sci.* 2013;28(3):957-964.

97. Norris JE. The effect of carbon dioxide laser surgery on the recurrence of keloids. *Plast Reconstr Surg.* 1991;87(1):44-49; discussion 50-53.

98. Stern JC, Lucente FE. Carbon dioxide laser excision of earlobe keloids. A prospective study and critical analysis of existing data. *Arch Otolaryngol Head Neck Surg.* 1989;115(9):1107-1111.

99. Wagner JA, Paasch U, Bodendorf MO, Simon JC, Grunewald S. Treatment of keloids and hypertrophic scars with the triple-mode Er: YAG laser: A pilot study. *Med Laser Appl.* 2011;26(1):10-15.

100. Choi JE, Oh GN, Kim JY, Seo SH, Ahn HH, Kye YC. Ablative fractional laser treatment for hypertrophic scars: Comparison between Er: YAG and CO2 fractional lasers. *J Dermatolog Treat.* 2014;25(4):299-303.

101. Azzam OA, Bassiouny DA, El-Hawary MS, El Maadawi ZM, Sobhi RM, El-Mesidy MS. Treatment of hypertrophic scars and keloids by fractional carbon dioxide laser: A clinical, histological, and immunohistochemical study. *Lasers Med Sci.* 2016;31(1):9-18.

102. Verhaeghe E, Ongenae K, Bostoen J, Lambert J. Nonablative fractional laser resurfacing for the treatment of hypertrophic scars: A randomized controlled trial. *Dermatol Surg.* 2013;39(3 Pt 1):426-434.

103. Kaushik SB, Alexis AF. Nonablative fractional laser resurfacing in skin of color: Evidence-based review. *J Clin Aesthet Dermatol.* 2017;10(6):51-67.

104. Shim HS, Jun DW, Kim SW, Jung SN, Kwon H. Low versus high fluence parameters in the treatment of facial laceration scars with a 1,550 nm fractional erbium-glass laser. *BioMed Res Int.* 2015;2015:825309.

105. Ha JM, Kim HS, Cho EB, et al. Comparison of the effectiveness of nonablative fractional laser versus pulsed-dye laser in thyroidectomy scar prevention. *Ann Dermatol.* 2014;26(5):615-620.

106. Shin J, Cho JT, Park SI, Jung SN. Combination therapy using non-ablative fractional laser and intralesional triamcinolone injection for hypertrophic scars and keloids treatment. *Int Wound J.* 2019;16(6):1450-1456.

107. Waibel JS, Wulkan AJ, Shumaker PR. Treatment of hypertrophic scars using laser and laser assisted corticosteroid delivery. *Lasers Surg Med.* 2013;45(3):135-140.

108. Braun SA, Schrumpf H, Buhren BA, Homey B, Gerber PA. Laser-assisted drug delivery: Mode of action and use in daily clinical practice. *J Dtsch Dermatol Ges.* 2016;14(5):480-488.

109. Kraeva E, Ho D, Jagdeo J. Successful treatment of keloid with fractionated carbon dioxide (CO2) laser and laser-assisted drug delivery of triamcinolone acetonide ointment in an African-American man. *J Drugs Dermatol.* 2017;16(9):925-927.

110. Mamalis A, Jagdeo J. Light-emitting diode–generated red light inhibits keloid fibroblast proliferation. *Dermatol Surg.* 2015;41(1):35-39.

111. Mamalis A, Koo E, Garcha M, Murphy WJ, Isseroff RR, Jagdeo J. High fluence light emitting diode-generated red light modulates characteristics associated with skin fibrosis. *J Biophotonics.* 2016;9(11-12):1167-1179.

112. Lev-Tov H, Mamalis A, Brody N, Siegel D, Jagdeo J. Inhibition of fibroblast proliferation in vitro using red light-emitting diodes. *Dermatol Surg.* 2013;39(8):1167-1170.

113. Barolet D, Boucher A. Prophylactic low-level light therapy for the treatment of hypertrophic scars and keloids: A case series. *Lasers Surg Med.* 2010;42(6):597-601.

114. Jagdeo J, Nguyen JK, Ho D, et al. Safety of light emitting diode-red light on human skin: Two randomized controlled trials. *J Biophotonics.* 2020;13(3):e201960014.

115. Mamalis A, Lev-Tov H, Nguyen DH, Jagdeo J. Laser and light-based treatment of Keloids–a review. *J Eur Acad Dermatol Venereol.* 2014;28(6):689-699.

116. Babalola O, Mamalis A, Lev-Tov H, Jagdeo J. The role of microRNAs in skin fibrosis. *Arch Dermatol. Res.* 2013;305(9):763-776.

117. de Planell-Saguer M, Rodicio MC. Analytical aspects of microRNA in diagnostics: A review. *Anal Chim Acta.* 2011;699(2):134-152.

118. Kashiyama K, Mitsutake N, Matsuse M, et al. miR-196a downregulation increases the expression of type I and III collagens in keloid fibroblasts. *J Invest Dermatol.* 2012;132(6):1597-1604.

119. Zhang J, Zhou Q, Wang H, et al. MicroRNA-130a has pro-fibroproliferative potential in hypertrophic scar by targeting CYLD. *Arch Biochem Biophys.* 2019;671:152-161.

12

Laser and Energy-Based Devices for the Treatment of Pigmented Lesions in Asians

Henry H. L. Chan

INTRODUCTION

Congenital and acquired pigmentary conditions are common among East and Southeast Asian populations (herein referred to as Asians). While laser and energy-based devices have been used successfully in many conditions (e.g., nevus of Ota, freckle, lentigo, and Hori's macules), for others responses can be more variable (e.g., café au lait patches, Becker's nevi, congenital melanocytic nevi, and melasma). Postinflammatory hyperpigmentation (PIH) is a common postlaser complication among Asians. This is particularly relevant given the fact that Asians tend to present with hyperpigmented lesions such as lentigines as the earliest cutaneous manifestation of photoaging, often with less wrinkling. Melasma is another common pigmentary condition that is frequently seen among Asians, in this case with a female predominance. This chapter will review the current literature pertaining to the use of laser and energy-based devices in the treatment of various pigmentary conditions among Asians (with a focus on East and Southeast Asian populations).

LASERS AND ENERGY-BASED DEVICES FOR THE TREATMENT OF CONGENITAL PIGMENTARY CONDITIONS

Café au Lait Patches or Macules (Fig. 12.1)

Café au lait patches or macules (CALMs) are brownish macules and patches characterized histologically by enlarged melanosomes and increase melanin content.

Previous studies demonstrated variable effects when Q-switched (QS) lasers were used for the treatment of café au lait patches and the response did not correlate with the histological subtypes.[1] Long-pulsed lasers without cooling have also been used with some success but recurrences can still occur. More recently, it has been proposed that morphological pattern can be related to clinical outcome with CALM lesions that have a jagged or ill-defined border being more responsive than those with smooth or well-defined borders.[2] A large-scale study looking at the use of QS Alexandrite laser among Chinese children with CALMs was recently published that indicated approximately 80% of patients had some degree of improvement and the number of treatments correlated with efficacy (rs = 0.26, $P < 0.0001$).[3] Shape of the lesion could be related (as the treatment effect was observed to be higher on lesions with an irregular shape and jagged edge) but this was not statistically significant. In a recent split lesion study, picosecond (PS) Alexandrite laser was found to be equally effective with QS lasers but with fewer adverse effects.[4]

In our practice, we use four different lasers (QS 532-nm neodymium-yttrium-aluminium-garnet (Nd:YAG), PS 532-nm Nd:YAG, PS Alexandrite 755 nm, and long-pulsed Alexandrite 755 nm) to perform test areas and assess the patient 4 weeks later before deciding which laser to proceed with. Patients and parents are warned in advance that if the lesion persists despite four or more treatments, further laser procedures may not be helpful. Another energy-based device that has also been used in the treatment of CALMs is cryomodulation, a new form of controlled cooling. Although early data

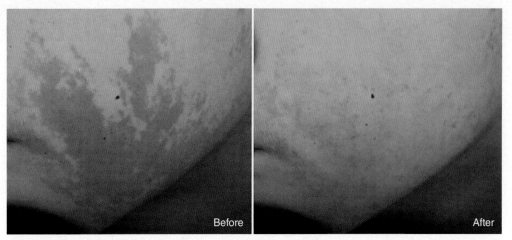

Fig. 12.1 Café au lait patches. Left: Café au lait patches before laser treatment. Right: 2 months post one treatment of 532-nm picosecond laser (0.43–0.85 J/cm^2 fluence, 3 Hz, 4 mm).

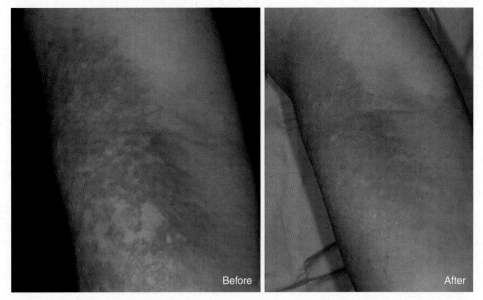

Fig. 12.2 Becker nevi. Left: Becker nevi before laser treatment. Right: 3 months post-11th nonablative fractional laser treatment (10–20 mJ, 8–10 passes).

are promising, clinical trials are warranted to further evaluate efficacy, safety, and relapse rates in a broad range of phototypes.[5]

Becker's Nevi (Fig. 12.2)

Becker's nevus is a pigmented hamartoma that presents clinically as a unilateral hyperpigmented patch with hypertrichosis usually located on the shoulder of male patients. The increase in pigmentation in Becker's nevus is due to greater melanin content in the basal layer and dermal melanophages may be present. A study comparing the use of Erbium:YAG laser to QS 1064-nm Nd:YAG laser in 22 patients after a follow up of 2 years demonstrated that the Erbium:YAG laser was significantly superior even after one treatment.[6] QS lasers have been used with some degree of success, but relapse is an issue;

other complications include hypo- and postinflammatory hyperpigmentation. Long-pulsed alexandrite or 1064 Nd:YAG laser with or without cooling have been used with some success not only to remove the pigmentation but also to improve the associated hypertrichosis.[7] Relapse, hypopigmentation, and texture changes are common complications and therefore combination therapy with nonablative fractional resurfacing have also been advocated with some degree of success.[8] Picosecond lasers have been used recently but relapse is a limitation.

Congenital Melanocytic Nevi (Fig. 12.3)

The use of lasers and energy-based devices for the treatment of congenital melanocytic nevi is controversial due to concerns about altering the appearance of melanocytic lesions and thereby confounding melanoma screening efforts. For Asians the risk of melanoma is lower than in the White population. For example, the incidence of melanoma among males is reported to be 55.8 per 100,000 in Australia compared with much lower incidence of 0.2 per 100,000 in Japan.[9,10] As a result, lasers are more commonly considered to be a therapeutic option. Earlier studies comparing the role of QS Ruby laser and normal-mode Ruby laser indicated normal-mode Ruby to be superior in terms of cosmetic outcome. Subtle microscopic scarring covering the underlying nevoid cells was proposed to be an important factor in the favorable results seen among cases treated with normal-mode ruby.[11] In the last decades, many other studies combined the use of a long-pulsed pigmented laser without cooling or an ablative laser, such as a carbon dioxide laser to remove the epidermal pigment to be followed immediately by QS lasers.[12,13] The intention was to allow the deeper component of the nevi to be treated and in doing so improve efficacy and reduce the number of treatment sessions. Side effects including erythema, relapse, hypopigmentation, and scarring have been reported.

Nonablative and ablative fractional resurfacing in conjunction with picosecond laser have also been used with some success.

More recently, surgical removal for small- and medium- size congenital melanocytic nevi followed by laser surgery to treat the scar or remove residual pigment has also been proposed. Initial retrospective data indicated comparable or even more superior results as compared with laser alone.[14]

Nevus of Ota (Fig. 12.4)

Nevus of Ota is a dermal melanocytic hamartoma that appears as a confluence of dusky blue and brown oval-shaped macules. The lesions are distributed in the skin and mucous membranes innervated by the first and

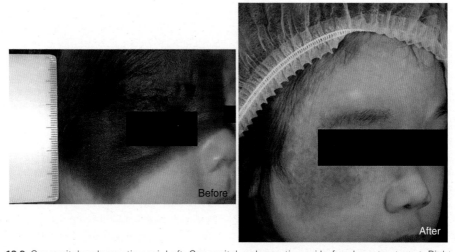

Fig. 12.3 Congenital melanocytic nevi. Left: Congenital melanocytic nevi before laser treatment. Right: Post-combined treatments with long-pulsed Alexandrite laser and pico alexandrite laser.

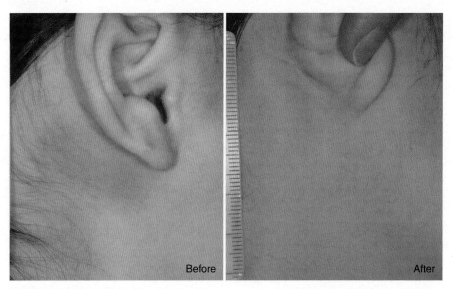

Fig. 12.4. Nevus of Ota. Left: Nevus of Ota before laser treatment. Right: 3 months after eighth treatment with picosecond laser (2.08–4.80 J/cm^2 fluence, 5–10 Hz, 2.3–3.5 mm).

second branches of the trigeminal nerve. Although lesions may present at birth, over 50% develop after 1 year of age. Among all congenital pigmentary lesions, nevus of Ota is most responsive to laser treatment. QS lasers were found to be effective and previous studies indicated that QS Ruby was the most effective as compared to QS Alexandrite and QS 1064-nm Nd:YAG lasers, with fewer treatment sessions.[15–17] At least three sessions were necessary to achieve improvement, and the number of treatment sessions rather than the interval of treatment was found to important in term of degree of clearing. Adverse effects include erythema, pigmentary changes including hypopigmentation and postinflammatory hyperpigmentation, texture changes, and relapse among 0.6% to 1.2% of patients. Early treatment is important not only to reduce the psychosocial impact associated with this condition, but also less treatment sessions and lower complication rate seen among younger age group.[18] Although laser fractional resurfacing has been reported to be effective, it has never gained popularity given the effectiveness of QS lasers. Picosecond Alexandrite laser has been shown to be associated with better efficacy, fewer complication, and less pain as compared with QS Alexandrite laser.[19] Given the fact that general anesthetic can be required, few treatments for children is important and therefore picosecond laser is the preferred choice of laser treatment for nevus of Ota.

THE USE OF LASERS AND ENERGY-BASED DEVICES FOR THE TREATMENT OF ACQUIRED PIGMENTARY CONDITIONS

Freckle and Solar Lentigo (Fig. 12.5)

Unlike the White population whereby photoaging often presents with wrinkling, for Asians, pigmentary conditions such as freckles and solar lentigines are more common manifestations of photoaging. Furthermore, for sociocultural reasons, skin lightening is frequently sought given that fair and even skin complexion has historically been considered to be a sign of beauty among Asian culture.

QS nanosecond (ns) lasers have been used with some success in the treatment of freckles and solar lentigines and while it can be most effective, the main risk among Asians is postinflammatory hyperpigmentation (PIH). This can occur in up to 20% of treated patients and solar lentigines that are erythematous carry a greater risk.[20] QS nanosecond lasers incur not only photothermal but also photomechanical effects. This can produce an excessive inflammatory reaction that presents as erythema and can result in PIH. Long-pulsed lasers and intense pulsed light source produce mainly photothermal effect and therefore lower risk of PIH. Previous studies comparing the use of QS nanosecond lasers and long-pulsed pigment lasers indicated a lower risk of PIH

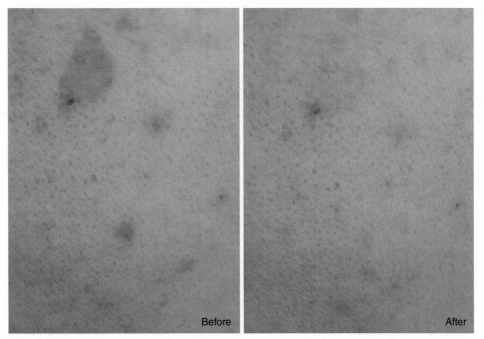

Fig. 12.5 Freckle and solar lentigo. Left: Freckle and solar lentigo before laser treatment. Right: 3 months post-second treatment with 532-nm picosecond laser (0.56–0.64 J/cm² fluence, 3 mm, 3 Hz, 1 pass).

among those treated with long-pulsed lasers.[21] The main disadvantage with long-pulsed pigmented lasers is that the clinical endpoint (ashen-grey appearance) is more subtle as compared with QS nanosecond lasers (immediate whitening). Furthermore, for light-color lesions, more treatment sessions are necessary for long-pulsed pigment lasers. A previous retrospective study comparing long-pulsed 532-nm Nd:YAG with contact cooling, QS ns 532-nm Nd:YAG, long-pulsed 595-nm dye laser with compression window, and long-pulsed Alexandrite laser for the treatment of freckles and lentigines among Asians found the long-pulsed 532-nm Nd:YAG laser with contact cooling and small spot size (3 mm) to be superior in terms of efficacy and complication rate.[22] Small spot size is important in the treatment of pigmented lesions in Asian skin as larger spot size devices such as intense pulsed light can result in collateral injury of surrounding skin causing dyspigmentation in a "footprint" pattern or, conversely, may result in undertreatment leading to lack of efficacy.

In recent years, picosecond lasers have also been advocated due to their efficacy and lower rate of PIH compared to nanosecond lasers. However, PIH can occur at a rate of approximately 5%.[23] Cryomodulation involving controlled cooling has recently been used an alternative means to treat such benign pigmentary conditions.

Melasma (Fig. 12.6)

Melasma is a common acquired pigmentary condition that presents with bilateral hyperpigmented patches affecting the centrofacial, malar. and/or mandibular area. It is particularly common among women of childbearing age with a multifactorial etiology that includes association with sun exposure, hormonal factors (worse during pregnancy and oral contraceptive use), and is characterized by melanocytic hyperactivity rather than melanocytic proliferation. First-line treatment consists of photoprotection and topical bleaching agents, including triple-combination topical therapy containing a hydroquinone, a retinoid, and a corticosteroid. Azelaic acid is also frequently used as a topical agent, especially in those who are not candidates for hydroquinone (e.g., from duration of use or sensitivity). Chemical peel and microdermabrasion have also been advocated with some degree of success. Oral tranexamic acid (250 mg twice daily) has been used in

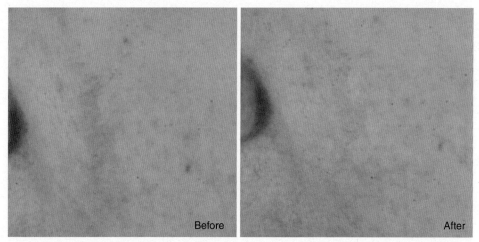

Before

After

Fig. 12.6 Melasma. Left: Melasma before laser treatment. Right: 1-month post-three laser treatments (first treatment: QS 1064 laser, second treatment: LP-Alex laser, third treatment: QS 1064 laser and LP-Alex laser).

recent years for moderate to severe melasma with some success. In a retrospective Singapore study involving 561 treated patients, 89.7% improved. 27.2% of patients relapsed after stopping medication with the medium relapse time being 7 months after cessation. Transient adverse effects including abdominal bloating and headache affected 7.1%. One patient developed deep vein thrombosis and was later diagnosed to have protein S deficiency.[24]

The use of lasers to treat melasma should be considered as a third-line treatment given the recurrence nature of the condition and side effects associated including PIH and hypopigmentation. Ablative laser resurfacing (CO_2 or Erbium-YAG lasers) with or without QS lasers were previously shown to be effective in resistant melasma but the side effects including PIH and potential infection made such an approach to be unpopular. 1550-nm Erbium glass nonablative fractional resurfacing was initially suggested to be effective but in the author's experience, about 10% of Asian subjects tend to worsen. 1927-nm fractional thulium was also used with some degree of success; in the author's experience, postinflammatory hyperpigmentation and worsening of melasma lesions occurs in 5% to 10% of the patients. Low-energy low-density 1927 diode laser in combination with pulsed dye 595-nm laser to treat not only the pigmentation but also the background erythema and telangiectasia has been advocated with moderate success. Whereas high-energy QS lasers had been reported to be associated with worsening of melasma, large spot size, low-energy QS laser has gained

much popularity in Asia. This approach is commonly referred to as laser toning and can be used in combination with microdermabrasion.[25,26] Both QS 755-nm Alexandrite or 1064-nm Nd:YAG lasers have been used with some success. Typically, four to eight treatment sessions at a treatment interval between 2 to 4 weeks is performed. Guttate hypopigmentation can occur and is related to the number of treatment sessions as well as energy used. In more recent years, picosecond lasers (755-mm Alexandrite or 1064-nm Nd:YAG) either fractionated approach or using large spot size, low-energy laser toning have also been shown to be effective with low adverse effects—mainly transient PIH.[27,28]

The Use of Laser for the Treatment of Acquired Bilateral Nevus of Ota-like Macules (ABNOM) (Fig. 12.7)

Acquired bilateral Nevus of Ota–like macules (ABNOM) or Hori macules, id an acquired pigmentary condition that presents as bilateral, symmetrical, dark brown to grayish-blue colored macules affecting the malar regions, lateral temples, eyelids, and forehead. Unlike nevus of Ota, ABNOM occurs later in life and does not involve the mucosal surfaces. Q-switched lasers had been used with good effect in the treatment of ABNOM. Previous work with the QS Ruby (fluence 7–10 J/cm² at a repetition rate of 1 Hz and spot size of 2–4 mm) indicated that complete clearance could be obtained in over 90% of patients and no recurrence was reported a mean

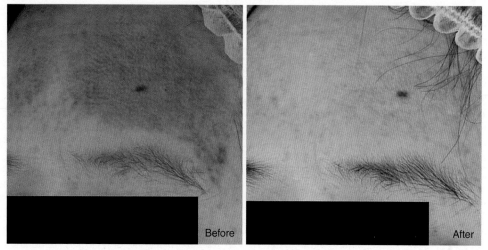

Fig. 12.7 Acquired bilateral nevus of Ota-like macules (ABNOM). Left: Acquired bilateral nevus of Ota-like macules before laser treatment. Right: Post-four treatment of QS Ruby laser (3.2–5.0 J/cm² fluence, 5 mm) and one treatment of Q-switched Alexandrite laser (5.5 J/cm² fluence, 5 Hz, 4 mm).

follow up of 2.5 years. Postinflammatory hyperpigmentation was common and affected 7% of patients. The QS 1064-nm Nd:YAG laser was also effective but with a greater degree of postinflammatory hyperpigmentation (50% to 73%).[29,30] Another retrospective analysis of 32 female Chinese patients treated with QS Alexandrite laser (755 nm, spot size 3 mm, 8 J/cm²) concluded that 80% of patients had more than 50% clearance (28% had complete clearance).[31] PIH occurred in 12.5% of the patients but resolved in all cases following treatment with hypopigmenting topical medication. In a recent retrospective study that examined the role of picosecond Alex laser in the treatment of dermal pigmentary conditions, among 8 nevus of Ota and 28 ABNOM patients treated, moderate to marked improvement was reported among 88.89% after one to four treatments. Transit pigmentary disturbance was only seen among three patients confirming the safety and efficacy of picosecond laser in the treatment of ABNOM.[32]

CONCLUSION

Lasers and energy-based devices can be used safely and effectively among Asians for the treatment of both congenital and acquired conditions. While some conditions such as freckle, lentigo, nevus of Ota, and ABNOM can be treated with a high degree of efficacy and safety, others can be more resistant with a greater risk of relapse or complication including café au lait patches, Becker nevi, congenital melanocytic nevi, and melasma. Picosecond lasers and cryomodulation are recent devices that allow clinicians to have more therapeutic options in the treatment of benign pigmentary conditions among Asians.

REFERENCES

1. Grossman MC, Anderson RR, Farinelli W, Flotte TJ, Grevelink JM. Treatment of cafe au lait macules with lasers. A clinicopathologic correlation. *Arch Dermatol.* 1995;131:1416-1420.
2. Belkin DA, Neckman JP, Jeon H, Friedman P, Geronemus RG. Response to laser treatment of cafe au lait macules based on morphologic features. *JAMA Dermatol.* 2017;153:1158-1161.
3. Zhang B, Chu Y, Xu Z, et al. Treatment of cafe-au-lait spots using Q-switched Alexandrite laser: Analysis of clinical characteristics of 471 children in mainland China. *Lasers Surg Med.* 2019;51:694-700.
4. Cen Q, Gu Y, Luo L, et al. Comparative effectiveness of 755-nm picosecond laser, 755- and 532-nm nanosecond lasers for treatment of cafe-au-lait macules (CALMs): A randomized, split-lesion clinical trial. *Lasers Surg Med.* 2021;53:435-442.
5. Chuang GS, Farinelli W, Anderson RR. Selective cryolysis of melanocytes: Critical temperature and exposure time to induce selective pigmentary loss in Yucatan pig skin. *Lasers Surg Med.* 2021;53:978-985.

6. Trelles MA, Allones I, Moreno-Arias GA, Velez M. Becker's naevus: A comparative study between erbium: YAG and Q-switched neodymium:YAG; clinical and histopathological findings. *Br J Dermatol.* 2005;152:308-313.

7. Wulkan AJ, McGraw T, Taylor M. Successful treatment of Becker's Nevus with long-pulsed 1064-nm Nd:YAG and 755-nm Alexandrite laser and review of the literature. *J Cosmet Laser Ther.* 2018;20:211-214.

8. Glaich AS, Goldberg LH, Dai T, Kunishige JH, Friedman PM. Fractional resurfacing: A new therapeutic modality for Becker's nevus. *Arch Dermatol.* 2007;143:1488-1490.

9. Garbe C, McLeod GR, Buettner PG. Time trends of cutaneous melanoma in Queensland, Australia and Central Europe. *Cancer.* 2000;89:1269-1278.

10. Tanaka H, Tsukuma H, Tomita S, et al. Time trends of incidence for cutaneous melanoma among the Japanese population: An analysis of Osaka Cancer Registry data, 1964-95. *J Epidemiol.* 1999;9:S129-S135.

11. Ueda S, Imayama S. Normal-mode Ruby laser for treating congenital nevi. *Arch Dermatol.* 1997;133:355-359.

12. Kono T, Nozaki M, Chan HH, Sasaki K, Kwon SG. Combined use of normal mode and Q-switched Ruby lasers in the treatment of congenital melanocytic naevi. *Br J Plast Surg.* 2001;54:640-643.

13. Al-Hadithy N, Al-Nakib K, Quaba A. Outcomes of 52 patients with congenital melanocytic naevi treated with ultrapulse carbon dioxide and frequency doubled Q-switched Nd-Yag laser. *J Plast Reconstr Aesthet Surg.* 2012;65:1019-1028.

14. Oh Y, Lee SH, Lim JM, Chung KY, Roh MR. Long-term outcomes of laser treatment for congenital melanocytic nevi. *J Am Acad Dermatol.* 2019;80:523-531.e12.

15. Kono T, Nozaki M, Chan HH, Mikashima Y. A retrospective study looking at the long-term complications of Q-switched ruby laser in the treatment of nevus of Ota. *Lasers Surg Med.* 2001;29:156-159.

16. Chan HH, King WW, Chan ES, et al. In vivo trial comparing patients' tolerance of Q-switched Alexandrite (QS Alex) and Q-switched neodymium:yttrium-aluminum-garnet (QS Nd:YAG) lasers in the treatment of nevus of Ota. *Lasers Surg Med.* 1999;24:24-28.

17. Chan HH, Ying SY, Ho WS, Kono T, King WW. An in vivo trial comparing the clinical efficacy and complications of Q-switched 755 nm Alexandrite and Q-switched 1064 nm Nd:YAG lasers in the treatment of nevus of Ota. *Dermatol Surg.* 2000;26:919-922.

18. Kono T, Chan HH, Ercocen AR, et al. Use of Q-switched ruby laser in the treatment of nevus of Ota in different age groups. *Lasers Surg Med.* 2003;32:391-395.

19. Ge Y, Yang Y, Guo L, et al. Comparison of a picosecond Alexandrite laser versus a Q-switched Alexandrite laser for the treatment of nevus of Ota: A randomized, split-lesion, controlled trial. *J Am Acad Dermatol.* 2020;83: 397-403.

20. Kang HJ, Na JI, Lee JH, Roh MR, Ko JY, Chang SE. Postinflammatory hyperpigmentation associated with treatment of solar lentigines using a Q-Switched 532-nm Nd: YAG laser: A multicenter survey. *J Dermatolog Treat.* 2017;28:447-451.

21. Chan HH, Fung WK, Ying SY, Kono T. An in vivo trial comparing the use of different types of 532 nm Nd:YAG lasers in the treatment of facial lentigines in Oriental patients. *Dermatol Surg.* 2000;26:743-749.

22. Ho SG, Chan NP, Yeung CK, Shek SY, Kono T, Chan HH. A retrospective analysis of the management of freckles and lentigines using four different pigment lasers on Asian skin. *J Cosmet Laser Ther.* 2012;14:74-80.

23. Kung KY, Shek SY, Yeung CK, Chan HH. Evaluation of the safety and efficacy of the dual wavelength picosecond laser for the treatment of benign pigmented lesions in Asians. *Lasers Surg Med.* 2019;51:14-22.

24. Lee HC, Thng TG, Goh CL. Oral tranexamic acid (TA) in the treatment of melasma: A retrospective analysis. *J Am Acad Dermatol.* 2016;75:385-392.

25. Omi T, Yamashita R, Kawana S, Sato S, Naito Z. Low fluence Q-switched Nd: YAG laser toning and Q-switched ruby laser in the treatment of melasma: a comparative split-face ultrastructural study. *Laser Ther.* 2012;21: 15-21.

26. Kauvar AN. Successful treatment of melasma using a combination of microdermabrasion and Q-switched Nd:YAG lasers. *Lasers Surg Med.* 2012;44:117-124.

27. Manuskiatti W, Yan C, Tantrapornpong P, Cembrano KAG, Techapichetvanich T, Wanitphakdeedecha R. A prospective, split-face, randomized study comparing a 755-nm picosecond laser with and without diffractive lens array in the treatment of melasma in Asians. *Lasers Surg Med.* 2021;53:95-103.

28. Wong CSM, Chan MWM, Shek SYN, Yeung CK, Chan HHL. Fractional 1064 nm picosecond laser in treatment of melasma and skin rejuvenation in Asians, a prospective study. *Lasers Surg Med.* 2021;53:1032-1042.

29. Kunachak S, Leelaudomlipi P, Sirikulchayanonta V. Q-Switched Ruby laser therapy of acquired bilateral nevus of Ota-like macules. *Dermatol Surg.* 1999;25: 938-941.

30. Polnikorn N, Tanrattanakorn S, Goldberg DJ. Treatment of Hori's nevus with the Q-switched Nd:YAG laser. *Dermatol Surg.* 2000;26:477-480.

31. Lam AY, Wong DS, Lam LK, Ho WS, Chan HH. A retrospective study on the efficacy and complications of Q-switched Alexandrite laser in the treatment of acquired bilateral nevus of Ota-like macules. *Dermatol Surg.* 2001;27:937-941; discussion 41-42.

32. Hu S, Yang CS, Chang SL, Huang YL, Lin YF, Lee MC. Efficacy and safety of the picosecond 755-nm Alexandrite laser for treatment of dermal pigmentation in Asians-a retrospective study. *Lasers Med Sci.* 2020;35:1377-1383.

13

Laser Hair Removal: Nuances and Best Practices for Skin of Color

Sultan B. AlSalem, Eliot F. Battle Jr.

SUMMARY AND KEY FEATURES:

- This chapter provides a comprehensive guide on laser hair removal/reduction (LHR) for skin of color patients. It discusses the principles of laser physics, LHR principles, and treatment expertise required for safe and effective laser hair removal. The chapter also highlights the importance of understanding the patient's skin type, hair type, and potential underlying conditions that could affect the treatment's success.
- LHR carries higher risks for pigmented skin due to increased epidermal melanin. Longer wavelength lasers in the near-infrared spectrum minimize potential epidermal injury with the 1064-nm Nd: YAG wavelength is established as safe for darker skin phototypes (IV-VI). For millisecond-range lasers, longer pulse durations and epidermal cooling

- unsure safety, and handpieces should correspond to area size and fluence.
- Laser wavelength should align with skin phototype and overall risk for pigmentation while treatment parameters should consider skin pigmentation, ancestry, phototype, and patient-specific factors. Informed consent, coupled with pre- and post-treatment photoprotection is essential.
- Another approach to LHR with the 1064-nm Nd: YAG laser is the use of a device with a fixed sub-millisecond pulse duration (requiring more pulses than traditional millisecond pulsed devices).
- Comparative and long-term studies of different approaches to LHR are warranted. Clinicians need to stay updated with new technologies to ensure optimal patient care.

SUMMARY

This chapter provides a comprehensive guide on laser hair removal for patients with skin of color. It discusses the principles of laser physics, laser hair removal principles, and treatment expertise required for safe and effective laser hair removal. The chapter also highlights the importance of understanding the patient's skin type, hair type, and potential underlying conditions that could affect the treatment's success.

INTRODUCTION

Unwanted hair growth is a common concern in most cultures, thus creating a need for techniques, instruments, and modalities to remove the hair safely and effectively. Until the creation of hair removal lasers, electrolysis was the only commonly used technique that created some level of hair removal permanency. But electrolysis is a tedious, time-consuming treatment, with an increased incidence in creating scarring and hyperpigmentation in patients with darker skin and curly hair.[1] Other conventional hair removal modalities include shaving, plucking, waxing, sugaring, and using chemical depilatories.[1] Although temporarily effective, many of these conventional hair removal treatments likewise have a higher incidence of skin irritation and inflammation, often leading to pseudofolliculitis barbae and hyperpigmentation, particularly in patients with darker skin with tightly curled hair.[1,2] Patients with darker skin and curly hair often had to accept these unwanted side effects because they had no acceptable option. Excessive hair growth in androgen-dependent areas (hirsutism) and excessive hair growth at any site on the body (hypertrichosis) are common concerns among patients with skin of color.[3,4] The above considerations led to the development of laser hair removal, which has become an increasingly popular, effective, and safe way to remove unwanted hair and dramatically improve the side effects of ingrown hair (pseudofolliculitis barbae and postinflammatory hyperpigmentation) in patients with skin of color.[5,6]

LASER HAIR REMOVAL PHYSICS

In 1996, Grossman, Dierickx, et al., through research at the Wellman Laboratories of Photomedicine at Harvard Medical School, using a Ruby laser introduced a viable treatment for unwanted hair for lighter-skin patients (skin phototypes I-III).[7,8]

Because of the higher level of permanency, speed of treatment, and skin improvement, laser hair removal quickly evolved to become one of the most sought-out cosmetic laser treatments. Because of the success of laser hair removal on lighter skin types, research subsequently focused on the development of hair removal lasers for darker skin types. Based on the early work of Dierickx, Battle, et al., research at The Wellman Center of Photomedicine at Harvard Medical School demonstrated that by combining longer wavelengths and longer pulse durations with aggressive skin cooling on a diode laser, they could safely and effectively treat patients with darker skin tones.[9–11] Although the diode laser was shown to be able to treat patients with skin of color, because of the inherent limitations of the diode wavelength, the laser was best suited to be limited to patients with skin types IV-V. Over time, the Nd:YAG wavelength laser was accepted as a safer wavelength to treat patients with darker skin types, particularly patients with skin phototype VI. The initial research of the use of Nd:YAG lasers on darker skin types was performed by Vic Ross at Scripps Labs and by Battle et al., at the Wellman Center of Photomedicine at Harvard Medical School. With the addition of the Nd:YAG laser, all patients, regardless of their skin color or ethnicity, could be safely and effectively treated. Twenty years after the initial research, and countless numbers of laser treatments in clinical practice, the Nd:YAG wavelength lasers are clearly regarded as the most appropriate laser

in terms of safety and efficacy in removing undesired hair from patients of color, especially those with skin phototypes V-VI. The diode laser and Alexandrite lasers (particularly the newer devices that combine multiple wavelengths or high-hertz treatments) can be safety used on intermediately pigmented skin types (e.g., IV-V), while the 1064-nm Nd:YAG is the safest wavelength for the full spectrum of skin of color. Table 13.1 compares different light and laser wavelengths in treating patients with skin of color.

To be able to safely perform laser hair removal on patients with skin of color, the laser practitioner must gain competency in laser physics, skin physiology, and laser treatment expertise.

The skin has three main skin absorption chromophores that are targeted in cosmetic laser treatments. The three targets are hemoglobin (blood), melanin (pigment), and water. For laser hair removal, the pigment in the hair shaft and hair bulb is the main chromophore. Some researchers have shown that the vascular plexus surrounding the lower portion of the hair bulb might also be an important target for laser hair removal. The foundation of laser light–based cosmetic therapy is based on the theory of selective photothermolysis that was proposed by Anderson and Parish at Harvard Medical School's Wellman Laboratory of Photomedicine.[12]

This theory simply states that by using the appropriate wavelength, pulse duration, and fluence, the thermal injury caused by lasers can be confined to the absorbing chromophore, therefore protecting the surrounding tissue.[12] To assure thermal damage confinement to only the chromophore, the pulse duration should be less than or equal to the thermal relaxation time (TRT; for additional laser terminology, see Table 13.2) of the targeted chromophore (hair shaft). The TRT of the hair shaft is estimated to be 10 to 100 ms, but the size dramatically varies from patient to patient and body area. Ethnicity has been shown to influence hair thickness. For specific cutaneous features in patients with skin of color, see Table 13.3.

Laser targets in follicles include the melanocytic external (outer) root sheath, the matrix, and the hair shaft. Permanent removal of hair is achieved once the laser thermally destroys the entire hair follicle including its progenitor stem cells. These stem cells are essential for hair growth and development. Animal (rodent) research studies have elucidated the split-fuse hypothesis. The

TABLE 13.1 Comparison of Different Light and Laser Sources with Corresponding Wavelength(s) and Indications in Different Skin Phototypes

Laser/Light Source	Wavelength(s)	Optical Depth	Epidermal Melanin Absorption	Skin of Color	Fitzpatrick Phototype	Comments
1 Intense Pulsed Light	Various (500–670 and 870–1400 nm)	-	Variable	Infrequently used	I, II, III, IV, V	Caution in skin of color; high rates of burns in FST IV-VI
2 Ruby	695 nanometers	+	High	Infrequently used	I, II, III	First laser used for hair removal. Not used in SOC due to complications such as dyspigmentation and burns
3 Alexandrite	755 nanometers	+ +	High	Infrequently used	I, II, III, (IV with caution)	Effective laser, higher risk of burns in SOC due to preferential absorption of melanin in epidermis
4 Diode	810 nanometers	+ + +	Moderate	Frequently used	I, II, III, IV, V	Appropriate for intermediate skin complexions; higher risk of burns in FST VI
5 Nd:YAG	1064 nanometers	+ + + +, Deepest	Low	Safest, frequently used	I, II, III, IV, V, VI	Safest laser for IV-VI. Requires more treatment sessions to achieve therapeutic outcomes than diode and Alexandrite lasers; laser of choice in FST VI

FST, Fitzpatrick Skin Type; *SOC,* skin of color.

theory identifies two stem cell populations; one is thought to be located at the proximal external root sheath (amelanotic and serves as a reservoir) and the second population is believed to be in the distal external root sheath.[13] In the mouse model, the location of the stem cells can be found within the hair follicle bulge region.[14] In humans, the bulge region is in the lower third of the external root sheath.

To achieve permanent hair reduction with lasers, a modified theory of selective photothermolysis is required to destroy the melanocytic hair shaft chromophore and the amelanotic hair follicle and stem cells. Low-powered lasers and devices may only have enough energy to impact the pigmented hair shaft and thus will produce only a delay in hair growth, which can last for months. The extended theory of selective photothermolysis in relation to laser hair removal basically states that to achieve permanent hair reduction, the thermal energy produced by the absorption of the laser light by the pigmented hair shaft must diffuse and destroy both the amelanotic hair follicle and the peripheral stem cells. To achieve this goal, longer pulse durations and adequate fluences are typically used to propagate thermal injury to the periphery of the hair follicle and surrounding stem cells.

HAIR REMOVAL LASER AND PARAMETER SELECTION

There is an increased risk for side effects when treating skin of color with lasers because the epidermal pigment competes for the laser energy that is intended for the hair shaft chromophore. This absorbed energy in the epidermis is naturally transferred into heat, which can cause epidermal thermal damage and result in blistering, discoloration, and scarring.

TABLE 13.2 Common Terms in Lasers and Laser Hair Removal

	Term	Definition
1	Thermal relaxation time (TRT)	TRT is the time needed for the target to dissipate about 63% of the incident thermal energy. It is related to size of chromophore and range from nanoseconds to milliseconds
2	Thermal damage time (TDT)	TDT is the time taken for the entire target along with the chromophore (e.g., melanin) and the surrounding target or structure (e.g., hair follicle), to cool by about 63% of the incident thermal energy. It includes cooling of both the chromophore and the entire target associated with it
3	Fluence	Amount of energy delivered per unit area (joules/cm^2)
4	Pulse duration	Duration of laser exposure in seconds
5	Spot size	Diameter through which the laser beam travels (millimeters)
	power	Amount of work performed per unit time (Watts, equal to joules per second)
6	Power density, intensity, irradiance	Measured power per area of spot size (Watts per square centimeter)
7	Selective photothermolysis	Localization of thermal injury to a specific target based on its absorption characteristics, the wavelength of light emitted, the duration of the pulse, and the amount of energy delivered
8	Extended theory of selective thermolysis	For nonuniformly pigmented targets the pulse duration is longer than the target thermal relaxation time
9	Scattering	A change in the direction of propagation of a photon resulting from imprecise absorption of laser energy by a biologic system that results in a diffuse effect on tissue
10	Absorption	The transfer of radiant energy into targeted tissues resulting in a change in tissue
11	Chromophore	A substance or molecule with selective light-absorbing properties, often to specific wavelengths
12	Beam	Radiant electromagnetic rays that may be convergent, divergent, or collimated (in parallel)

TABLE 13.3 Cutaneous Features of Skin of Color

1. Higher activity of melanocytes
2. Increased epidermal melanin
3. Increased prevalence of pigmentary disorders
4. Variations in hair structure and morphology

Available hair removal lasers include the long-pulsed Alexandrite (755 nm), long-pulsed diode (810 nm), and the long-pulsed (millisecond range) and short-pulsed (microsecond range) Nd:YAG (1064 nm). Of these options, the long-pulsed 1064-nm Nd:YAG laser is the gold standard for treating darker skin, particularly skin phototypes V and VI, while the long-pulsed 810-nm diode[11] can be used in intermediately pigmented complexions (e.g., phototypes IV-V). In addition, the 650-microsecond 1064-nm Nd:YAG laser has been used safely on skin of color (phototypes IV-VI) and may be considered an alternative to longer-pulsed 1064-nm lasers. The shorter pulse (sub-millisecond or microsecond) laser obviates the need for active cooling or use of gels and may confer higher tolerability (less pain associated with treatment). One to two additional pulses to areas of persistent hair may be required to achieve the desired reduction when using the 650-microsecond pulsed laser. Long-term efficacy studies to confirm the duration of hair reduction are warranted.

Across the infrared spectrum, melanin absorption decreases as infrared wavelengths increase. The Nd:YAG wavelength has the lowest melanin absorption as compared to the other wavelengths used for laser hair removal (diode & Alexandrite). The highest melanin absorption is the Alexandrite wavelength with the diode wavelength between the Nd:YAG and the Alexandrite wavelength (see Table 13.1).

To safely treat skin of color, minimizing collateral thermal injury to the epidermis is a key goal. The Nd:YAG wavelength is safer than the diode wavelength to treat darker skin types.[15] The longer wavelength of the Nd:YAG minimizes epidermal melanin absorption with the appropriate laser energy depth penetration to target the dermal hair follicular unit. When the Nd:YAG lasers are combined with aggressive skin cooling and pulse durations $\geq$30 ms, they can safely treat Fitzpatrick Skin Types VI.[16] Most of the FDA-approved Nd:YAG wavelength lasers incorporate efficient epidermal cooling. The higher safety of Nd:YAG's longer wavelength in skin of color is associated with a slight reduction in efficacy because of reduced melanin absorption compared to the 810-nm or 755-nm wavelengths.[16,17] A comparative study conducted by Galadari showed a 35% reduction in hair at 12 months after six treatments with the Nd:YAG lasers compared with a 40% reduction observed with the diode laser after a comparable number of treatments and similar follow-up period.[16]

Diode lasers equipped with chill-tip technology have been used for laser hair removal in skin of color. In a prospective observational study of 55 patients undergoing, Tulpule et al. evaluated the efficacy and safety of the 810-nm diode laser equipped with chill-tip technology over 2 years.[18] The study reported the majority (37 out of 55, 67.3%) of patients having skin phototype IV; the most common site was the chin (23 out of 55), with the average growth reduction at the end of three sessions (61.25%). Notably, four (8%) patients had short-term adverse effects including superficial burns, postinflammatory hyperpigmentation, and acneiform eruptions, while none of the patients developed long-term adverse effects.[18]

In a study conducted by Aldraibi et al., examining the use of the Alexandrite laser in 31 patients (skin types IV to VI) showed an average hair reduction of 35.4% at 6 months with a high rate of hyperpigmentation (48.4% at 1 week). In this study, pretreatment and short-term postlaser treatment with a super-potent topical steroid improved erythema, crusting, and dyspigmentation caused by the laser.[19]

As our understanding of lasers improves, newer technologies are being introduced. One example is a new generation 1064-nm Nd:YAG laser with cold-air cooling that obviates the need for an external cooling medium (e.g., a gel). Another approach to laser hair removal with the 1064-nm Nd:YAG laser is the use of a device with a fixed sub-millisecond pulse duration. The theory behind this sub-millisecond (650 microsecond, or 0.65 millisecond) technology is related to the thermal relaxation time of skin, which is thought to be slightly less than 1 millisecond.[20] Thus, a pulse duration that is less than the thermal relaxation time of skin suggests less dissipation of heat to the surrounding skin. In addition to the advantages of 1064-nm Nd:YAG laser, this 650-microsecond laser does not require direct epidermal cooling during treatment. Treatment can be done for all skin phototypes safely with minimal pain or discomfort.

Other approaches to laser hair removal may include a combination of wavelengths such as the 1064-nm Nd:YAG and the 755-nm Alexandrite lasers. In a recent prospective randomized trial of 36 patients (phototypes I–IV) comparing laser-directed hair removal with the Alexandrite, the Nd:YAG, or a blended simultaneous combination of both wavelengths, showed greater than 50% reduction in hair in 40%, 24%, and 60% of subjects on the lower extremity, respectively.[21] In contrast, using the same criteria, but applied to patients receiving axillary hair removal, the rates for those achieving more than 50% reduction at 2 months posttreatment were 20% (Alexandrite), 25% (Nd:YAG), and 24% (Alexandrite-Nd:YAG blend).[21] Most subjects (82%) were of phototypes of less than IV, and therefore, evidence for safety in higher skin phototypes is currently lacking. Likewise, Lehavit et al. conducted a retrospective cohort study among 11 males Fitzpatrick (FST) III-V who underwent laser hair removal with a laser device able to simultaneously deliver pulsed wavelengths of 755, 810, and 1064 nanometers and showed an overall meaningful reduction in mean hairs (3.4 out of 4) based on the Global Aesthetic Improvement Scale (GAIS).[22] These studies show the potential added benefit of simultaneously blended lasers that emit certain wavelengths for purposes of hair removal; however, large-scale safety studies are required.

Similarly, certain devices may be able to generate multiple wavelengths to allow the treating clinician to select the appropriate option for specific patients. Although this addition is beneficial, caution should be implemented to avoid inadvertent use of the technology.

Some diode and Alexandrite lasers use a different approach to improve their safety in treating skin of color. Some have large cooling plates and utilize a scanning technique. Some lasers suction the skin into the handpiece, changing the skin's optics, allowing for the use of safer lower fluences. Other lasers use a constant motion technique, allowing them to use lower safer fluences with shorter diode and alexandrite wavelengths.

The main cause for laser hair removal side effects is thermal damage. Epidermal-dermal separation (blisters) occur when the epidermis surpasses 45 °C.[23] Keeping the epidermis under 45 °C dramatically reduces the risk for thermal-induced side effects. Longer pulse durations also are safer for skin of color because of the thermokinetic selectivity theory.[24] This theory states that smaller structures (epidermal melanin) will lose heat faster than larger structures (dermal hair follicle).[24] The quicker dissipation of epidermal melanin heat in comparison to the much larger hair follicle serves as a protective mechanism for the epidermis.[24]

Darker skin types have melanosomes that are more evenly distributed throughout the epidermis. Epidermal melanin competes for the same laser light that is intended to target the hair shaft. The light absorbed by the epidermal pigment is transferred into heat, and if the epidermal heat surpasses 43 °C, it can produce unwanted events and side effects like erythema, blistering, and postinflammatory hyperpigmentation. Removing the undesired epidermal heat from the epidermis through aggressive skin cooling is an essential ingredient to be able to safely and effectively treat skin of color.

Cooling of the epidermis can be achieved by many methods including cooling by direct contact or noncontact cooling by utilizing cold-air cryogen spray. Cooling can also be categorized as precooling, parallel cooling, and postcooling. Precooling is cooling the skin immediately prior to the laser pulse. Parallel cooling is cooling the skin during the laser pulse and is usually achieved by using a sapphire glass cooling plate. Postcooling is cooling the skin after the laser pulse. Appropriate skin cooling, to remove the unwanted heat from the epidermis, is an essential component to safely treat skin of color. But there are limits to cooling, and excessive cooling of skin of color is not without risk of side effects. Excessive skin cooling that can be observed in coolant-induced injuries can lead to blistering and discoloration. Cryogen spray can reach temperatures as low as –26 °C and can produce both hypopigmentation and hyperpigmentation if not optimized.

CHOOSING APPROPRIATE LASER PARAMETERS AND TEST SPOTS

Many laser devices are currently available; however, differences exist including recommended settings or protocol(s) depending on the type of laser and manufacturer. Additionally, manufacturers may propose slightly different mechanisms for laser hair removal. Despite these differences, laser hair removal devices ultimately induce heat within hairs leading to destruction of germinative cells.

Clinicians and patients benefit from test spots. They allow the clinician to detect the endpoint in that specific patient and gain their confidence while the patient sees visible hair reduction without burns or resultant dyspigmentation and feels minimal discomfort, all of which improve patient compliance and overall satisfaction.

Wavelength. As discussed, the target chromophore for lasers in hair removal is melanin, which can be found in the hair shaft, the outer-root sheath, and within the matrix of hair. Melanin may be targeted by wavelengths produced from Ruby, Alexandrite, diode, and Nd:YAG in addition to intense pulsed light. For patients with skin of color, with a general Fitzpatrick phototype of IV or more, the safest recommended laser with modest efficacy is the 1064-nm Nd:YAG followed by the diode laser that is more efficacious than the former.

Spot size. It is defined as the diameter (in millimeters) of the laser ray or beam. The larger the spot area or size, the greater the depth of penetration for that laser. As the laser ray penetrates through the dermis, scatter from dermal components (e.g., collagen) occurs and these scattered rays do not contribute to the treatment. Small spot sizes scatter more. Thus, larger spot sizes are preferable. In addition, in laser hair removal a larger area or spot size is preferable because a smaller area at the same fluence would increase the risk of injury to the epidermis. In addition, a larger spot size allows for a lower number of pulses compared to the smaller spot sizes.

Pulse width or duration. The duration of the pulses given in any laser defines the pulse duration. Based on the diameter of terminal hairs, the thermal relaxation time (TRT) has been estimated to be about 100 milliseconds. However, due to the three-dimensional configuration of the chromophore (melanin) within hair follicles it may be difficult to quantify the actual TRT of the collective hair follicle. The expanded photothermolysis theory proposed the concept of thermal damage time (TDT), which is longer than the TRT. Sub-millisecond pulses may also be effective at removing hairs but may not be as efficacious for permanent hair removal.

Fluence. Fluence is the total amount of energy delivered in a treatment area, in joules per square centimeter (J/cm^2). Using higher fluences achieves better permanent hair removal. However, with higher fluences the risk for side effects increases. Recommendations for specific fluences are typically provided by the laser device manufacturer. In addition, it is vital to determine the optimal fluence for the individual patient based on realizing desired clinical endpoints including perifollicular edema and erythema. Thus, for experienced operators, the highest fluence that achieves these clinical endpoints without causing untoward side effects is carefully chosen.

PATIENT SELECTION AND CONSULTATION

Hair provides multiple benefits, including sun protection, added external sensation, reduction of friction at flexures, and aesthetic appearance. Some individuals may be culturally compelled to maintain certain hair practices. It is always important to verify with the patient the treatment location and goals of the patient. It is equally important to set reasonable expectations for your patient to avoid any unnecessary outcomes and establish a realistic plan with the patient.

The anatomical location of unwanted hair is a useful consideration. Some areas may respond differently compared to others. For example, success rates for underarm laser hair removal are higher than hairs of the lip. Similarly, certain regions of hair are influenced by hormones. Certain hair types are more susceptible to laser, such as dark and coarse hairs as opposed to fine, white, or red or vellus hairs.

It is essential to identify patients at increased risk for hair growth, such as those who may have endocrinological disorders (such as polycystic ovarian syndrome [PCOS] or hyperandrogenism). These patients may be more resistant to laser hair removal and may require additional treatments. Patients with endocrinological disorders must be diagnosed and treated appropriately to prevent recurrence and increase success rates.

LASER TREATMENT

Pretreatment considerations include avoidance of tanning, wearing protective attire, and sunscreen and excessive sun exposure for 4 to 6 weeks. In the past, patients have been instructed to avoid waxing or electrolysis about 6 weeks before the first treatment and during the whole treatment duration. But this recommendation is controversial and under additional research consideration since the target for laser hair removal is the hair bulb, which is not impacted by waxing or electrolysis. Al-Haddab et al. compared immediate preshaving versus prewaxing in a clinical trial of 20 healthy females (Fitzpatrick IV-V) undergoing axillary hair removal using the long-pulsed Alexandrite laser; the trial showed minimal difference in LHR efficacy between preshaving and prewaxing.[25] Some clinicians opt to use bleaching topicals to prevent hyperpigmentation with certain higher-risk lasers, but this is uncommon with current advancements and when selecting appropriate lasers for the right patient. Shaving is appropriate on the day of treatment (long hairs may lead to blistering due to generated heat within the hair at the surface). Patients should inform the clinician if they are on medications (especially photosensitizers) including tetracycline antibiotics, strong topical retinoids, gold therapy, or oral isotretinoin. Contraindications for laser hair removal include patient refusal, therapy with gold, herbal treatment such as St. John's Wort, and active signs of inflammation. Although pregnancy is not an absolute contraindication for LHR, treatment consideration is best done after delivery. In recent years, systemic isotretinoin has been the subject of controversial debate and most clinicians currently allow laser hair removal while on oral isotretinoin. Importantly, it is beneficial to understand if the patient has specific goals for hair removal to be attained within a specific timeframe (e.g., a deadline such as a wedding). As with any procedure, a complete discussion of the benefits, risks, and alternatives to laser hair removal and written informed consent should be obtained and documented. Additional pearls in laser hair removal for patients with skin of color are summarized in Table 13.4.

Immediately preprocedure, the patient should cleanse the affected area and remove any reflective objects. Topical anesthetics are not used by many clinicians because of the possible masking of pain that would lead to potential burns. The space should be relatively free of mirrors or other reflective surfaces. The lens of the laser should be thoroughly cleaned based on the manufacturer's recommendation. All staff and the patient involved in the laser procedure must have appropriate eye protection that covers the specific wavelengths used

TABLE 13.4   Clinical Pearls for Laser Hair Removal in Skin of Color

1. Select appropriate wavelength of laser according to skin phototype and other predictors of dyspigmentation from laser-induced thermal injury (e.g., constitutive pigmentation or history of postinflammatory hyperpigmentation).
2. Select optimal laser parameters according to the patient's phototype, constitutive pigmentation, and response to test spots or previous treatments.
3. For lasers in the millisecond range, longer pulse durations and epidermal cooling are recommended for safety in skin of color.
4. The 650-microsecond-pulsed 1064-nm Nd:YAG laser is a safe alternative to traditional millisecond-pulsed lasers in skin of color, but additional pulses may be required to achieve the desired clinical endpoint. (Comparative and long-term studies are lacking).
5. Larger handpieces are used for greater surface areas with lower fluences, while smaller handpieces are employed for smaller areas such as the lip using higher fluences.
6. Pre-and posttreatment photoprotection is paramount.

before the treatment starts. Blindness is a real possibility and may occur if the eyes receive laser exposure inadvertently. As such, when treating near the eyes, intraocular eye shields and avoidance of the ocular orbit are recommended. Similarly, caution should be implemented when treatments for hair removal involve important structures such as the reproductive organs when treating the groin. Before starting the procedure, it is important to check all equipment involved to ensure the systems are working as planned. A skilled clinician will be able to modulate the following five parameters safely and effectively: wavelength (laser type), pulse width (or duration), spot size (in millimeters), fluence (also known as energy density or energy per unit area, J/cm^2), and cooling if applicable to each patient. The treating clinician should start with the lowest recommended manufacturers' settings in the first treatment or test spot. Subsequent treatment settings can be adjusted according to the patient's response and tolerance to the laser and based on the presence or absence of side effects. The parameters vary according to the phototype of the patient (which is influenced by ancestry), location of treatment, the density of hair, hair thickness and

the number of anagen hairs, and intensity of the color of hairs.

Posttreatment instructions include minimizing sun exposure and application of a soothing moisturizer with sunscreen (SPF 30 or higher) for 6 weeks after treatment and throughout treatment. Immediately after laser hair removal, tenderness, erythema, and or wheals may arise, and this quickly improves within minutes to hours. Swelling may be alleviated by the use of ice packs applied for 10 to 15 minutes posttreatment. Avoidance of scrubbing and irritating the area is encouraged. Minimizing waxing and avoidance of electrolysis should be discussed with the patient while shaving or clipping is permitted. In certain instances, exuberant reactions may occur including oozing and scabbing with resultant crusts and patients should be reminded of this possibility. When this occurs, patients should avoid picking or removing the crusts, and antihistamines and gentle topical corticosteroids may be needed such as hydrocortisone 2.5% ointment. Finally, patients may apply light nonirritating makeup after treatments if the area is not irritated or crusted.

LASER-INDUCED SIDE EFFECTS

Lasers represent a major advancement in modern medicine, and appropriate and inappropriate use may be associated with unwanted side effects. It is crucial to educate patients on these risks and how to best minimize them by implementing certain guidelines for every treated patient. Importantly, in the United States, laser hair removal is one of the commonest procedures performed and the potential for complications is considerable. Many procedures are done by nonphysicians and physician extenders (e.g., physician assistants, nurse practitioners, estheticians).[26] Additionally, in the United States LHR has been cited as the most common procedure (44 out of 69 cases, from 2012 to 2020) that resulted in litigation[26] and in 71% (49 out of 69) of cases involved nonphysician operators.[26] In about half of the litigation cases, the cases are won in favor of the litigating (plaintiff) party, with an average indemnity of $320,975.[26] Fortunately, many of these side effects are preventable and uncommonly occur. Importantly, patients should be informed of all possible side effects of LHR as well as other risks, benefits and alternatives of the procedure should be fully discussed and documented. The goal of laser treatment is to induce change (in the form of heat) in target tissues while minimizing the heating of the surrounding tissues.

Burns are a feared side effect of laser or light removal. Several light and laser hair removal associated burns have been reported.[27,28] Most burns that occur after laser or light-based procedures are first-degree burns. Second-degree burns are less likely, but possible. Burns can be easily prevented by appropriate device selection, conservative parameters, and tailoring the treatments for the correct type of patient. Pulse stacking or excessive overlapping of pulses should be avoided.[29] In addition, appropriate history and physical examination can lower the chances of developing burns in a patient. For example, historical considerations may include use of irritating skin care products (and prescribed medications such as retinoids) or presence of makeup. The latter should be carefully washed, and the skin cleansed before laser hair removal. Feared complications of burns may include dyspigmentation, infection, and scarring. Importantly, a patient who experiences a burn is less likely to return to the treating clinician.

Dyschromia refers to changes in the color in the laser-treated area. They are common pigmentary changes that occur after laser hair removal. Hyperpigmentation is usually transient and more common than hypopigmentation, which may have a more protracted course. Risks of dyschromia increase with increasing phototypes (e.g., risk is higher in FST V compared to FST III). Generally, risk of dyschromia is higher with shorter wavelength lasers, compared to low risk in longer wavelength lasers such as the Nd:YAG. Weisberg and Greenbaum reported a case series of seven patients including patients with phototype IV undergoing laser hair removal with the 755-nm Alexandrite laser equipped with a dynamic cooling device that developed patterned dyschromia at treated sites while none of the patients developed permanent pigmentary changes.[30] Interestingly, most of the cases had characteristic erythematous-to-hyperpigmented scaly ring-like patches on treated areas that initially resulted in hyperpigmentation followed by hypopigmentation followed by normalization of pigment over weeks to months (range 2 weeks to 6 months) after treatment.[30] Similarly, Alajlan reported a case series of 15 patients treated with the same laser (755 nm with built-in cryogen) resulting in similar crescent-like hyperpigmentation.[31] The authors of both studies suggested that the most likely cause of this patterned dyschromia in their cohorts was related to aberrations in cooling or malfunction of the built-in cryogen.[30,31]

Posttreatment folliculitis is an uncommon self-limited side effect of laser hair removal.[32] It has been suggested that it occurs in higher frequency in those who have coarse hairs, pilli multigemini, or have previously developed folliculitis to shaving.[32] In such patients with a history of laser-induced folliculitis, appropriate prophylactic topical corticosteroids, and antibiotics may be considered.

Paradoxical hypertrichosis (PH) is an uncommon (pooled prevalence of 3%, range 1% to 6%) occurrence that involves undesired growth of terminal hairs at laser hair removal treatment sites.[33] Cases typically involve females with ethnic skin with a recent report showing skin type III and IV being the most common type involved in such cases.[33] Interestingly, most reported cases occurred on the face and the neck.[33] Interestingly, PH may be seen at sites away from the treated area.[33,34] The typical patient that develops PH would be someone who undergoes laser or light-related removal of vellus hairs, and the treatment paradoxically triggers terminal hair growth. When this complication occurs, continuation of treatment with the same treatment (but more aggressive settings) is recommended.

Hirsutism refers to unwanted excess hair on surfaces that are normally hairless and under androgenic control.[35] This diagnosis is made in females or children who exhibit adult, male-pattern hypertrichosis.[35] For example, women with hirsutism may present with coarse terminal hairs on the lower cheeks, chin, upper lip, and/or the chest. As discussed previously, identification of concomitant signs of hyperandrogenism and necessary work up to exclude underlying conditions (e.g., PCOS) is vital. Complete history and physical examination coupled with select testing would identify causes, which should be managed before or concomitantly with hair treatments with lasers.

Hypertrichosis is a condition of excessive hair growth at sites of normally appearing terminal hairs. Mechanisms of hypertrichosis include increased conversion of vellus to terminal hairs, hair-cycle alterations, and increased hair-follicle density.[35] It should not be confused with paradoxical hypertrichosis, which is secondary to laser treatment of hair intended for removal but leads to the surprising excessive growth in treated areas as discussed previously. Hypertrichosis may be genetically predetermined or due to conditions (such as porphyria cutanea tarda, thyroidal dysfunction, nutritional alterations, or inflammatory or neoplastic conditions), or due to medications (e.g., cyclosporine, phenytoin, minoxidil, prednisolone).[35]

HAIR-ASSOCIATED DISORDERS TREATED WITH LASER HAIR REMOVAL

Pseudofolliculitis barbae (PFB) is a common hair-associated condition in skin of color, involving hair-bearing areas of the face and other sites where hair is removed among men and women.[36] Shaving exacerbates the condition and postinflammatory hyperpigmentation is a common associated feature. In severe cases, scarring can occur.[36] PFB presents with perifollicular inflammatory papules, pustules, and sometimes nodules.[36] The advent of laser-directed hair removal has transformed the care for patients who suffer from this condition. Depending on the severity, the device, and patient-specific factors, treatments may require approximately 6 to 8 sessions for clinically significant hair reduction and resolution of PFB. Occupational or cultural behaviors that require a clean-shaven appearance may be a factor in influencing the development of PFB. Other factors associated with PFB include inappropriate choice of instrument or technique used by affected individuals. For example, shaving against the direction that hairs grow and using multiple blades at once have been shown to exacerbate PFB. Patients should be instructed on the best practices if shaving is required, with appropriate recommendations on perishaving practices such as using a soothing shaving cream, application of appropriate topical antibiotic, or gentle topical corticosteroids such as 1% hydrocortisone to minimize super infection and irritation respectively.

Acne keloidalis nuchae (AKN) is a common, chronic hair follicle–associated condition in patients with skin of color.[37] AKN presents with follicular papules or nodules that become indurated or keloidal, on the occipital scalp and nape of the neck. Pustules may also be present in some cases. It can result in scarring alopecia if not treated appropriately.[37] Multiple lasers can be employed to treat AKN in addition to medical or surgical management.[37–40] In patients with skin of color, the safest option for hair removal in the treatment of AKN is the 1064-nm Nd:YAG laser wavelength. Careful consideration of laser-directed hair removal in the scalp should include discussion with the patient about the risk of permanent hair loss in treated areas given that reduction in hair densities is expected with treatment.

CONCLUSION

Laser hair removal in skin of color requires an approach that targets melanin in the hair follicle while minimizing absorption by the competing chromophore of epidermal melanin. To that end, longer wavelength lasers in the near-infrared spectrum can be used effectively, with the 1064-nm Nd:YAG being the safest for patients with melanin-rich skin. In intermediate skin phototypes, the diode and Alexandrite lasers can be used for greater efficacy, albeit with a greater risk of complications than the 1064-nm Nd:YAG. Conservative fluences, epidermal cooling, and photoprotection are important strategies for safest outcomes. Patient selection and initial consultation are essential to establish a safe and effective treatment plan that is personalized for the patient. Understanding laser-light physics and determinants of laser-assisted hair removal allows the clinician to maximize efficacy while maintaining safety, especially in darker-skinned patients. As new technologies are introduced, the clinician should remain up to date with the latest advances to deliver the best care for patients with skin of color.

REFERENCES

1. Rosenfield RL. Clinical practice. Hirsutism. *N Engl J Med.* 2005;353(24):2578-2588. doi:10.1056/NEJMcp033496.
2. Ogunbiyi A. Pseudofolliculitis barbae; current treatment options. *Clin Cosmet Investig Dermatol.* 2019;12:241-247. doi:10.2147/CCID.S149250.
3. Afifi L, Saeed L, Pasch LA, et al. Association of ethnicity, Fitzpatrick skin type, and hirsutism: A retrospective cross-sectional study of women with polycystic ovarian syndrome. *Int J Womens Dermatol.* 2017;3(1):37-43. doi:10.1016/j.ijwd.2017.01.006.
4. Barth JH, Wilkinson JD, Dawber RP. Prepubertal hypertrichosis: Normal or abnormal? *Arch Dis Child.* 1988;63(6):666-668. doi:10.1136/adc.63.6.666.
5. Dorgham NA, Dorgham DA. Lasers for reduction of unwanted hair in skin of colour: A systematic review and meta-analysis. *J Eur Acad Dermatol Venereol.* 2020;34(5):948-955. doi:10.1111/jdv.15995.
6. Battle EF. Advances in laser hair removal in skin of color. *J Drugs Dermatol.* 2011;10(11):1235-1239.
7. Dierickx CC, Grossman MC, Farinelli WA, Anderson RR. Permanent hair removal by normal-mode ruby laser. *Arch Dermatol.* 1998;134(7):837-842. doi:10.1001/archderm.134.7.837.
8. Grossman MC, Dierickx C, Farinelli W, Flotte T, Anderson RR. Damage to hair follicles by normal-mode ruby laser pulses. *J Am Acad Dermatol.* 1996;35(6):889-894. doi:10.1016/s0190-9622(96)90111-5.
9. Dierickx CC, Anderson RR, Campos VB, Grossman MC. *Effective, Long-Term Hair Removal Using A Pulsed High-Power Diode Laser.* Pleasanton, CA: Coherent Medical; 1999.

10. Battle EF, Anderson RR. *Study of Very Long-Pulsed (100ms) High-Powered Diode Laser for Hair Reduction on All Skin Types*. Santa Clara, CA: Coherent Medical; 2000.
11. Battle EF. Very long-pulsed (20-200 ms) diode laser for hair removal on all skin types. *Lasers Surg Med Suppl*. 2000;12:21.
12. Anderson RR, Parrish JA. Selective photothermolysis: precise microsurgery by selective absorption of pulsed radiation. *Science*. 1983;220(4596):524-527. doi:10.1126/science.6836297.
13. Commo S, Gaillard O, Bernard BA. The human hair follicle contains two distinct K19 positive compartments in the outer root sheath: A unifying hypothesis for stem cell reservoir? *Differentiation*. 2000;66(4-5):157-164. doi:10.1046/j.1432-0436.2000.660401.x.
14. Cotsarelis G, Sun TT, Lavker RM. Label-retaining cells reside in the bulge area of pilosebaceous unit: Implications for follicular stem cells, hair cycle, and skin carcinogenesis. *Cell*. 1990;61(7):1329-1337. doi:10.1016/0092-8674(90)90696-c.
15. Alster TS, Bryan H, Williams CM. Long-pulsed Nd:YAG laser-assisted hair removal in pigmented skin: A clinical and histological evaluation. *Arch Dermatol*. 2001;137(7):885-889.
16. Galadari I. Comparative evaluation of different hair removal lasers in skin types IV, V, and VI. *Int J Dermatol*. 2003;42(1):68-70.i:10.1046/j.1365-4362.2003.01744.x.
17. Bouzari N, Tabatabai H, Abbasi Z, Firooz A, Dowlati Y. Laser hair removal: Comparison of long-pulsed Nd:YAG, long-pulsed Alexandrite, and long-pulsed diode lasers. *Dermatol Surg*. 2004;30(4 Pt 1):498-502. doi:10.1111/j.1524-4725.2004.30163.x.
18. Tulpule MS, Bhide DS, Bharatia P, Rathod NU. 810 nm diode laser for hair reduction with chill-tip technology: Prospective observational analysis of 55 patients of Fitzpatrick skin types III, IV,V. *J Cosmet Laser Ther*. 2020;22(2):65-69. doi:10.1080/14764172.2020.1726961.
19. Aldraibi MS, Touma DJ, Khachemoune A. Hair removal with the 3-msec Alexandrite laser in patients with skin types IV-VI: Efficacy, safety, and the role of topical corticosteroids in preventing side effects. *J Drugs Dermatol*. 2007;6(1):60-66.
20. Walsh JT, Flotte TJ, Anderson RR, Deutsch TF. Pulsed CO2 laser tissue ablation: Effect of tissue type and pulse duration on thermal damage. *Lasers Surg Med*. 1988;8(2):108-118. doi:10.1002/lsm.1900080204.
21. Ross EV, Domankevitz Y. Hair removal with blended 755/1064 nm laser energy. *Lasers Surg Med*. 2021;53(8):1020-1025. doi:10.1002/lsm.23381.
22. Lehavit A, Eran G, Moshe L, Assi L. A combined triple-wavelength (755nm, 810nm, and 1063nm) laser device for hair removal: Efficacy and safety study. *J Drugs Dermatol*. 2020;19(5):515-518. doi:10.36849/JDD.2020.4735.
23. Arora S, Kar BR. Reduction of blister formation time in suction blister epidermal grafting in vitiligo patients using a household hair dryer. *J Cutan Aesthet Surg*. 2016;9(4):232-235. doi:10.4103/0974-2077.197045.
24. Fuchs M. Thermokinetic selectivity—a new highly effective method for permanent hair removal: Experience with the LPIR Alexandrite laser. *Derm Prakt Dermatologie*. 1997;5:1.
25. Al-Haddab M, Al-Khawajah N, Al-Ala´a A, Al-Majed H, Al-Shamlan Y, Al-Abdely M. The effect of waxing versus shaving on the efficacy of laser hair removal. *Dermatol Surg*. 2017;43(4):548-552. doi:10.1097/DSS.0000000000001025.
26. Khalifian S, Vazirnia A, Mohan GC, Thompson KV, Jalian HR, Avram MM. Causes of injury and litigation in cutaneous laser surgery: an update from 2012 to 2020. *Dermatol Surg*. 2022;48(3):315-319. doi:10.1097/DSS.0000000000003375.
27. Balyen L. Inadvertent macular burns and consecutive psychological depression secondary to Alexandrite laser epilation: A case report. *Saudi J Ophthalmol*. 2019;33(1):105-108. doi:10.1016/j.sjopt.2018.03.006.
28. Kacar SD, Ozuguz P, Demir M, Karaca S. An uncommon cause of laser burns: The problem may be the use of gel. *J Cosmet Laser Ther*. 2014;16(2):104-105. doi:10.3109/14764172.2013.877748.
29. Willey A, Anderson RR, Azpiazu JL, et al. Complications of laser dermatologic surgery. *Lasers Surg Med*. 2006;38(1):1-15. doi:10.1002/lsm.20286.
30. Weisberg NK, Greenbaum SS. Pigmentary changes after Alexandrite laser hair removal. *Dermatol Surg*. 2003;29(4):415-419. doi:10.1046/j.1524-4725.2003.29098.x.
31. Alajlan A. Crescent-shaped hyperpigmentation following laser hair removal: Case series of fifteen patients. *Lasers Surg Med*. 2021;53(3):333-336. doi:10.1002/lsm.23296.
32. Schuler A, Veenstra J, Tisack A. Folliculitis induced by laser hair removal: proposed mechanism and treatment. *J Clin Aesthet Dermatol*. 2020;13(5):34-36.
33. Snast I, Kaftory R, Lapidoth M, Levi A. Paradoxical hypertrichosis associated with laser and light therapy for hair removal: a systematic review and meta-analysis. *Am J Clin Dermatol*. 2021;22(5):615-624. doi:10.1007/s40257-021-00611-w.
34. Rasheed AI. Uncommonly reported side effects of hair removal by long pulsed-Alexandrite laser. *J Cosmet Dermatol*. 2009;8(4):267-274. doi:10.1111/j.1473-2165.2009.00465.x.

35. Wendelin DS, Pope DN, Mallory SB. Hypertrichosis. *J Am Acad Dermatol.* 2003;48(2):161-179; quiz 180. doi:10.1067/mjd.2003.100.

36. Coley MK, Alexis AF. Managing common dermatoses in skin of color. *Semin Cutan Med Surg.* 2009;28(2):63-70. doi:10.1016/j.sder.2009.04.006.

37. Maranda EL, Simmons BJ, Nguyen AH, Lim VM, Keri JE. Treatment of acne keloidalis nuchae: A systematic review of the literature. *Dermatol Ther (Heidelb).* 2016;6(3): 363-378. doi:10.1007/s13555-016-0134-5.

38. Esmat SM, Abdel Hay RM, Abu Zeid OM, Hosni HN. The efficacy of laser-assisted hair removal in the treatment of

acne keloidalis nuchae; a pilot study. *Eur J Dermatol.* 2012;22(5):645-650. doi:10.1684/ejd.2012.1830.

39. Tawfik A, Osman MA, Rashwan I. A novel treatment of acne keloidalis nuchae by long-pulsed Alexandrite laser. *Dermatol Surg.* 2018;44(3):413-420. doi:10.1097/DSS.0000000000001336.

40. Woo DK, Treyger G, Henderson M, Huggins RH, Jackson-Richards D, Hamzavi I. Prospective controlled trial for the treatment of acne keloidalis nuchae with a long-pulsed neodymium-doped yttrium-aluminum-garnet laser. *J Cutan Med Surg.* 2018;22(2):236-238. doi:10.1177/1203475417739846.

14

Skin Resurfacing: Nuances and Best Practices for Skin of Color

Elise D. Martin, Gilly Munavalli

SUMMARY AND KEY FEATURES

- Anatomic and physiologic characteristics in skin of color translate clinically to difference in the aging process as well as a greater propensity for pigmentary alterations and abnormal scarring.
- The higher risk of pigmentary alteration associated with resurfacing in skin of color largely prohibits use of fully ablative resurfacing. However, advances in laser technology with the development of ablative fractional and nonablative fractional lasers introduced alternative safe and effective options for laser resurfacing in patients with skin of color.
- Though fractional and nonablative lasers can be used safely on skin of color, the risk of dyspigmentation still exists—albeit typically less significant and more transient.

- Melanin absorption extends across many wavelengths peaking in the ultraviolet range and decreasing as wavelengths lengthen. Longer wavelength lasers are less efficiently absorbed by completing epidermal melanin and therefore safer in patients with skin of color.
- Radiofrequency and ultrasound devices are excellent and safe alternatives to lasers for rejuvenation and aging in patients with skin of color.
- Even when using a laser deemed safe for use in darker skin, selection of proper treatment parameters is crucial to avoid complications. In general, use of conservative density and fluence settings, proper cooling, and greater intervals between treatments is prudent.
- Topical agents including sunscreen, corticosteroids, and hydroquinone are helpful pre- and post-laser treatment adjuncts.

INTRODUCTION

As the United States population continues to diversify, it is imperative for medical providers be prepared to best meet the needs of all patients. Demographics have shifted with a growing non-White population.[1] Between 1990 and 2000, Hispanics, Black/African-Americans, and Asians all demonstrated growth rates ranging from 12% to 40%, while the growth rate of non-Hispanic White population was a marginal 2%.[2] According to the United States Census Bureau, this growth is projected to continue with Black/African-American, Hispanic, Asian, and multiracial individuals anticipated to comprise more than half of the United States population by 2044.[3]

In the field of dermatology, Black/African-American, Asian, Hispanic, and multiracial individuals, collectively referred to as patients with skin of color (SOC), are increasingly constituting the already rapidly expanding cosmetic procedure market.[4] Cosmetic procedures in the United States, both surgical and nonsurgical, increased more than 30% between 2010 and 2016. Importantly, an increasing number of these procedures were performed in patients of SOC, as procedures in non-White patients also rose from 19% to 25%.[5] Cosmetic procedures have garnered more interest across all skin types, but particularly in SOC patients with increased availability of safe technologies and options for darker skin types.[6,7]

Despite a growing SOC population seeking dermatologic care and cosmetic procedures, education and literature regarding SOC in dermatology is limited.[6] SOC patients most often can be categorized into Fitzpatrick skin phototypes III through VI. Physiologic differences exist between lighter and darker skin with important treatment implications, particularly with use of laser and light devices. Despite these differences, most of the current literature regarding laser procedures addresses only Fitzpatrick type I–II skin types. Laser protocols are largely based on clinical experience predominantly in lighter skin types.[8] Of the finite laser studies in non-White patients, the majority are in Asian or type III–IV skin types.[9] There is a paucity of studies examining laser procedures in type V and VI skin.[7] Perhaps even fewer studies discuss darker skin types in the setting of laser resurfacing, particularly as early resurfacing lasers were contraindicated in skin types IV–VI.[7] With information on laser resurfacing in darker skin types lacking, providers may have trepidation with performing resurfacing procedures in SOC patients, or worse, treat SOC patients inappropriately with consequential adverse effects.[10] This chapter aims to reduce this knowledge gap by discussing nuances and best practices for laser resurfacing in skin of color.

ANATOMIC AND PHYSIOLOGIC DIFFERENCES IN SKIN OF COLOR

Melanocytes

Differences in skin color between lighter and darker skin types can be attributed to variation in distribution and size of melanosomes as melanocyte number is identical.[7] In darker skin types, melanosomes are larger, denser, and more singly dispersed.[7,11] These differences allow for greater photoprotection against UV radiation in darker skin types.[11,12] Studies have shown types V and VI skin to possess an inherent sun protection factor (SPF) of 13.4.[13–15] Consequently, individuals of SOC are less likely to develop skin cancer and generally demonstrate delayed, less discernable photoaging.[7,11] Though

useful for photoprotection, the increased melanin in SOC can become problematic when treating with lasers. When utilizing lasers with a target chromophore of melanin, the increased melanin in the epidermis of SOC can compete with the true target and absorb more energy than intended.

Though melanocyte number remains the same across skin types, melanocytes in darker skin types demonstrate increased reactivity.[16] In SOC, trauma, light, or other inciting injury or inflammatory event may lead to a labile melanocyte response with a tendency for resultant pigmentary alteration, most commonly hyperpigmentation.[7,16]

Fibroblasts

Melanocytes and melanosomes are not the only histologic and physiologic variance between skin types. Fibroblasts are larger, more numerous, and more reactive in SOC.[7,16–18] Greater numbers of fibroblasts have been noted in Black female facial skin compared to White female facial skin.[18] Additionally, fibroblasts in Black skin tend to be larger and often multinucleate amidst tightly arranged, smaller collagen bundles.[16,17] Not only more numerous and larger, fibroblasts in SOC exhibit increased reactivity that translates clinically to the increased incidence of hypertrophic and keloidal scarring in darker skin types.[7,16,17] This tendency toward abnormal scarring must be considered when treating with lasers inducing iatrogenic dermal injury.[7]

Aging

As mentioned previously, increased melanin in SOC confers increased photoprotection and, in turn, delayed photoaging. Signs of aging may develop 10 to 20 years later in SOC individuals compared to Whites.[19,20] The aging process in SOC is not only delayed compared to White individuals, but also distinct in its morphology. Photoaging in SOC presents more commonly with pigmentary irregularities rather than rhytids.[1,12] Pigmentary changes appear earlier in SOC compared to Whites, while wrinkles appear later.[9] Additionally, aging in SOC patients, particularly Black/African-American individuals, tends to manifest as increased skin laxity and volume depletion, while in White individuals rhytids are more prototypical.[21–23] Aging skin and facial structure varies across ethnicities.[24] For example, there is a greater inclination towards mid- and lower-facial aging in Black patients.[25,26] These morphological differences in aging across skin types render distinct cosmetic concerns in SOC necessitating disparate therapeutic approaches.

COMPLICATION CONCERNS IN SKIN OF COLOR

Pigmentary Aberrations

As briefly discussed prior, patients of SOC are more subject to pigmentary alterations, which may be secondary to direct melanosome disruption as well as postinflammatory effects.[9] Reactive melanocytes in SOC patients increases the risk of pigmentary alterations. Postinflammatory hyperpigmentation (PIH) has been reported as the third most common diagnosis in Black patients presenting to a dermatologist.[14] Histologically, PIH correlates with pigmentary incontinence secondary to inflammation and disruption at the dermal–epidermal junction. In turn, greater dermal–epidermal junction inflammation and disruption increases the risk of PIH.[1] This is well demonstrated in lichenoid dermatitis such as lichen planus characterized by inflammation nearly obscuring of the dermal–epidermal junction with resultant pigmentary incontinence, clinically observable with marked PIH.[27]

In the setting of laser treatment, disruption of the dermal–epidermal junction is most commonly attributed to bulk heating.[28] As melanin has a broad absorption spectrum (250–1200 nm), it can be targeted by all visible light and near infrared dermatologic lasers.[29] This can become problematic when increased melanin in the epidermis of SOC competes with the intended chromophore target of the laser in use.[12] Lasers transmit energy (in the form of photons) that, when nonspecifically or unintentionally absorbed by the increased melanin in the basal epidermis of SOC patients, leads to bulk heating and thermal injury with associated risk of pigmentary changes.[29] Hence, it would follow that higher epidermal melanin content, as in SOC, is associated with an increased risk of pigmentary complications when utilizing lasers that target melanin. This concept is important clinically as any sun exposure preceding laser treatment induces increased epidermal melanin, heightening the risk of dyspigmentation.[12]

It is not surprising, therefore, that while transient hyperpigmentation is the most common side effect after laser resurfacing, the incidence of this complication is significantly higher in skin types IV–VI.[29] Reported incidence of PIH from resurfacing in SOC patients ranges widely from 4% to 90% depending on the choice of laser and settings.[7,30,31]

Though hyperpigmentation is exceedingly more common, hypopigmentation can occur as well. Hypopigmentation can even result from 1064-nm laser toning, which entails very low-fluence, high-frequency, repetitive treatments.[32] Hypopigmentation tends to present later, even 6 months or more postprocedure. Additionally, hypopigmentation is less transient and more recalcitrant to treatment compared to hyperpigmentation.[29] Clinically, the etiology of hypopigmentation after laser procedures can be difficult to discern. Though easily attributed to the frequent concomitant use of retinoids or hydroquinone, hypopigmentation secondary to these topical medications typically resolves with discontinuation of application.[33]

Unintended epidermal absorption not only can cause epidermal injury, but also decreases the amount of energy reaching the laser's intended target. With inadequate energy reaching the target, efficacy is lost and the patient has an unsatisfactory clinical result. Additional potential adverse effects beyond dyspigmentation include textural changes, focal atrophy, and scarring.[29] Test spots can be considered to assess for these alterations prior to more extensive treatment.[6]

Keloidal and Hypertrophic Scarring

As discussed prior, darker skin exhibits a more exuberant fibroblastic response. Accordingly, SOC patients are more prone to abnormal scarring in response to injury with development of hypertrophic and keloid scars.[7] This must be taken into consideration, particularly in patients of African and Asian ancestry, when performing laser resurfacing involving dermal injury.[9] The risk of hypertrophic and keloidal scarring can be anticipated by predicting the degree of dermal injury and identifying patients' personal and family history of abnormal scarring.[10]

NUANCES AND BEST PRACTICES FOR SKIN OF COLOR

Patient Selection

As with any medical procedure, a thorough history and physical exam is an essential first step in determining if a patient may be a candidate for laser surgery.

Contraindications including active cutaneous infection, recent sun exposure, current isotretinoin use, history of photosensitivity disorders, history of keloidal scarring, and history of body dysmorphic disorder must be recognized and discussed. An additional measure paramount in preparation for laser or other cosmetic surgery is ensuring and establishing of realistic patient expectations. Standardized photographs at baseline can aid in this task. Treatment options and their associated risks must be elucidated.[12]

Laser Selection
Ablative Lasers

Long the gold standard for skin resurfacing, ablative lasers, including carbon dioxide (CO_2) and erbium-doped yttrium aluminum garnet (Er:YAG), allow for excellent clinical results. However, these results are not achieved without considerable downtime and significant risk of potential side effects.[12] The risk of potential side effects with ablative resurfacing, including dyschromia and scarring, is universal but heightened in patients of SOC.[12,23] The increased risk of adverse effects when performing ablative laser resurfacing in SOC demands extreme caution in efforts to avoid pigmentary complications.[34,35] The higher risk of pigmentary aberrations in skin types IV–VI is widely accepted, though studies in types V–VI skin are limited.[6] These risks have established traditional fully ablative laser resurfacing largely contraindicated in SOC patients.[36] However, advances

in laser technology with the development of ablative fractional (AFL) and nonablative fractional lasers (NAFLs) introduced alternative safe and effective treatments for laser resurfacing in SOC patients.[7,28]

Fractional Lasers

In fractional photothermolysis, laser energy is concentrated to microscopic treatment zones (MTZ) with intervening untreated skin. A fixed percentage of skin undergoes laser-induced thermal injury, while the surrounding skin serves as a reservoir allowing for rapid healing. This mechanism of laser-energy delivery allows for clinical results comparable to fully ablative resurfacing without as significant downtime or side effect profile.[12] While fully ablative laser treatment induces nonspecific thermal damage and bulk tissue heating with total disruption of the dermal–epidermal junction, fractional-laser treatment spares the dermal–epidermal junction in zones of untreated skin. This translates clinically as a reduced risk of PIH with fractional laser treatment.[1]

Incorporation of this tissue-sparing laser technology, AFL have been utilized successfully and safely in patients of SOC, particularly in Asian patients (Figs. 14.1 and 14.2). One study found fractional CO_2 ablative laser treatment in Chinese patients to improve skin texture, laxity, rhytids, enlarged pores, and acne scarring.[37] Others have similarly supported AFL resurfacing in Asian patients as an effective treatment modality for atrophic scarring and photoaging.[1]

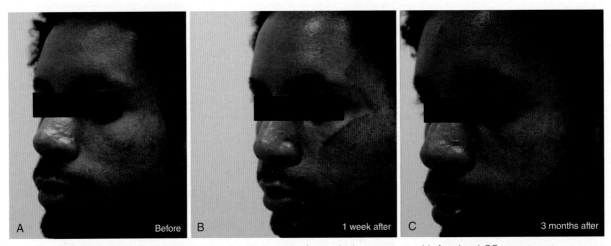

Fig. 14.1. (A) Acne scarring before and (B) 1 week after a single treatment with fractional CO_2; treatment parameters using 15 mj/m2, 10% density, and 75 Hz, (C) 3 months after the laser resurfacing. (*Photo courtesy P. Kosari, MD*)

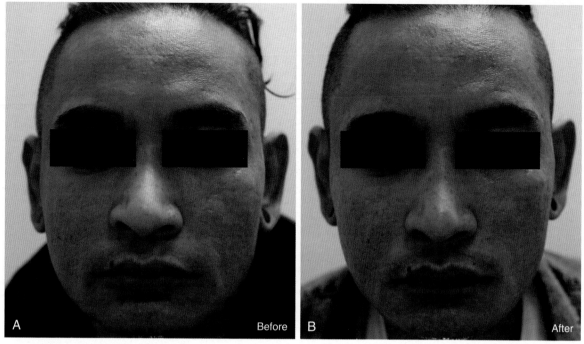

Fig. 14.2. Mild acne scarring treated with fractional CO_2 resurfacing (A) before and (B) 3 months after treatment. (*Photo courtesy P. Kosari, MD*)

AFL resurfacing, though preferable to fully ablative resurfacing in terms of its safety profile, must be prudently practiced. Though decreased, the risk of dyspigmentation still exists in AFL surgery with rates of PIH reported from 50% to 92%.[37–39] Importantly, PIH from fractional laser treatment is typically less significant and more transient than PIH from NAFL.[33,40] One study found the rate of PIH after fractional CO_2 treatment in Chinese patients to diminish with time, from 55.5% at 1 month to 11.1% at 6 months.[12] Careful patient selection for AFL resurfacing is essential, as younger patients with acne scarring or mild photodamage may be less willing to undergo the downtime and accept the possible dyspigmentation risks compared to elderly patients with advanced facial aging.[1]

Nonablative Lasers

Nonablative lasers prove to be yet another treatment alternative with shorter recovery time and reduced risk of adverse effects compared to both fully and fractional ablative lasers. Though unable to achieve as dramatic of clinical result as ablative lasers, nonablative lasers provides patients, particularly of SOC, with a safe option

for resurfacing.[9] In Asian patients, NAFL is considered by some as the treatment of choice for atrophic scarring and photorejuventation.[1]

Through dermal heating, which can also be fractionally delivered with some devices, nonablative lasers allow for improvement in texture, scarring, and rhytids with less downtime and a more favorable side effect profile compared to ablative lasers.[8,12] Nonablative lasers fall in the mid-infrared portion of the electromagnetic spectrum, thus targeting water rather than melanin, but also not producing the epidermal destruction seen with ablative lasers.[9] Wavelengths of lasers such as 1320-nm neodymium-doped yttrium aluminum garnet (Nd:YAG), 1450-nm diode, and 1540-nm erbium-glass (Er:glass) fall in this optimal range to target water while sparing the epidermis.[8] Both of these characteristics are advantageous when used for remodeling in SOC patients. The rate of PIH development in SOC patients undergoing nonablative laser treatment in multiple studies is notably low or nonexistent. Some find these lasers, particularly 1440-nm diode and 1927-nm thulium, especially helpful in treating the unique characteristics of photoaging, predominant pigmentary changes with less significant wrinkling, seen in SOC.[41,42]

Multiple studies have evaluated use of NAFL in Asian patients. Low-energy, low-density NAFL using a fractionated diode laser is effective for early signs of enlarged pore size, textural changes, and dyspigmentation.[41] More significant photoaging can be improved with a low-density 1550-nm laser, while dyspigmentation along with lentigines and macular seborrheic keratoses are best addressed with a 1927-nm thulium laser.[42,43] Additionally, NAFL can reduce periorbital and forehead rhytids with efficacy nearing that seen with ablative fractional laser resurfacing.[44,45]

Studies in darker phototypes are limited, but with promising data. Fractional 1440-nm diode has improved pore size and skin texture without PIH development in types IV and VI skin.[46] Similarly, one study comparing NAFL with AFL CO_2 resurfacing for acne scarring in patients with skin types up to V found NAFL to be superior in reducing pore size.[47]

Though superior in terms of safety profile, nonablative lasers are limited in the degree of clinical improvement that can be achieved in comparison to ablative lasers.[27,48] However, NAFL seems to be superior to traditional nonablative laser treatment for wrinkle reduction.[28] Additionally, NAFL is superior to other modalities for certain indications, such as chemical reconstruction of skin scars (CROSS) for rolling scars.[49] Altogether, nonablative laser resurfacing is a beneficial option for SOC patients to achieve satisfactory clinical results without the unacceptable side effect profile of both fully and fractionated ablative lasers.

Visible and Near-Infrared Lasers

Nonablative lasers, with wavelengths falling in the mid-infrared range, do not target melanin as a chromophore, an advantage when treating melanin-rich SOC.[30] However, melanin is absorbed broadly by lasers with wavelengths in the visible and near infrared range. While the range of melanin absorption extends across many wavelengths, it peaks in the ultraviolet range and decreases as wavelengths lengthen.[8,36] Additionally, longer wavelength lasers penetrate deeper into the dermis up to 1300 nm.[50] Thus, longer wavelength lasers, such as a 1064-nm Nd:YAG, are less efficiently absorbed by the competing epidermal melanin and therefore safer in SOC patients.[6,7,50] Resurfacing with both microsecond and long-pulsed 1064-nm Nd:YAG laser has been shown to be effective in skin types III–VI with low risk of complications.[4,7] When treating with visible or near-infrared lasers, safest treatments are performed with longer wavelength lasers, longer pulse durations, and appropriate cooling.[28]

Intense-pulsed light (IPL), a polychromatic light with wavelengths (500–1200 nm) ranging over the visible and near-infrared spectrum, must be utilized judiciously in SOC, if at all.[6,51] IPL wavelengths extensively overlap with sections of the spectrum strongly absorbed by melanin, increasing the risk of unintended epidermal absorption in SOC. Hence, IPL settings must be adjusted to allow only for longer wavelengths when treating SOC. This has been done successfully as studies describes the efficacy of IPL treatment in Asian patients for facial lentigines, skin texture, and photoaging with negligible adverse effects.[52,53]

Other Energy Devices

Radiofrequency and ultrasound devices are excellent alternatives to lasers, particularly for rejuvenation and aging in SOC patients (Table 14.1). Radiofrequency delivers an electric current that generates heat in the dermis secondary to tissue impedance.[54–57] Fractional radiofrequency can be performed through use of radiofrequency microneedling (RFMN), which incorporates microneedles that mechanically penetrate the epidermis while delivering radiofrequency currents to the dermis.[58,59] On the other hand, high-intensity focused ultrasound (HIFU) transmits acoustic energy-inducing vibrations that cause coagulative necrosis beneath the epidermis.[51]

Melanin is not a chromophore target of these devices, which is ideal for treatment in SOC.[7] Additionally, radiofrequency and ultrasound devices focus their

TABLE 14.1	**Device Options for Specific Rejuvenation concerns**	
Rejuvenation Concern	**Device Options**
Mild rhytids	Fractional resurfacing
Moderate rhytids	Fractional resurfacing, radiofrequency microneedling, Nd:YAG 1064 nm
Acne scars	Fractional resurfacing, radiofrequency microneedling
Skin tightening	Radiofrequency microneedling, high-intensity focused ultrasound

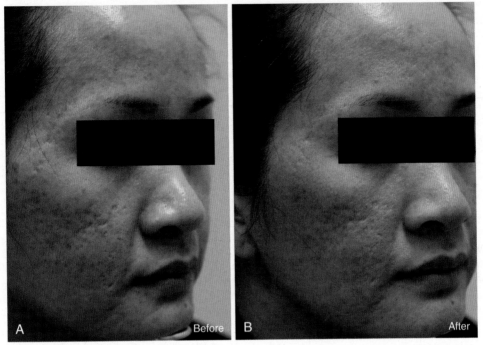

Fig. 14.3. Mild to moderate acne scarring (A) before and (B) 2 months after 2 treatments with radiofrequency microneedling.

energy in the dermis to induce collagen contraction and remodeling, sparing the epidermis.[11] While RFMN does partially disrupt the epidermis, portions of the epidermis are left intact, allowing for quicker healing. Additionally, unlike lasers, RFMN does not induce thermal activation of melanocytes.[60] These characteristics decrease the risk of epidermal injury and subsequent pigmentary alterations, making these devices safe in all skin types.[7,8] However, with improper operator technique, thermal epidermal injury is possible and can be detrimental.[7] Cooling must be utilized during monopolar radiofrequency treatment to protect darker skin types from epidermal injury.[8,12]

Through nonspecific dermal damage, radiofrequency and ultrasound devices provoke collagen contraction and remodeling with subsequent clinically apparent skin tightening.[11,12,59] In fact, fractional radiofrequency has shown durable improvement in periorbital rhytids and superior efficacy for nasolabial, perioral, jawline, and neck rhytids in comparison to fractional Er:YAG resurfacing.[61] RFMN can also be efficacious for acne scarring (Fig. 14.3), without disruption of the epidermis. These devices may be of great

benefit in aging SOC patients as they are both safe and address skin laxity, a common presentation of aging in SOC. Studies observing SOC patients have demonstrated skin tightening devices to be efficacious.[62]

Laser Practice Nuances

Even when using a laser deemed safe for use in darker skin, selection of proper treatment parameters is crucial to avoid complications.[8,63] Herein we will discuss general parameter and practice considerations, though these must be adjusted on a case-by-case basis in light of the individual patient and laser at use (Box 14.1).

Settings

Fluence. Related to laser energy, fluence is the measure of energy per cm^2, while power describes the rate of energy delivery.[51] Energy and fluence are important factors as melanin-targeting lasers deliver energy that is absorbed exceptionally efficiently in melanin-rich darker skin. Fluence settings should therefore be minimized to limit damage to surrounding tissue while still achieving clinical effect.[8] Studies assessing the impact of fluence on PIH development

Box 14.1   General Practice Considerations for Resurfacing in Skin of Color

Low fluence
Low density
Less passes
Increased pre- and postoperative cooling
Avoid pulse stacking
Use of a test spot
Increased total number of treatments
Increased interval between treatments

when performing nonablative resurfacing in SOC patients are discordant. Some describe higher fluences to be associated with increased PIH incidence, while others have found no statistically significant relationship.[30,64] Even when PIH did occur in these studies, the complication rate was low and self-limited with complete resolution.[64] Nevertheless, to avoid potential complications in SOC, particularly in areas at high risk of dyspigmentation such as infraorbital skin, fluences should be set conservatively.[8,47]

Density. Density, or the percentage of skin surface subject to laser-energy delivery by fractional lasers, is arguably the most important parameter to consider when performing laser resurfacing in SOC. In general, higher-density settings are more efficacious and require less treatment sessions.[51] However, these results do not come without increased risk, particularly in SOC patients. Few studies of resurfacing in types IV–VI skin found no difference in efficacy or risk of PIH at varying densities. One split-face trial of 1550 nm resurfacing in types IV–VI skin observed greater improvement and more pain with higher-density treatment, but there was no significant difference in PIH development between high and low densities.[65]

However, the majority of studies describe the importance of lower-density settings to reduce occurrence of PIH.[1,6,7,12,27,66,67] Density settings should be more conservative when treating skin types I–III.[9] Many identify treatment density as a stronger factor than energy contributing to PIH development.[9,27,66] One study found high-energy and low-density settings to be less likely to cause PIH than low-energy and high-density settings, though results were not statistically significant.[27] In general, higher-density settings correlated with increased incidence of PIH when treating forearms of Chinese patients with 1540-nm Er:glass. However, within groups

with identical densities, those treated with higher energy also had increased rates of PIH, highlighting the importance of both of these parameters.[27]

The impact of density can be observed histologically, as high-density fractional resurfacing results in a significantly greater inflammatory infiltrate compared to low- and moderate-density treatments.[68] Increasing density from 10% to 20% has increased prolonged PIH from an average 50.5 days to 62.5 days.[67] In Asian patients, a greater number of low-density treatments performed at further intervals achieved similar results with less PIH development.[1] Similarly, one study compared a series of three NAFR treatments comprised of eight passes of a low-density treatment to a series of six NAFR treatments comprised of four passes at half of the density of the first group. The groups demonstrated equivalent clinically efficacy, but those treated with less passes at a lower density had a significantly lower rate of complications.[43] Though beneficial in preventing adverse effects, low-density and low-energy settings do inevitably mandate the need for longer series of treatments to achieve desired efficacy.[69–71] In general, use of lower densities, more numerous treatments, and sufficient recovery periods between treatments are practice strategies to achieve the optimal results while minimizing complications.[1,43]

Other practice recommendations. When performing ablative resurfacing, avoidance of pulse stacking and significant overlap reduces the risk of scarring.[8] Between each laser pass, partially desiccated tissue should be removed. If only a single pass is performed, remnant desiccated tissue can remain to act as a biologic wound dressing.[72] Additionally, as in all skin types, fully ablative resurfacing in nonfacial skin, particularly the neck and chest, must be either avoided or performed with extreme caution as these areas have few pilosebaceous units for reepithelization.[73] However, with proper technique and settings, NAFL and low-density AFL can be effective and performed safely on nonfacial skin.[74,75]

In general, reducing inflammation aids to prevent PIH. This can be achieved by increasing the interval between treatments to allow for resolution of inflammation prior to the next session.[27] Furthermore, development of PIH is an indication to lengthen the duration between sessions.[9] PIH can also be attributed to bulk heating. Methods to avoid bulk heating include widening treatment intervals, decreasing the number of passes, and increasing cooling preoperatively, postoperatively, and between passes.[6,9,27,66,68] Particularly when employing contact cooling, slow treatment speed and increased time between passes maximizes cooling.[7] Adequate cooling is essential when treating smaller surface areas as smaller sites are more prone to bulk heating.[27]

Given the complexity of selecting a laser and its respective settings for safe treatment in SOC patients, use of a test spot and conservative settings is prudent to avoid complications.[76] Ideally, treatment should be planned 2 to 3 weeks after performing a test spot for adequate time to evaluate the skin's response.[36]

Pre- and Posttreatment Recommendations

Sunscreen. Regular sunscreen use after laser treatment is widely recommended. Some suggest sunscreen with a sun protective factor (SPF) of 30 or greater should be applied for several weeks prior to treatment and reinitiated as soon as able postoperatively.[77] Use of sunscreen has been shown to be protective against PIH development after ablative fractional resurfacing.[78] One split-face study in type IV skin found starting sunscreen application 1 day after ablative resurfacing to have decreased rates of PIH compared to use of petroleum only.[31] Sun protection and avoidance should be continued in the weeks following treatment.[1] In SOC patients, this recommendation must be especially emphasized. A gap in public knowledge exists regarding sunscreen use in darker skin types, and rates of sunscreen use is lower in these populations.[6,10] For patients of SOC who regularly use sunscreen, vitamin D supplementation may be necessary.[10,79]

Topical corticosteroids. Pre- and postoperative topical corticosteroids is recommended, particularly in the setting of posttreatment edema or erythema.[6,7] Corticosteroids are thought to suppress cell activity and consequentially melanin production.[80] Clinically, clobetasol ointment use in Asian patients undergoing ablative fractional resurfacing minimized PIH development.[81] Though generally recommended and beneficial for preventing PIH, topical corticosteroids may delay wound healing and increase infection risk.[31]

Hydroquinone and other topical agents. The use of hydroquinone or other bleaching topicals to prevent PIH in SOC patients undergoing laser resurfacing is debated. Studies are conflicting on the efficacy of prophylactic hydroquinone for the prevention of PIH.[6] If hydroquinone is utilized, it should be applied over 2 to 4 weeks prior to laser treatment and resumed posttreatment for a 4-week course.[7] It should be avoided in the

week immediately following laser treatment in efforts to avoid potential irritation.[82]

Hydroquinone can also be utilized for the treatment of PIH if this complication were to occur. One study of both ablative and nonablative fractional resurfacing in primarily type IV skin found all cases of PIH resolved with use of hydroquinone 4% or 6% with retinoic acid, glycolic acid, or kojic acid in 6 to 8 weeks in addition to strict sun avoidance.[47]

Other prophylactic topical agents with debated efficacy include tretinoin and glycolic acid.[83] Retinoic acid may speed reepithelization when used preoperatively and reduce melanin production when used postoperatively.[84] However, it does not appear to decrease the incidence of PIH development.[8]

CONCLUSION

Resurfacing in SOC patients, formerly an unconceivable option given its unacceptable rate of complications, can now be performed safely and efficaciously with advances in laser technology. However, structural and functional differences of darker skin increase certain risks of these procedures, particularly dyspigmentation. Laser surgeons must be cognizant of these risks and practice cautiously with intentionality when performing laser resurfacing in skin of color patients.

REFERENCES

1. Wat H, Wu DC, Chan HH. Fractional resurfacing in the Asian patient: Current state of the art. *Lasers Surg Med.* 2017;49(1):45-59. doi:10.1002/lsm.22579.
2. Taylor SC, Cook-Bolden F. Defining skin of color. *Cutis.* 2002;69(6):435-437.
3. Colby SL, Ortman JM. Projections of the size and composition of the U.S. Population: 2014 to 2060. *Curr Popul Rep.* 2015:25-1143. Available at: https://www.census.gov/content/dam/Census/library/publications/2015/demo/p25-1143.pdf.
4. Roberts WE, Henry M, Burgess C, Saedi N, Chilukuri S, Campbell-Chambers DA. Laser treatment of skin of color for medical and aesthetic uses with a new 650-microsecond Nd:YAG 1064nm laser. *J Drugs Dermatol.* 2019;18(4):s135-s137.
5. *Cosmetic Surgery National Data Bank Statistics 2016.* The American Society for Aesthetic Plastic Surgery; 2017. Available at: https://www.surgery.org/sites/default/files/ASAPS-Stats2016.pdf.

6. Adotama P, Papac N, Alexis A, Wysong A, Collins L. Common dermatologic procedures and the associated complications unique to skin of color. *Dermatol Surg.* 2021;47(3):355-359. doi:10.1097/DSS.0000000000002813.

7. Alexis AF. Lasers and light-based therapies in ethnic skin: Treatment options and recommendations for Fitzpatrick skin types V and VI. *Br J Dermatol.* 2013;169 suppl 3: 91-97. doi:10.1111/bjd.12526.

8. Bhatt N, Alster TS. Laser surgery in dark skin. *Dermatol Surg.* 2008;34(2):184-195. doi:10.1111/j.1524-4725.2007.34036.x.

9. Kaushik SB, Alexis AF. Non-ablative fractional laser resurfacing in skin of color: Evidence-based review. *J Clin Aesthet Dermatol.* 2017;10(6):51-67.

10. Alexis AF, Few J, Callender VD, et al. Myths and knowledge gaps in the aesthetic treatment of patients with skin of color. *J Drugs Dermatol.* 2019;18(7):616-622.

11. Awosika O, Burgess CM, Grimes PE. Considerations when treating cosmetic concerns in men of color. *Dermatol Surg.* 2017;43 suppl 2:S140-S150. doi:10.1097/DSS.0000000000001376.

12. Chan HL, Ho S. Laser treatment of ethnic skin. In: Hruza GJ, Tanzi EL, eds. *Lasers and Lights.* Elsevier; 2018:125-144.

13. Al-Jamal MS, Griffith JL, Lim HW. Photoprotection in ethnic skin. *Dermatologica Sinica.* 2104;32(4):217-224.

14. Halder RM, Grimes PE, McLaurin CI, Kress MA, Kenney Jr JA. Incidence of common dermatoses in a predominantly Black dermatologic practice. *Cutis.* 1983;32(4):388-390.

15. Kaidbey KH, Agin PP, Sayre RM, Kligman AM. Photoprotection by melanin—a comparison of Black and Caucasian skin. *J Am Acad Dermatol.* 1979;1(3):249-260. doi:10.1016/s0190-9622(79)70018-1.

16. Taylor SC. Skin of color: Biology, structure, function, and implications for dermatologic disease. *J Am Acad Dermatol.* 2002;46(2 Suppl Understanding):S41-S62. doi:10.1067/mjd.2002.120790.

17. Butler PD, Longaker MT, Yang GP. Current progress in keloid research and treatment. *J Am Coll Surg.* 2008; 206(4):731-741. doi:10.1016/j.jamcollsurg.2007.12.001.

18. Montagna W, Carlisle K. The architecture of Black and White facial skin. *J Am Acad Dermatol.* 1991;24(6 Pt 1): 929-937. doi:10.1016/0190-9622(91)70148-u.

19. Alexis AF, Grimes P, Boyd C, et al. Racial and ethnic differences in self-assessed facial aging in women: Results from a multinational study. *Dermatol Surg.* 2019;45(12): 1635-1648. doi:10.1097/DSS.0000000000002237.

20. Rossi AM, Eviatar J, Green JB, et al. Signs of facial aging in men in a diverse, multinational study: Timing and preventive behaviors. *Dermatol Surg.* 2017;43 suppl 2: S210-S220. doi:10.1097/DSS.0000000000001293.

21. Boyd CM. Approaches to the aging face in African American patients. *Facial Plast Surg Clin North Am.* 2002;10(4):377-380. doi:10.1016/s1064-7406(02)00037-8.

22. Burgess C, Awosika O. Ethnic and gender considerations in the use of facial injectables: African-American patients. *Plast Reconstr Surg.* 2015;136(suppl 5):28S-31S. doi:10.1097/PRS.0000000000001813.

23. Davis EC, Callender VD. Aesthetic dermatology for aging ethnic skin. *Dermatol Surg.* 2011;37(7):901-917. doi:10.1111/j.1524-4725.2011.02007.x.

24. Talakoub L, Wesley NO. Differences in perceptions of beauty and cosmetic procedures performed in ethnic patients. *Semin Cutan Med Surg.* 2009;28(2):115-129. doi:10.1016/j.sder.2009.05.001.

25. Hamilton TK, Burgess CM. Considerations for the use of injectable poly-L-lactic acid in people of color. *J Drugs Dermatol.* 2010;9(5):451-456.

26. Harris MO. The aging face in patients of color: minimally invasive surgical facial rejuvenation-a targeted approach. *Dermatol Ther.* 2004;17(2):206-211. doi:10.1111/j.1396-0296.2004.04021.x.

27. Chan HH, Manstein D, Yu CS, Shek S, Kono T, Wei WI. The prevalence and risk factors of post-inflammatory hyperpigmentation after fractional resurfacing in Asians. *Lasers Surg Med.* 2007;39(5):381-385. doi:10.1002/lsm.20512.

28. Battle Jr EF, Soden Jr CE. The use of lasers in darker skin types. *Semin Cutan Med Surg.* 2009;28(2):130-140. doi:10.1016/j.sder.2009.04.003.

29. Bhatt N, Alster TS. Laser surgery in dark skin. *Dermatol Surg.* 2008;34(2):184-195. doi:10.1111/j.1524-4725.2007.34036.x.

30. Clark CM, Silverberg JI, Alexis AF. A retrospective chart review to assess the safety of non-ablative fractional laser resurfacing in Fitzpatrick skin types IV to VI. *J Drugs Dermatol.* 2013;12(4):428-431.

31. Manuskiatti W, Iamphonrat T, Wanitphakdeedecha R, Eimpunth S. Comparison of fractional erbium-doped yttrium aluminum garnet and carbon dioxide lasers in resurfacing of atrophic acne scars in Asians. *Dermatol Surg.* 2013;39(1 Pt 1):111-120. doi:10.1111/dsu.12030.

32. Shah SD, Aurangabadkar SJ. Laser toning in melasma. *J Cutan Aesthet Surg.* 2019;12(2):76-84. doi:10.4103/JCAS.JCAS_179_18.

33. Metelitsa AI, Alster TS. Fractionated laser skin resurfacing treatment complications: a review. *Dermatol Surg.* 2010;36(3):299-306. doi:10.1111/j.1524-4725.2009.01434.x.

34. Goh CL, Khoo L. Laser skin resurfacing treatment outcome of facial scars and wrinkles in Asians with skin type III/IV with the unipulse CO2 laser system. *Singapore Med J.* 2002;43:28-32.

35. Prado A, Andrades P, Danilla S, et al. Full-face carbon dioxide laser resurfacing: a 10-year follow-up descriptive study. *Plast Reconstr Surg.* 2008;121:983-993.

36. Battle Jr EF. Cosmetic laser treatments for skin of color: A focus on safety and efficacy. *J Drugs Dermatol*. 2011; 10(1):35-38.

37. Chan NP, Ho SG, Yeung CK, Shek SY, Chan HH. Fractional ablative carbon dioxide laser resurfacing for skin rejuvenation and acne scars in Asians. *Lasers Surg Med*. 2010;42(9):615-623. doi:10.1002/lsm.20974.

38. Huang L. A new modality for fractional CO2 laser resurfacing for acne scars in Asians. *Lasers Med Sci*. 2013;28(2):627-632. doi:10.1007/s10103-012-1120-5.

39. Manuskiatti W, Triwongwaranat D, Varothai S, Eimpunth S, Wanitphakdeedecha R. Efficacy and safety of a carbon-dioxide ablative fractional resurfacing device for treatment of atrophic acne scars in Asians. *J Am Acad Dermatol*. 2010;63(2):274-283. doi:10.1016/j.jaad.2009.08.051.

40. Graber EM, Tanzi EL, Alster TS. Side effects and complications of fractional laser photothermolysis: Experience with 961 treatments. *Dermatol Surg*. 2008;34(3):301-307. doi:10.1111/j.1524-4725.2007.34062.x.

41. Marmon S, Shek SY, Yeung CK, Chan NP, Chan JC, Chan HH. Evaluating the safety and efficacy of the 1,440-nm laser in the treatment of photodamage in Asian skin. *Lasers Surg Med*. 2014;46(5):375-379. doi:10.1002/lsm.22242.

42. Polder KD, Mithani A, Harrison A, Bruce S. Treatment of macular seborrheic keratoses using a novel 1927-nm fractional thulium fiber laser. *Dermatol Surg*. 2012;38(7 Pt 1): 1025-1031. doi:10.1111/j.1524-4725.2012.02427.x.

43. Chan NP, Ho SG, Yeung CK, Shek SY, Chan HH. The use of non-ablative fractional resurfacing in Asian acne scar patients. *Lasers Surg Med*. 2010;42(10):710-715. doi:10.1002/lsm.20976.

44. Moon HR, Yun WJ, Lee YJ, Lee MW, Chang S. A prospective, randomized, double-blind comparison of an ablative fractional 2940-nm erbium-doped yttrium aluminum garnet laser with a non-ablative fractional 1550-nm erbium-doped glass laser for the treatment of photoaged Asian skin. *J Dermatolog Treat*. 2015;26(6):551-557. doi:10.3109/09546634.2014.999020.

45. Wattanakrai P, Pootongkam S, Rojhirunsakool S. Periorbital rejuvenation with fractional 1,550-nm ytterbium/erbium fiber laser and variable square pulse 2,940-nm erbium:YAG laser in Asians: A comparison study. *Dermatol Surg*. 2012; 38(4):610-622. doi:10.1111/j.1524-4725.2011.02298.x.

46. Saedi N, Petrell K, Arndt K, Dover J. Evaluating facial pores and skin texture after low-energy non-ablative fractional 1440-nm laser treatments. *J Am Acad Dermatol*. 2013;68(1):113-118. doi:10.1016/j.jaad.2012.08.041.

47. Alajlan AM, Alsuwaidan SN. Acne scars in ethnic skin treated with both non-ablative fractional 1,550 nm and ablative fractional CO2 lasers: Comparative retrospective analysis with recommended guidelines. *Lasers Surg Med*. 2011;43(8):787-791. doi:10.1002/lsm.21092.

48. Izikson L. Laser photorejuvenation of Asian and ethnic skin. *J Cosmet Laser Ther*. 2008;10(3):161-166. doi:10.1080/14764170802308427.

49. Kim HJ, Kim TG, Kwon YS, Park JM, Lee JH. Comparison of a 1,550 nm Erbium: glass fractional laser and a chemical reconstruction of skin scars (CROSS) method in the treatment of acne scars: A simultaneous split-face trial. *Lasers Surg Med*. 2009;41(8):545-549. doi:10.1002/lsm.20796.

50. Tanzi EL, Lupton JR, Alster TS. Lasers in dermatology: Four decades of progress. *J Am Acad Dermatol*. 2003;49(1): 1-34. doi:10.1067/mjd.2003.582.

51. Bolognia J, Schaffer JV, Cerroni L, eds. *Dermatology*. 4th ed. Elsevier; 2018.

52. Negishi K, Tezuka Y, Kushikata N, Wakamatsu S. Photorejuvenation for Asian skin by intense pulsed light. *Dermatol Surg*. 2001;27(7):627-632. doi:10.1046/j.1524-4725.2001.01002.x.

53. Tanaka Y, Tsunemi Y, Kawashima M. Objective assessment of intensive targeted treatment for solar lentigines using intense pulsed light with wavelengths between 500 and 635 nm. *Lasers Surg Med*. 2016;48(1):30-35. doi:10.1002/lsm.22433.

54. Rongsaard N, Rummaneethorn P. Comparison of a fractional bipolar radiofrequency device and a fractional erbium-doped glass 1,550-nm device for the treatment of atrophic acne scars: A randomized split-face clinical study. *Dermatol Surg*. 2014;40(1):14-21. doi:10.1111/dsu.12372.

55. Qin X, Li H, Jian X, Yu B. Evaluation of the efficacy and safety of fractional bipolar radiofrequency with high-energy strategy for treatment of acne scars in Chinese. *J Cosmet Laser Ther*. 2015;17(5):237-245. doi:10.3109/14764172.2015.1007070.

56. Yeung CK, Chan NP, Shek SY, Chan HH. Evaluation of combined fractional radiofrequency and fractional laser treatment for acne scars in Asians. *Lasers Surg Med*. 2012; 44(8):622-630. doi:10.1002/lsm.22063.

57. Zhang Z, Fei Y, Chen X, Lu W, Chen J. Comparison of a fractional microplasma radio frequency technology and carbon dioxide fractional laser for the treatment of atrophic acne scars: A randomized split-face clinical study. *Dermatol Surg*. 2013;39(4):559-566. doi:10.1111/dsu.12103.

58. Munavalli G, Childs J, Ross EV. Radiofrequency microneedling. *Adv Cosmet Surg*. 2020;3(1):25-38.

59. Tan MG, Jo CE, Chapas A, Khetarpal S, Dover JS. Radiofrequency microneedling: A comprehensive and critical review. *Dermatol Surg*. 2021;47(6):755-761. doi:10.1097/DSS.0000000000002972.

60. Cohen BE, Elbuluk N. Microneedling in skin of color: a review of uses and efficacy. *J Am Acad Dermatol*. 2016; 74(2):348-355. doi:10.1016/j.jaad.2015.09.024.

61. Serdar ZA, Tatlıparmak A. Comparison of efficacy and safety of fractional radiofrequency and fractional Er:YAG laser in facial and neck wrinkles: Six-year experience with 333 patients. *Dermatol Ther.* 2019;32(5):e13054. doi:10.1111/dth.13054.

62. Woolery-Lloyd H, Viera MH, Valins W. Laser therapy in Black skin. *Facial Plast Surg Clin North Am.* 2011;19(2): 405-416. doi:10.1016/j.fsc.2011.05.007.

63. Tanzi EL, Alster TS. Cutaneous laser surgery in darker skin phototypes. *Cutis.* 2004;73(1):21-30.

64. Mahmoud BH, Srivastava D, Janiga JJ, Yang JJ, Lim HW, Ozog DM. Safety and efficacy of erbium-doped yttrium aluminum garnet fractionated laser for treatment of acne scars in type IV to VI skin. *Dermatol Surg.* 2010;36(5): 602-609. doi:10.1111/j.1524-4725.2010.01513.x.

65. Alexis AF, Coley MK, Nijhawan RI, et al. Non-ablative fractional laser resurfacing for acne scarring in patients with Fitzpatrick skin phototypes·IV-VI. *Dermatol Surg.* 2016;42(3):392-402. doi:10.1097/DSS.0000000000000640.

66. Kono T, Chan HH, Groff WF, et al. Prospective direct comparison study of fractional resurfacing using different fluences and densities for skin rejuvenation in Asians. *Lasers Surg Med.* 2007;39(4):311-314. doi:10.1002/lsm.20484.

67. Yuan XH, Zhong SX, Li SS. Comparison study of fractional carbon dioxide laser resurfacing using different fluences and densities for acne scars in Asians: A randomized split-face trial. *Dermatol Surg.* 2014;40(5): 545-552. doi:10.1111/dsu.12467.

68. Manstein D, Herron GS, Sink RK, Tanner H, Anderson RR. Fractional photothermolysis: A new concept for cutaneous remodeling using microscopic patterns of thermal injury. *Lasers Surg Med.* 2004;34(5):426-438. doi:10.1002/lsm.20048.

69. Laubach HJ, Tannous Z, Anderson RR, Manstein D. Skin responses to fractional photothermolysis. *Lasers Surg Med.* 2006;38(2):142-149. doi:10.1002/lsm.20254.

70. Nouveau-Richard S, Yang Z, Mac-Mary S, et al. Skin ageing: A comparison between Chinese and European populations. A pilot study. *J Dermatol Sci.* 2005;40(3):187-193. doi:10.1016/j.jdermsci.2005.06.006.

71. Tsukahara K, Fujimura T, Yoshida Y, et al. Comparison of age-related changes in wrinkling and sagging of the skin in Caucasian females and in Japanese females. *J Cosmet Sci.* 2004;55(4):351-371.

72. Alster T, Hirsch R. Single-pass CO2 laser skin resurfacing of light and dark skin: Extended experience with 52 patients. *J Cosmet Laser Ther.* 2003;5(1):39-42.

73. Alster TS, Lupton JR. Prevention and treatment of side effects and complications of cutaneous laser resurfacing. *Plast Reconstr Surg.* 2002;109(1):308-318. doi:10.1097/00006534-200201000-00048.

74. Oram Y, Akkaya AD. Neck rejuvenation with fractional CO2 laser: Long-term results. *J Clin Aesthet Dermatol.* 2014;7(8):23-29.

75. Preissig J, Hamilton K, Markus R. Current laser resurfacing technologies: A review that delves beneath the surface. *Semin Plast Surg.* 2012;26(3):109-116. doi:10.1055/s-0032-1329413.

76. Downie JB. Esthetic considerations for ethnic skin. *Semin Cutan Med Surg.* 2006;25(3):158-162. doi:10.1016/j.sder.2006.06.009.

77. Alster TS. Preoperative patient considerations. In: Alster TS, ed. *Manual of Cutaneous Laser Techniques.* 2nd ed. Philadelphia, PA: Lippincott Williams & Wilkins; 2000:13-32.

78. Wanitphakdeedecha R, Phuardchantuk R, Manuskiatti W. The use of sunscreen starting on the first day after ablative fractional skin resurfacing. *J Eur Acad Dermatol Venereol.* 2014;28(11):1522-1528. doi:10.1111/jdv.12332.

79. Tseng M, Giri V, Bruner DW, Giovannucci E. Prevalence and correlates of vitamin D status in African American men. *BMC Public Health.* 2009;9:191. doi:10.1186/1471-2458-9-191.

80. Tomita Y, Maeda K, Tagami H. Melanocyte-stimulating properties of arachidonic acid metabolites: Possible role in postinflammatory pigmentation. *Pigment Cell Res.* 1992;5(5 Pt 2):357-361. doi:10.1111/j.1600-0749.1992.tb00562.x.

81. Cheyasak N, Manuskiatti W, Maneeprasopchoke P, Wanitphakdeedecha R. Topical corticosteroids minimise the risk of postinflammatory hyper-pigmentation after ablative fractional CO2 laser resurfacing in Asians. *Acta Derm Venereol.* 2015;95(2):201-205. doi:10.2340/00015555-1899.

82. Alexis AF. Fractional laser resurfacing of acne scarring in patients with Fitzpatrick skin types IV-VI. *J Drugs Dermatol.* 2011;10(suppl 12):s6-s7.

83. West TB, Alster TS. Effect of pretreatment on the incidence of hyperpigmentation following cutaneous CO2 laser resurfacing. *Dermatol Surg.* 1999;25(1):15-17. doi:10.1046/j.1524-4725.1999.08123.x.

84. McDonald WS, Beasley D, Jones C. Retinoic acid and CO2 laser resurfacing. *Plast Reconstr Surg.* 1999;104(7):2229-2238. doi:10.1097/00006534-199912000-00044.

15

Chemical Peels: Nuances and Best Practices for Skin of Color

Pearl E. Grimes

SUMMARY AND KEY FEATURES

- Chemical peels are efficacious and safe in skin of color.
- As you increase the depth of the peeling agent increases, there is an increase in the likelihood of experiencing complications.
- Priming the skin prior to peeling optimizes outcomes.
- Superficial peels are often best in skin of color.

INTRODUCTION

Chemical peeling involves the topical application of wounding agents to the skin to induce controlled injury to the epidermis and dermis with subsequent organized regeneration and repair of the skin. The early history of chemical peeling encompasses an Egyptian tradition of using alpha hydroxy acids in sour milk to enhance the beauty and texture of the skin. Other agents used included alabaster, animal oils, and salt.[1] The science of chemical peeling has undergone substantial advances in the last century. Fox, Hebra, Unna, and Stegman pioneered many of the fundamental concepts currently used for chemical peeling in dermatology.[2,3]

Peeling procedures are currently used in all skin types for facial resurfacing and rejuvenation. There has been enormous growth in the frequency of cosmetic procedures, including chemical peels, in darker-skinned racial-ethnic groups. Darker-skinned individuals represent the majority of the global population and include Africans, Afro Caribbeans, Hispanics, East and South Asians, Middle Easterners, Malaysians, Aleuts, Eskimos, and Pacific Islanders. Moreover, Census Bureau data

project that by the year 2045, people of color will represent the majority of the U.S. population.[4] Recent 2020 survey data from the American Society of Plastic Surgeons (ASPS) reported that people of color constituted 34% of all cosmetic procedures performed, compared to 20% in 2005. Hispanics accounted for 13%, African Americans 11%, Asian Americans 8%, and others 2%. Of those surveyed, chemical peels were performed in 931,473 individuals and in 28% of subjects with skin of color.[5] These numbers continue to grow.

MORPHOLOGIC AND STRUCTURAL DIFFERENCES IN SKIN OF COLOR

The unique structural, aging, and pigmentary differences significantly influence the choice of the peeling agent and the depth of peeling. Myriad morphologic features define pigmented skin.[6–8] There are no quantitative differences in melanocytes among various racial-ethnic groups. The melanocytes of darker-skinned individuals, in particular Black skin, produce more epidermal melanin. In addition, melanosomes are often large and singly dispersed within melanocytes and keratinocytes throughout the epidermis. However, in Whites and Asians, melanosomes are limited to the basal and lower Malpighian layer of the epidermis. They are smaller and often aggregated and membrane bound. Dark skin demonstrates significantly greater intrinsic photoprotection compared to white skin. On average, five times as much ultraviolet light reaches the upper dermis of White compared to Black skin. The increased epidermal melanin of Black skin serves as a significant filter for blocking ultraviolet light transmission and provides a natural sun protective factor of 13.1 compared to 3.4 for White skin.[9] Other features of deeply pigmented skin include a more compact stratum corneum, increased epidermal lipids, and large, active, binucleated, and multinucleated dermal fibroblasts.[6–8] This increased activity of fibroblasts may predispose patients to keloids and hypertrophic scars.

Clinical features of photodamage, aging skin, actinic keratosis, rhytids, and skin malignancies are less common problems in deeply pigmented skin.[10–12] In a detailed comparison of skin aging in different racial-ethnic groups, Black/African-American women in different age groups of 20–24, 40–44, and 60–64 (Fitzpatrick V and VI) were compared to similar groupings of White women. Biopsies were taken from photo-exposed facial skin and arms and photo-protected buttock skin. Elastosis was marked in the photo-exposed skin of the White women in the 40-plus age group but relatively absent in Black/African-American skin.[13]

Darker skin types are frequently plagued with dyschromias because of the labile response of cutaneous melanocytes. In a survey of 2000 Black patients seeking dermatology care in a private practice in Washington, DC, the third most commonly cited skin disorders following acne and eczema were pigmentary problems other than vitiligo.[14] Similarly, in a series of Hispanic patients, pigmentary disorders were the third most common reason for seeking dermatologic treatment.[15] In addition, in 1412 patients visiting an urban dermatology clinic, dyschromias were the most common diagnosis in Black patients.[16] Cosmetic issues of concern may also differ in darker versus lighter skin types. In a survey assessing issues of cosmetic concern in 100 women of color, the most commonly cited problems were dark spots or blotchy skin, texturally rough skin, oily skin, and increased sensitivity to topical products. Wrinkles and photodamage were significantly less frequent issues of concern when compared to an age-matched White population of 141 women.[17]

INDICATIONS AND PEEL SELECTION

The indications for peeling procedures differ in darker racial-ethnic groups compared to lighter skin types (Table 15.1). Key indications in darker skin include disorders of hyperpigmentation such as postinflammatory

TABLE 15.1   Summary of Clinical Features, Peeling Indications, and Types of Peels Commonly Used in Lighter Skin Types (Fitzpatrick I-III) Versus Skin of Color (IV-VI)

	Skin Types I-III	Skin Types IV-VI
Clinical Features	Coarse and Fine Wrinkles Laxity Solar Keratoses Sallowness Mild to Moderate Pigmentary Changes	Minimal Wrinkling Jowl Formation Minimal Solar Keratoses Hypertrophic Scarring Moderate to Severe Hyperpigmentation
Indications	Rhytids Solar Keratoses Acne Vulgaris Hyperpigmentation Scarring	Hyperpigmentation Acne vulgaris Textural Changes Pseudofolliculitis barbae Fine Wrinkles Acne Scarring Laxity
Peels	Superficial Medium Depth Deep	Superficial Medium Depth

hyperpigmentation and melasma, texturally rough skin, oily skin, acne vulgaris, and pseudofolliculitis barbae. Peels can also improve fine lines and mild laxity. In contrast, primary indications in lighter skin types (Fitzpatrick I-III) are rhytids, photodamage, solar elastosis, acne vulgaris, textural changes, scarring, and dyschromia.

Chemical peels are classified as superficial (very light and light), medium depth, and deep peeling (Fig. 15.1). Choosing the appropriate peeling agent most often varies with the skin type of the individual and the condition being treated as complications and side effects are often commiserate with the depth of the peel. Superficial peels target the stratum corneum to the papillary dermis.[18] Commonly used agents include alpha hydroxy acids, salicylic acid, tretinoin, Jessner's solution, and lower concentrations of trichloroacetic acid (TCA). They are most often used to treat hyperpigmentation, mild photodamage, and acne vulgaris. Medium-depth peels penetrate to the upper-reticular dermis and include TCA 35% to 50% and phenol 88%. Indications include mild to moderate rhytids and photodamage, hyperpigmentation, acne scars, and premalignant lesions. Deep peels penetrate the mid-reticular dermis and typically use variations of the Baker–Gordon phenol formula. Phenol peeling is most often used for severe rhytids and photodamage, scarring, premalignant lesions, and hyperpigmentation. It is optimal for skin types I and II; however, in darker skin types, phenol peels can induce severe post-peel erythema and prolonged hypo- and hyperpigmentation. In general, it should be avoided in skin types V and VI.

Given the structural, physiologic, and aging differences in skin of color, a review of published databases suggest that optimal peeling outcomes in skin of color can be achieved utilizing the spectrum of superficial peeling agents, while simultaneously minimizing complications.

PATIENT EVALUATION AND PEEL PRIMING

A detailed history and cutaneous examination should be performed in all patients before chemical peeling. Any history of cutaneous or systemic illnesses, including hypertrophic scars and keloids, smoking, or surgeries that could impact the peel procedure and healing, should be documented and discussed with the patient. Medications should be reviewed with a focus on those that can cause or exacerbate pigmentary disorders and scarring. The benefits and risks of the procedure should be reviewed in depth and the patient should sign an informed consent. The primary issues of cosmetic concern to be addressed by the peeling procedure should be reviewed and patients with unrealistic expectations should be addressed with extreme care and caution. Peels may be best avoided in such individuals.

General pre- and post-peel care includes optimal photoprotection, lighteners, exfoliants, antioxidants, and if indicated, antiviral therapy. Any preexisting history of herpes simplex viral infections should be reviewed and the frequency of flaring should be obtained. Pretreatment with valacyclovir 500 mg, acyclovir 400 mg, or

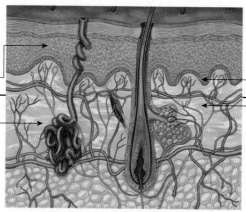

Superficial very light
Glycolic acid 20–50%
Salicylic acid 20–50%
TCA 10–20%
Tretinoin
Stratum spinosum

Superficial light
TCA 20–30%
Jessner's solution
Glycolic acid 70%

Medium depth
TCA 35–40%
Jessner's/TCA 35%
70% glycolic-TCA
Solid co2/TCA
88% phenol
Upper-reticular dermis

Deep peels
Unoccluded or occluded baker's phenol peel
TCA>50%
Mid-reticular dermis

Fig. 15.1 Cross section of skin illustrating the depth and peeling for superficial, medium, and deep peels.

TABLE 15.2   Priming the Skin for Peeling: Pre- and Post-Peel Care

Pre-Peel Care	Post-Peel Care
Lighteners *(hydroquinone 4% or higher formulations, kojic acid; arbutin, azelaic acid, cysteamine; tranexamic acid 2%–5%; niacinamide, combination formulas):* Begin 2–4 weeks prior to peeling procedure	**Lighteners:** If no irritation, resume after 2–7 days post procedure
Exfoliants: *(Alpha hydroxy acid, 10%–20% glycolic acid, retinoids)* Discontinue 7–10 days prior to peeling unless a deeper peel is desired.	**Exfoliants:** Resume in 2–7 days post peel
	Antioxidants: Resume 2–7 days post procedure
Antioxidants *(Vitamin A, Vitamin C, Vitamin E, niacinamide, ferulic acid);* Daily	**Antiviral Therapy:** Discontinue 7 days post procedure
Antiviral Therapy *(if indicated) (valacyclovir, famciclovir, acyclovir):* Begin 2 days prior to procedure and can discontinue 7–10 days	**Broad Spectrum and Visible Light Photoprotection:** Daily
	Bland Cleansers and Moisturizers: 1–7 days post procedure
Broad Spectrum and Visible Light Photoprotection: Daily	**Topical Corticosteroids (low-mid potency):** 1–7 days post procedure for moderate post-peel irritation

famciclovir 500 mg twice daily can be initiated beginning 2 days prior to peeling for a total of 7 to 10 days (Table 15.2). Detailed photographs including frontal and lateral images should always be taken prior to and after peeling procedures.

Priming the skin for peeling often varies with the condition being treated. The prepeel priming protocol can differ for photodamage, disorders of hyperpigmentation (melasma and postinflammatory hyperpigmentation), acne vulgaris, and other conditions. The skin is usually prepped for 2 to 4 weeks with a topical lightener to reduce epidermal melanin (Table 15.2). Commonly used lightening agents include hydroquinone 4%, higher-compounded formulations of 5% to 10%, azelaic acid 15% to 20%, kojic acid formulations, cysteamine, tranexamic acid 3% to 5%, or other combination lightening agents. The use of topical lighteners is paramount when treating dyschromias in skin of color. Lighteners can be used up until the day before peeling if it does not contain a retinoid and can be resumed postoperatively after evidence of irritation subsides. Use of broad-spectrum sunscreens are mandatory before and after peeling. Recent studies have documented persistent hyperpigmentation induced by visible light exposure.[19] Hence, tinted sunscreens providing additional visible light protection are preferred.

Use of topical retinoids (tretinoin, tazarotene, adapalene, retinols) thin the stratum corneum and enhance epidermal turnover. These effects are evident 2 to 6 weeks following daily use and also reduce epidermal melanin and expedite epidermal healing. Retinoids enhance the penetration and depth of chemical peeling and often optimize the effects of chemical peeling in Fitzpatrick skin types I through III. They are used until 1 to 2 days prior to peeling in lighter skin types and resumed postoperatively after all evidence of peeling and desquamation subsides. In contrast to photodamage, when treating conditions such as melasma, postinflammatory hyperpigmentation, and acne vulgaris, retinoids should either be discontinued 1 or 2 weeks before peeling or completely eliminated from the peeling prep to avoid post-peel complications such as moderate to severe erythema, crusting, and desquamation. Postinflammatory hyperpigmentation and/or hypopigmentation and scarring are sequalae of the aforementioned reactions.

CHEMICAL PEELING AGENTS

Alpha Hydroxy Acids
Glycolic Acid

Glycolic acid is the most frequently used alpha hydroxy acid for chemical peeling. Concentrations for peeling range from 20% to 70% and correlate with the depth of peeling. Glycolic acid peels work by causing epidermolysis, decreased corneocyte cohesion, keratinocyte plugging, as well as melanin dispersion. The efficacy of glycolic acid peeling has been documented for facial hyperpigmentation, photodamage, acne vulgaris, and actinic keratoses.

Numerous studies have reported the efficacy of glycolic acid peels in darker racial-ethnic groups.[18] Nineteen Black patients with postinflammatory hyperpigmentation were treated with glycolic acid peeling.[20] The control group was treated with a 2% hydroquinone/10% glycolic acid formulation twice daily and tretinoin 0.05% at bedtime, whereas the active peel group received the same topical regimen plus a series of six serial glycolic acid peels. Although not statistically significant, greater improvement was noted in the chemical peel group. In another study, 30 Indian patients (skin types III-V) with postinflammatory hyperpigmentation were randomly assigned to two groups of 15 patients each. One group received serial glycolic peeling (30% x3, 50% x3) and a topical modified Kligman regimen. The other group received treatment with the modified Kligman regimen alone. Statistically significant greater improvement was noted for the peel group at 12 and 21 weeks. Side effects included erythema, burning, and desquamation in 73%. The investigators reported no long-term complications.[21]

Glycolic peels have also been used in skin of color for treatment of melasma. The safety and efficacy of a series of glycolic acid facial peels were investigated in 25 Indian women. Patients were treated with 50% glycolic acid peels monthly for 3 months. Improvement was noted in 91% with maximal clearing occurring in patients with epidermal melasma.[22] In another study of 80 Indian women with melasma, the efficacy of glycolic acid peeling with a series of three 30% glycolic peels and three 40% peels in combination with a modified Kligman bleaching regimen (hydroquinone 5%, hydrocortisone acetate 1%, and tretinoin 0.05%) was compared to the use of the modified Kligman formulation alone.[23] Both groups showed a statistically significant improvement in the Melasma Area of Severity Index (MASI) score at 21 weeks. However, maximal improvement occurred in the group treated with the series of glycolic acid peels in combination with the topical bleaching regimen. Side effects included mild burning, erythema, and transient postinflammatory hyperpigmentation.

Prior to peeling, the skin is cleansed with 70% isopropyl alcohol or acetone using cotton balls or 2x2 gauze. The peeling agent can then be applied using cotton-tip swabs or 2x2 gauze. In general, the peel is left in place for 3 to 5 minutes, then neutralized with 10% sodium bicarbonate solution. A handheld fan should be used to mitigate any burning, stinging, or discomfort caused by the peel. The patient should be closely monitored during the procedure. Concentrations can be titrated from 20% to 35%, to 50%, and finally 70% if indicated. Some patients may not tolerate the higher concentrations due to side effects.

In general, glycolic acid peels and other alpha hydroxy acids are well tolerated in darker racial-ethnic groups (Fig. 15.2) Glycolic acid peels are most advantageous when treating darker skin types with sensitive skin. Contraindications include product sensitivity, hypersensitivity reactions, and increased sensitivity to ultraviolet light. Hypopigmentation, hyperpigmentation, and scarring can occur with aggressive use of glycolic acid, particularly with higher strength formulations. Complications can be minimized by gradual titration of concentrations from lower concentrations to higher strength formulation.

Lactic Acid

Lactic acid represents another alpha hydroxy acid demonstrating efficacy for acne vulgaris and hyperpigmentation disorders. It decreases corneocyte adhesion and stratum corneum thickness. In a study of 20 patients with melasma, 92% lactic acid was applied for six peeling sessions. There was a significant reduction in MASI scoring.[24] In addition, the efficacy and safety of 40% glycolic acid peeling was compared to 60% lactic acid peeling in 112 patients (skin types IV and V) with epidermal melasma. Both groups showed comparable efficacy in MASI score reduction. However, the group treated with lactic acid experienced significantly fewer side effects.[25]

Mandelic Acid

Mandelic acid is one of the largest of the alpha hydroxy acid peels. It penetrates the epidermis uniformly and more slowly compared to other alpha hydroxy peels. In a retrospective study of chemical peeling in 473 patients, 42 subjects with skin of color were treated with mandelic acid. None experienced side effects.[26] Forty-four Indian patients with skin types IV and V with acne vulgaris, postacne scarring, and hyperpigmentation were treated with either glycolic acid 35% peeling or a combination salicylic acid 20% and 10% mandelic acid peeling. The combination peel had higher efficacy for active acne lesions and postinflammatory hyperpigmentation.[27] This combination mandelic acid/salicylic acid peel used for acne, pigmentary disorders, and scarring has few side effects in darker skin types.

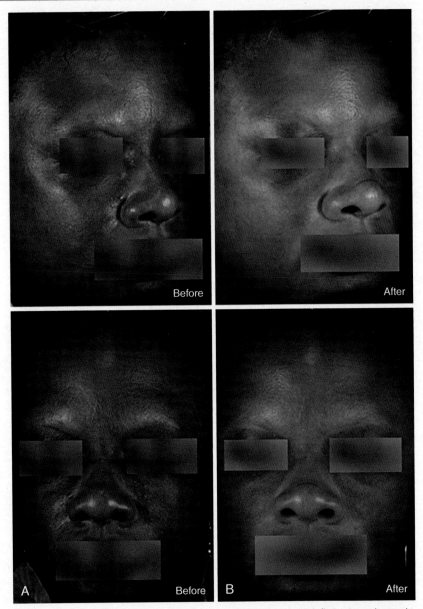

Fig. 15.2 African female with acne vulgaris, enlarged pores, scarring, and postinflammatory hyperpigmentation. Treated with a series of salicylic (3) acid 20% and glycolic (3) acid 35% peeling (A, before; B, after).

Salicylic Acid Peeling

Salicylic acid is a beta hydroxy acid that has been formulated in a hydroethanolic vehicle at concentrations of 20% and 30% for use as a superficial peeling agent. It is a lipophilic agent that removes intercellular lipids and has antimicrobial, sebostatic, and anti-inflammatory effects. Multiple formulations including combination formulas are commercially available including 10%, 20%, and 30% ethanol-based concentrations.

Salicylic acid is commonly used for acne vulgaris, hyperpigmentation, oily skin, textural changes, and pseudofolliculitis barbae. Its lipophilic effects make it an excellent option for patients with oily skin and acne vulgaris. Twenty-five patients with skin types V and VI were treated with a series of salicylic acid peels.[28] Conditions treated included acne vulgaris, postinflammatory hyperpigmentation, oily skin with textural changes, and melasma. Patients were pretreated for 2 weeks with hydroquinone 4%, followed by a series of two 20% and three 30% salicylic acid peels performed biweekly. Moderate to significant improvement was observed in 88%. Minimal to mild side effects occurred in 16%. Three patients experienced hyperpigmentation that resolved in 7 to 14 days. In another study, 35 Korean patients with facial acne were treated biweekly for 12 weeks with 30% salicylic acid peels.[29] Both inflammatory and noninflammatory lesions were significantly improved. In general, the peel was well tolerated with few side effects. In a study of 40 Indian patients with mild to moderate facial acne, 30% salicylic acid was compared to Jessner's solution peeling.[30] Six peels were performed for each group. Thirty percent salicylic acid peels were more effective than Jessner's solution for treatment of noninflammatory acne lesions.

Salicylic acid peels are performed at 2- to 4-week intervals. The face is thoroughly cleansed with alcohol and/or acetone to remove oils. The peel is then applied using wedge sponges, 2x2 gauze, or cotton-tipped applicators. A total of two to three coats of salicylic acid is usually applied and left on for 3 to 5 minutes. Most patients experience some mild burning and stinging during the procedure. A white precipitate, representing crystallization of the salicylic acid, begins to form at 30 seconds to 1 minute following peel application. This should not be confused with frosting or whitening of the skin, which represents protein agglutination. Frosting usually indicates that the patient will observe some crusting and peeling following the procedure. This may be appropriate when treating photodamage. However, it is best to have minimal to no frosting when treating other conditions as complications may ensue in darker skin. After 3 to 5 minutes, the face is thoroughly rinsed with tap water and a bland cleanser is used to remove any residual salicylic acid precipitate.

Salicylic acid peeling can be used safely in all racial-ethnic groups and skin types. It has an excellent safety profile and provides substantial efficacy for acne vulgaris, oily skin, enlarged pores, and hyperpigmentation (Fig. 15.3). Given its limited depth of peeling, it has minimal efficacy in patients with moderate to significant photodamage. Contraindications include unrealistic patient expectations, salicylate hypersensitivity/allergy,

acute viral infection, acute facial dermatitis, inflammation, and pregnancy.

Tretinoin Peeling

The efficacy of tretinoin for fine and coarse lines and the dyschromia of photodamage well documented. Tretinoin increases epidermal thickness, improves stratum corneum compactness, and decreases epidermal melanin. Other studies document its ability to increase collagen types I, III, and VII as well as the reorganization of dermal collagen.

Several studies have assessed the efficacy of tretinoin peels.[31,32] In an investigation of tretinoin peels in 15 women, peels were performed twice weekly in concentrations of 1% to 5%. The peel solution was left in contact with the skin for 6 to 8 hours. Three of the treated patients were classified as skin type IV. Improvement in skin texture and appearance and histologic assessments showed a decrease in stratum corneum thickness, as well as an increase in the thickness of the epidermis. There were no reported side effects.[32] In a subsequent study, 10 Indian women with melasma were treated weekly in a split-face trial in which 70% glycolic acid was applied to one side of the face and 1% tretinoin to the opposite side.[33] A significant reduction in the modified MASI score was noted at 6 and 12 weeks on both sides of the face. There was no difference between responses for each peel, suggesting that tretinoin peels are well tolerated in darker-skinned patients with melasma. Thirty melasma patients were randomized for peeling with either 5% or 10% tretinoin. Fifty percent of subjects were skin type IV. Peels were performed at baseline, 2, 4, and 6 weeks.[34] There was a significant reduction in the MASI score with no difference in efficacy of the 5% and 10% peel.

After thorough cleaning of the face with alcohol and acetone, two coats of the tretinoin peeling agent are applied to the full face and allowed to dry. The patient is instructed to wash the face in 4 to 8 hours. Peeling usually ensues in 48 hours and may last for 3 to 5 days. Bland cleansers and moisturizers are used daily until peeling subsides and routine skin care is resumed.

Tretinoin peels are extremely well tolerated in skin types IV through VI. It has become one of the most popular peels performed in my practice (Fig. 15.4). However, additional studies are necessary to situate tretinoin in our overall hierarchy of superficial peeling agents. Contraindications include hypersensitivity,

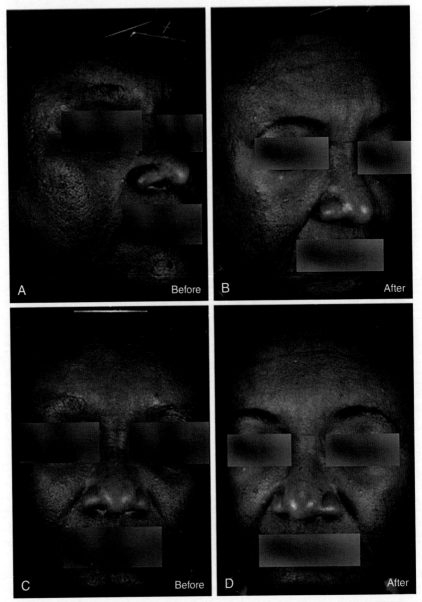

Fig. 15.3 African American female with skin type VI treated with salicylic (3) acid peeling 20% (A, right-side before; B, right-side after; C, frontal before; D, frontal after).

pregnancy, and dermatitis with side effects of erythema, crusting, and postinflammatory pigmentation.

Jessner's Solution

Jessner's solution contains 14% resorcinol, 14% salicylic acid, and 14% lactic acid in 95% ethanol. Modified Jessner's formulations replace resorcinol often with

citric acid. It is a lipophilic compound that disrupts intercellular lipids, decreases corneocyte adhesion, and induces intercellular and intracellular edema.[18] Jessner's solution has been used alone for superficial peeling or in combination with TCA 35% to achieve a medium-depth peel. Increasing the number of coats applied to the treated area increases the depth and reaction

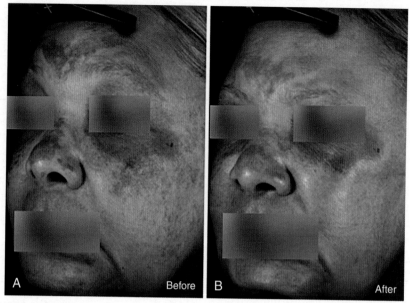

Fig. 15.4 Severe melasma (A, baseline) treated with a series of three proprietary salicylic acid/tretinoin 2.5% (B, after treatment).

induced by the Jessner's peel. These peels are well tolerated with minimal side effects.

As with glycolic acid and salicylic acid peels, Jessner's peels are most commonly used as adjunctive therapy for moderate to severe facial dyschromias, acne, oily skin, texturally rough skin, fine wrinkles, and pseudofolliculitis barbae. The efficacy of Jessner's solution was compared to 70% glycolic acid in a split-face study of 16 patients. Of the total group, five were skin type IV, three were V, and one was VI. There was no statistically significant difference in improvement between the two groups. The investigator did not report an increased frequency of side effects in patients of skin types IV-VI.[35] In a randomized, double-blind, split-face study of 36 patients (skin types IV and V) with acne vulgaris and post-acne hyperpigmentation, split faces received either Jessner's solution or salicylic acid.[36] Subjects were treated weekly for a total of three sessions. Both Jessner's solution and salicylic acid were equally effective in treating acne vulgaris and post-acne hyperpigmentation.

Skin priming for Jessner's peel is similar to other superficial peels. The skin is usually degreased prior to peeling with alcohol followed by a mild acetone scrub. After cleansing, the solution is applied to the face using a 2x2 gauze, cotton-tipped applicators, or a sable brush.

For superficial peeling, two coats are usually applied. Additional coats can be applied if a deeper peel is desired. Jessner's peels have an excellent safety profile for all skin types with minimal down time. Side effects are similar to other superficial peeling agents.

Trichloroacetic Acid Peeling

TCA is considered the gold standard for peeling. Concentrations of 10% to 30 % are used for superficial peeling and higher concentrations of 35% to 40% for medium depth peeling. Combinations of 70% glycolic/TCA 35% and Jessner's/TCA 35% are also used for medium-depth. TCA precipitates epidermal proteins, causing sloughing and necrosis of the treated area. The extent of wounding is concentration dependent. TCA concentrations are correctly formulated using a weight-in-volume (W/V) method.[37] In contrast to alpha hydroxy acids, salicylic acid, or tretinoin peeling, there is a substantially smaller window of safety when using TCA peeling in darker skin types. Indications for superficial TCA peeling include hyperpigmentation, mild photodamage, and rhytids. Medium-depth TCA peeling can be used to treat actinic keratoses, thin seborrheic keratoses, mild to moderate photoaging, moderate to severe rhytids, scarring, and hyperpigmentation.

A comparative study in 30 Indian patients assessed the efficacy of 15% TCA versus 35% glycolic acid for treatment of melasma. There was no statistically significant difference between the two groups.[38] However, subjects treated with TCA experienced more post-peel side effects interfering with their daily activities. A recent study compared the efficacy of 30% glycolic acid, 15% TCA, and 92% lactic acid in 90 patients with melasma. Subjects were equally split in two groups. Peels were performed every 2 weeks for 12 weeks. Both TCA and glycolic were equally efficacious and both were superior to lactic acid. However, the incidence of adverse effects was maximum in the TCA peel group followed by glycolic acid and lactic acid.[39]

TCA peeling for dark skin can safely be used in concentrations of 10% to 15% and less common instances of 20%. Retinoids significantly increase the depth of TCA peeling. Hence, unless a deeper, more aggressive peel is desired, retinoids should be discontinued for at least 7 to 10 days or longer prior to peeling. Prior to application of the TCA peel, the face should be thoroughly cleansed and degreased with alcohol, or hibiclens, followed by acetone. TCA is applied using a cotton-tipped applicator or a 2x2 gauze. Several coats are sequentially applied to the forehead, bilateral cheeks, upper lip, and chin area. The skin is monitored closely for a level I (erythema and mild patchy areas of white frosting) or level II (diffuse white frosting and erythema) frost. The face can be rinsed to control any further reactions.

TCA peeling should be used with care and caution in darker skin types. Side effects of TCA peeling include persistent postinflammatory hyperpigmentation, hypopigmentation, and scarring. TCA is versatile and can be used as a superficial, medium-depth, or deep peel. Superficial peeling is best for darker skin type as deeper peels can be fraught with greater side effects in darker racial-ethnic groups.

Miscellaneous Peeling Agents

Several new peeling agents are commercially available. They include B-lipohydroxy acids and pyruvic acid. B-lipohydroxy acid is a derivative of salicylic acid with an additional fatty acid chain. It has increased lipophilicity compared to salicylic acid and has shown moderate efficacy in patients with acne vulgaris.[40] Pyruvic acid is a carboxylic acid that penetrates rapidly and deeply through the skin. It has keratolytic, antimicrobial, and sebostatic

TABLE 15.3   Marketed Proprietary Combination Peels and Manufacturers

PROPRIETARY PEELS	
Peel	Ingredients
Micropeel Plus 20 and 30[1]	20%/30% Salicylic acid • 3% Glycolic acid • Alcohol
Melanage Micropeel[2]	1% Tretinoin • 10% Azelaic acid • 10% Lactic acid • 10% Retinol
Vitalize Peel[3]	10% Salicylic acid • 10% Lactic acid • 10% Resorcinol • 10% Retinol
Vi Peel	10%–12% TCA • 10%–12% Phenol • 10%–12% Salicylic acid • 0.4% Tretinoin
Cosmelon Peel[4]	8% Hydroquinone • Retinoic acid • Azelaic acid • Kojic acid • Arbutin • Phytic acid • Ascorbic acid

[1]SkinCeuticals; [2]Young Pharmaceuticals, Inc.; [3]SkinMedica; [4]Mesoestetics.

properties. It is effective for treating photodamage, acne, acne scarring, and hyperpigmentation. There are minimal data on its use in darker racial-ethnic groups.

Combination Proprietary Peels

Several proprietary peels are commonly used in patients with skin of color. These proprietary formulations frequently contain lighteners and combinations of multiple ingredients. Indications for these marketed peels include melasma, postinflammatory hyperpigmentation, acne vulgaris, textural changes, photodamage, and pseudofolliculitis barbae (Table 15.3). Seventeen subjects with moderate to severe hyperpigmentation (Fitzpatrick skin types III-VI) received a series of three Vitalize® peels monthly for 12 weeks. Fourteen subjects completed the study. There was a statistically significant reduction in appearance of overall hyperpigmentation, photodamage, and skin tone unevenness at 8 and 12 weeks. The peel was well tolerated with minimal side effects.[41]

CONCLUSIONS

Chemical peeling procedures have increased in popularity in darker racial-ethnic individuals comprising skin types IV-VI in the last decade. Serial superficial peeling agents are most often used in skin of color and offer substantial benefits for postinflammatory hyperpigmentation, melasma, acne, pseudofolliculitis barbae, oily skin, and texturally rough skin. When selecting a peeling agent, the benefits of the procedure should always substantially outweigh any associated risks or complications. Superficial peels with appropriate titration of concentrations are generally safe and efficacious for darker-skinned patients. However, given the labile nature of melanocytes of darker-complexioned individuals, medium-depth and deep peels are more likely to induce substantial complications and side effects.

REFERENCES

1. Bryan CP, Smith GE. *Ancient Egyptian Medicine: The Papyrus Ebers*. Ares Publishers; 1974.
2. Hebra F, Kaposi M. *On diseases of the skin, including the exanthemata*. New Sydenham Society; 1866.
3. Stegman SJ. A comparative histologic study of the effects of three peeling agents and dermabrasion on normal and sundamaged skin. *Aesthetic Plast Surg*. 1982:6(3):123-135. Available at: https://doi.org/10.1007/BF01570631.
4. Vespa J, Medina L, Armstrong DM. *Demographic Turning Points for the United States: Population Projections for 2020 to 2060. Current Population Reports*. U.S. Census Bureau; 2020:P25-P1144. Available at: https://www.census.gov/library/publications/2020/demo/p25-1144.html
5. American Society of Plastic Surgeons. *2020 Plastic Surgery Statistics Report*. ASPS Public Relations; 2020. Available at: https://www.plasticsurgery.org/documents/News/Statistics/2020/plastic-surgery-statistics-full-report-2020.pdf Available at: https://www.plasticsurgery.org/news/plastic-surgery-statistics?sub=2020+Plastic+Surgery+Statistics.
6. Taylor SC. Skin of color: Biology, structure, function, and implications for dermatologic disease. *J Am Acad Dermatol*. 2002;46(2 suppl Understanding):S41-S62. Available at: https://doi.org/10.1067/mjd.2002.120790.
7. Alexis AF, Obioha JO. Ethnicity and aging skin. *J Drugs Dermatol*. 2017;16(6):s77-s80.
8. Grimes PE, Sherrod Q. Structural and physiologic differences in the skin of darker racial ethnic groups. In: *Aesthetics and Cosmetic Surgery for Darker Skin Types*. New York: Lippincott Williams & Wilkins; 2008:15-26.
9. Kaidbey KH, Agin PP, Sayre RM, Kligman AM. Photoprotection by melanin—a comparison of Black and Caucasian skin. *J Am Acad Dermatol*. 1979;1(3):249-260. Available at: https://doi.org/10.1016/s0190-9622(79)70018-1.
10. Lim JT, Tham, SN. Glycolic acid peels in the treatment of melasma among Asian women. *Dermatol Surg*. 1997; 23(3):177-179. Available at: https://doi.org/10.1111/j.1524-4725.1997.tb00016.x.
11. Fajuyigbe D, Young, AR. The impact of skin colour on human photobiological responses. *Pigment Cell Melanoma Res*. 2016;29:607-618. Available at: https://doi.org/10.1111/pcmr.12511.
12. Rijken F, Bruijnzeel PLB, van Weelden H, Kiekens RCM. Responses of Black and White skin to solar-simulating radiation: differences in DNA photodamage, infiltrating neutrophils, proteolytic enzymes induced, keratinocyte activation, and IL-10 expression. *J Invest Dermatol*. 2004;122(6):1448-1455. Available at: https://doi.org/10.1111/j.0022-202X.2004.22609.x.
13. Osborne R, Tamura M, Jarrold B, et al. Multiethnic comparison of facial skin aging. *J Am Acad Dermatol*. 2018; 79(3 suppl 1):AB196.
14. Halder RM, Grimes PE, McLaurin CI, Kress MA, Kenney Jr JA. Incidence of common dermatoses in a predominantly black dermatologic practice. *Cutis*. 1983;32(4):388-390.
15. Sanchez MR. Cutaneous diseases in Latinos. *Dermatol Clin*. 2003;21(4):689-697. Available at: https://doi.org/10.1016/s0733-8635(03)00087-1.
16. Alexis AF, Sergay AB, Taylor SC. Common dermatologic disorders in skin of color: A comparative practice survey. *Cutis*. 2007;80(5):387-394.
17. Grimes PE. Agents for ethnic skin peeling. *Dermatol Ther*. 2000;13(2):159-164. Available at: https://doi.org/10.1046/j.1529-8019.2000.00019.x.
18. Grimes P, Tosti A, De Padova MP. Chemical peels in dark skin. In: *Color Atlas of Chemical Peels*. 2nd ed. Springer; 2012.
19. Dumbuya H, Grimes PE, Lynch S, et al. Impact of iron-oxide containing formulations against visible light-induced skin pigmentation in skin of color individuals. *J Drugs Dermatol*. 2020;19(7):712-717. Available at: https://doi.org/10.36849/JDD.2020.5032.
20. Burns RL, Prevost-Blank PL, Lawry MA, Lawry TB, Faria DT, Fivenson DP. Glycolic acid peels for postinflammatory hyperpigmentation in black patients. A comparative study. *Dermatol Surg*. 1997;23(3):171-175. Available at: https://doi.org/10.1111/j.1524-4725.1997.tb00014.x.
21. Sarkar R, Parmar NV, Kapoor S. Treatment of postinflammatory hyperpigmentation with a combination of glycolic acid peels and a topical regimen in dark-skinned patients: a comparative study. *Dermatol Surg*. 2017;43(4):566-573. Available at: https://doi.org/10.1097/DSS.0000000000001007.
22. Javaheri SM, Handa S, Kaur I, Kumar B. Safety and efficacy of glycolic acid facial peel in Indian women with melasma. *Int J Dermatol*. 2001;40(5):354-357. Available at: https://doi.org/10.1046/j.1365-4362.2001.01149.x.
23. Sarkar R, Kaur C, Bhalla M, Kanwar AJ. The combination of glycolic acid peels with a topical regimen in the

treatment of melasma in dark-skinned patients: A comparative study. *Dermatol Surg.* 2002;28(9):828-832. Available at: https://doi.org/10.1046/j.1524-4725.2002.02034.x.

24. Sharquie KE, Al-Tikreety MM, Al-Mashhadani SA. Lactic acid as a new therapeutic peeling agent in melasma. *Dermatol Surg.* 2005;31(2):149-154. Available at: https://doi.org/10.1111/j.1524-4725.2005.31035.

25. Hafeez A, Shaukat S, Sanai M, Ahmad T, Aman S. Comparison of the efficacy and safety of 40% glycolic acid and 60% lactic acid chemical peel in treatment of epidermal melasma. *J Pak Assoc Dermatol.* 2019;29(2): 176-181.

26. Vemula S, Maymone MBC, Secemsky EA, et al. Assessing the safety of superficial chemical peels in darker skin: A retrospective study. *J Am Acad Dermatol.* 2018;79(3): 508-513.e502. Available at: https://doi.org/10.1016/j.jaad.2018.02.064.

27. Garg VK, Sinha S, Sarkar R. Glycolic acid peels versus salicylic–mandelic acid peels in active acne vulgaris and post-acne scarring and hyperpigmentation: A comparative study. *Dermatol Surg.* 2009;35(1):59-65. Available at: https://doi.org/10.1111/j.1524-4725.2008.34383.x.

28. Grimes PE. The safety and efficacy of salicylic acid chemical peels in darker racial-ethnic groups. *Dermatol Surg.* 1999;25(1):18-22. Available at: https://doi.org/10.1046/j.1524-4725.1999.08145.x.

29. Lee HS, Kim IH. Salicylic acid peels for the treatment of acne vulgaris in Asian patients. *Dermatol Surg.* 2003; 29(12):1196-1199. Available at: https://doi.org/10.1111/j.1524-4725.2003.29384.x.

30. Dayal S, Amrani A, Sahu P, Jain VK. Jessner's solution vs. 30% salicylic acid peels: a comparative study of the efficacy and safety in mild-to-moderate acne vulgaris. *J Cosmet Dermatol.* 2017;16(1):43-51. Available at: https://doi.org/10.1111/jocd.12266.

31. Sumita JM, Leonardi GR, Bagatin E. Tretinoin peel: A critical review. *An Bras Dermatol.* 2017;92(3):363-366. Available at: https://doi.org/10.1590/abd1806-4841.201755325.

32. Cucé LC, Bertino MC, Scattone L, Birkenhauer MC. Tretinoin peeling. *Dermatol Surg.* 2001;27(1):12-14.

33. Khunger N, Sarkar R, Jain RK. Tretinoin peels versus glycolic acid peels in the treatment of Melasma in dark-skinned patients. *Dermatol Surg.* 2004;30:756-760; discussion 760.

34. Magalhães GM, Borges MFM, Queiroz ARC, Capp AA, Pedrosa SV, Diniz MS. Double-blind randomized study of 5% and 10% retinoic acid peels in the treatment of melasma: Clinical evaluation and impact on the quality of life. *Surg Cosmet Dermatol.* 2011;3(1):17-22.

35. Lawrence N, Cox SE, Brody HJ. Treatment of melasma with Jessner's solution versus glycolic acid: A comparison of clinical efficacy and evaluation of the predictive ability of Wood's light examination. *J Am Acad Dermatol.* 1997;36(4):589-593. Available at: https://doi.org/10.1016/s0190-9622(97)70248-2.

36. How KN, Lim PY, Wan Ahmad Kammal WSL, Shamsudin N. Efficacy and safety of Jessner's solution peel in comparison with salicylic acid 30% peel in the management of patients with acne vulgaris and postacne hyperpigmentation with skin of color: A randomized, double-blinded, split-face, controlled trial. *Int J Dermatol.* 2020;59(7): 804-812. Available at: https://doi.org/10.1111/ijd.14948.

37. Harmon CB, Hadley M, Tristani P. Trichloroacetic acid. In: Tosti A, Grimes P, De Padova M, eds. *Color Atlas of Chemical Peels.* Berlin, Heidelberg: Springer; 2012. Available at: https://doi.org/10.1007/978-3-642-20270-4_5.

38. Puri N. Comparative study of 15% TCA peel versus 35% glycolic acid peel for the treatment of melasma. *Indian Dermatol Online J.* 2012;3(2):109-113. Available at: https://doi.org/10.4103/2229-5178.96702.

39. Sahu P, Dayal S. Most worthwhile superficial chemical peel for melasma of skin of color: Authors' experience of glycolic, trichloroacetic acid, and lactic peel. *Dermatol Ther.* 2021;34(1):e14693. Available at: https://doi.org/10.1111/dth.14693.

40. Zeichner JA. The use of lipohydroxy acid in skin care and acne treatment. *J Clin Aesthet Dermatol.* 2016;9(11):40-43.

41. Downie J, Schneider K, Goberdhan L, Makino ET, Mehta RC. Combination of in-office chemical peels with a topical comprehensive pigmentation control product in skin of color subjects with facial hyperpigmentation. *J Drugs Dermatol.* 2017;16(4):301-306.

16

Body Contouring: Racial/Ethnic Considerations and Expert Techniques for Optimal Outcomes

Nazanin Saedi, Rosannah Marie Velasquez

SUMMARY AND KEY FEATURES

- Noninvasive body contouring seeks to provide fat removal with a safer profile, less downtime, and minimal discomfort when compared to the gold standard of liposuction.
- Modalities for noninvasive body contouring include cryolipolysis, lipid-selective

- wavelengths of laser lights, ultrasound, and radiofrequency.
- Current literature reveals the FDA-approved noninvasive body contouring modalities all have a safe profile with no increased risk of hyperpigmentation after treatments in skin of color.

INTRODUCTION

One of the most common cosmetic concerns is excess fat, and the desire for the "perfect body" is ubiquitous among all ethnicities, albeit with cultural and individual variations in the ideal image. The gold standard for body contouring remains fat removal through liposuction; however, many patients are averse to seeking invasive intervention due to downtime, pain, infection risk, and anesthetic concerns. Noninvasive body contouring has sought to fill this void for patients desiring results with a safer profile, less downtime, and minimal discomfort. Modalities for noninvasive body contouring include cryolipolysis, lipid-selective wavelengths of laser lights, ultrasound, and radiofrequency. It is important to remind patients that body contouring is not meant to be a treatment for weight loss and does not replace diet or exercise.

As we evaluate patients for these noninvasive techniques, it is important for us to recognize any special considerations for patients with skin of color given the propensity for hyperpigmentation. The Skin of Color Society defines skin of color as individuals of Hispanic, Latino, Asian, African, Native American, Pacific Island descent, and mixtures thereof.[1] According to the US Census by 2060, Hispanics, Asians, Black/African-American, and other individuals of color will represent approximately 57% of the US population.[2] From 2000 to 2010, the Hispanic, Asian, and Black/African-American populations grew by 43%, 43.3%, and 12.3%, respectively, and are projected to be 27.5%, 9.1%, and 15% of the nation's population in 2060, respectively.[2,3]

CRYOLIPOLYSIS

Coolsculpting (Zeltiq, Pleasanton, CA) is the FDA-approved noninvasive procedure intended to break down adipocytes through controlled cooling at the surface of the skin.[4] It remains the most commonly used device for noninvasive fat reduction. Treatment areas approved include the visible fat bulges in the submental area, submandibular area, thighs, abdomen, flanks, bra fat, back fat, underneath the buttocks (aka the "banana roll"), and upper arms.[4] In addition to treating fat, the device is approved to improve the appearance of lax tissue in the submental area.[4] Cryolipolysis is contraindicated in patients with history of cryoglobulinemia, paroxysmal cold hemoglobinuria, and cold agglutinin disease.[4] Most studies that have been performed using cryolipolysis are in the White population, although there have been a few studies on Asian populations.[5] In the Asian populations, there appears to be a similar safety profile as to the White population with no reported pigmentary disorders after treatment.[6,7] Henry Chan et al., specifically studied cryolipolysis in the Chinese population.[8] In the study, two groups received treatment of either the abdomen or flanks. One group of 21 patients received one treatment, and the second group of 12 patients received two treatments on average 3 months apart. They found cryolipolysis was an effective treatment in the Chinese with the greatest improvement after the first treatment and lesser improvement after the second treatment. All patients reported transient pain and numbness with resolution of all symptoms within 3 weeks. Other adverse events reported were redness in five patients and bruising in two patients, all which resolved within 1 week.[8] Paradoxical adipose hyperplasia (PAH) is an adverse effect that has unclear pathogenesis and has been reported to be a greater risk in males and the Hispanic/Latino population.[9] As of 2015, 473 PAH events were reported to Zeltiq in 291 patients in over 2 million treatment cycles throughout the world.[10] Of the reported cases, 42% were men. If we consider that men make up approximately 15% of CoolSculpting patients in these data, this makes the incidence of PAH approximately three times higher than expected.[10] In a retrospective chart review from May 2013 to May 2016, Kelly et al., found all 11 cases at their center were of Hispanic background (eight men and three women).[11] Hispanic men receiving treatment of the abdomen with a large applicator seemed to be at increased risk of PAH, but this could not be statistically confirmed. A bias noted by Kelly is that their center is in a community with a majority represented by the Hispanic population.[11] Patients will typically present with a painless, firm, well-demarcated, and visually appreciable tissue growth in the area treated 3 to 9 months after treatment.[9] Ho et al., hypothesizes that some adipocytes may be "naturally selected" for survival due to their inherent tolerance to cryolipolysis and a

resulting hyperplasia of these adipocytes occurs.[9] If PAH occurs, the treatment of choice is liposuction.[9]

LIPID-SELECTIVE WAVELENGTHS OF LASER LIGHT

SculpSure (Cynosure, Westford, MA) is a noninvasive 1060-nm laser body contouring system intended to permanently eliminate adipocytes through noninvasive lipolysis.[12] The device is FDA-approved for treatment of the submental area, abdomen, flanks, back, and inner and outer thighs. Ideal patients should have a body mass index (BMI) <30 for any body treatments and a BMI <49 for treatment of the submental area.[12] Katz et al., performed a study in 49 patients treating one flank to assess safety and efficacy of the 1060 nm laser in fat reduction.[13] Patients included in this study represented all skin types, with 65% having Fitzpatrick skin types I–III. No patients from this study withdrew or were discontinued due to an adverse event. Mild adverse events were reported by 83%, moderate adverse events reported by 17%, and no severe adverse events were reported. The most common adverse event in the safety analysis was treatment discomfort in 71% of patients. Other adverse events reported included transient edema, blistering, erythema, pain and bruising, and subcutaneous nodules or hardness. There were no reports of hypopigmentation and hyperpigmentation. Katz concluded that the 1060-nm laser was safe and effective with a statistically significant fat reduction in the treated side.[13]

ULTRASOUND

Cavitation-Based Lower-Frequency Nonthermal Ultrasound

UltraShape (Syneron/Candela Inc, Irvine, CA) is a noninvasive procedure using low-frequency (~220 kHz) focused, pulsed ultrasound energy to selectively destroy adipocytes.[14] The device is FDA approved for treating the abdominal region.[14] In the phase II clinical trial that was conducted, there were 164 patients from five centers included—two in Japan, two in the United States, and one in the United Kingdom.[15] While there was no mention of skin type in the trial, there were no adverse effects in regard to pigmentary disorders reported. Shek et al., later performed a study looking at UltraShape in treating 53 Asian patients and discovered that this modality seemed to be less effective in Southern Asians.[16] The suggested hypothesis for this difference in efficacy seems to be due to their smaller body figures and less voluminous adipocytes. In this patient population, no adverse effects regarding pigmentary disorders were reported.[16]

Thermal-Focused Ultrasound

LipoSonix (Beijing VCA Laser Technology, Beijing, China) is a noninvasive procedure that quickly raises the local temperature in a focused area within the subcutaneous tissue to >56°C.[17] The quick heating results in a coagulative necrosis and almost immediate cell death of adipocytes with no damage to surrounding tissue. The device is FDA approved for treatment of waist, abdomen, and thigh circumference. While there are limited studies on this modality, Jewell et al., completed a randomized control trial of 180 patients of which 13% were non-White and reported no specific adverse events related to skin of color.[18] In the study, 5 out of 12 patients failed to complete treatment due to pain. Procedural pain was the most common adverse event reported in 90% of actively treated patients and postprocedural pain in 57% of actively treated patients. The second most common adverse event in 66% of patients was bruising/ecchymosis. Edema and swelling was the only other adverse event reported in 9% of patients.[18]

RADIOFREQUENCY

Radiofrequency (RF) energy has been used for over a century for a multitude of medical applications including electrodessication, electrocoagulation, cardiac ablation, and neoplasm of eradication.[19] RF energy is harnessed to deliver heat to dermal structures such as fat.

Vanquish (BTL Aesthetics, Prague CR) is a noninvasive, noncontact selective RF technology that disrupts adipocytes through selective heating.[20] Adipose tissue contains dipoles and when RF is applied it induces rapid oscillation of charged molecules, leading to friction between molecules in the adipose tissue and ultimately heat-induced apoptosis.[21,22] The difference in impedance of skin (low impedance) and fat (high impedance) allows the device to focus on the high-impedance adipose tissue while minimizing risk to the epidermis, dermis, and muscle layers.[21,22] The device is FDA-approved with no BMI limits for treatment of the entire abdominal area and inner and outer thighs.[20] Suh et al.,

performed a retrospective study on 12 patients in South Korea who each received five treatments to the abdomen and no adverse events were reported in regard to pigmentary disorders.[21] The only adverse event reported in this study was in one patient who complained of hyperesthesia on the abdomen right after the third and fourth sessions. The hyperesthesia resolved within 3 days after the session and was not associated with any erythema, burn, or abdominal discomfort.[21]

VelaShape (Syneron Medical Ltd., Yokneam, Israel) is a noninvasive treatment that combines infrared light (IR), bipolar RF energy, and vacuum.[23] The device causes deep heating of the adipocytes, the surrounding connective tissue, and underlying dermal collagen fibers. While there is no adipocyte apoptosis, there is induction of collagen denaturation and neocollagenesis.[24] The device is FDA approved for temporary reduction in the appearance of cellulite and temporary reduction of thigh and abdominal circumferences in an ideal patient with BMI <30.[23] Brightman et al., performed a nonrandomized clinical trial treating 29 patients with skin types I–V with VelaShape.[24] There were no reported complications or differences in efficacy in darker skin types. However, it was noted that when treating darker skin types, superficial heating occurred quicker than in lighter skin types resulting in occasional decreases in the IR with these patients, but the clinical endpoint was still achieved.[24]

CONCLUSION

The growing demand for noninvasive body contouring and our ever-increasing population of skin of color patients puts into perspective the limited studies we have including and reporting skin of color. Based on current literature, our FDA-approved noninvasive body contouring modalities all have a safe profile with no increased risk of hyperpigmentation after treatments in skin of color. There are certain adverse events that may occur more frequently in different ethnicities such as PAH with cryolipolysis and we need to have a better understanding of the pathology. Overall, more studies need to be done tailored to include patients with skin of color in order to have a more complete evaluation of these patient populations. Additionally, more studies still need to be done in the future and as new modalities emerge it is of utmost importance that we recognize responses in different skin types.

REFERENCES

1. Skin of Color Society. April 23, 2021. Available at: https://skinofcolorsociety.org/about-socs/our-mission/.

2. Vespa J, Medina L, Armstrong DM. Demographic turning points for the United States: Population projections for 2020 to 2060 population estimates and projections current population reports. 2020. April 23, 2021. Available at: www.census.gov/library/publications/2020/demo/p25-1144.html.

3. Humes KR, Jones NA, Ramirez RR. *Overview of Race and Hispanic Origin*: 2010 Census Briefs; 2010. April 23, 2021. Available at: www.whitehouse.gov/omb.

4. About CoolSculpting ® Introduction; 2019. April 23, 2021. Available at: www.CoolSculpting.com.

5. Stevens WG, Pietrzak LK, Spring MA. Broad overview of a clinical and commercial experience with CoolSculpting. *Aesthet Surg J*. 2013;33(6):835-846. doi:10.1177/1090820X13494757.

6. Putra IB, Jusuf NK, Dewi NK. Utilisation of cryolipolysis among Asians: A review on efficacy and safety. *Open Access Maced J Med Sci*. 2019;7(9):1548-1554. doi:10.3889/oamjms.2019.318.

7. Oh CH, Shim JS, Bae KL, Chang JH. Clinical application of cryolipolysis in Asian patients for subcutaneous fat reduction and body contouring. *Arch Plast Surg*. 2020;47(1):62-69. doi:10.5999/aps.2019.01305.

8. Shek SY, Chan NPY, Chan HH. Non-invasive cryolipolysis for body contouring in Chinese-a first commercial experience. *Lasers Surg Med*. 2012;44(2):125-130. doi:10.1002/lsm.21145.

9. Ho D, Jagdeo J. A systematic review of paradoxical adipose hyperplasia (PAH) post-cryolipolysis. *J Drugs Dermatol*. 2017;16(1):62-67.

10. Sasaki GH. Reply: Cryolipolysis for fat reduction and body contouring: Safety and efficacy of current treatment paradigms. *Plast Reconstr Surg*. 2016;137(3):640e-641e. doi:10.1097/01.prs.0000479983.49996.c0.

11. Kelly ME, Rodríguez-Feliz J, Torres C, Kelly E. Treatment of paradoxical adipose hyperplasia following cryolipolysis: A single-center experience. *Plast Reconstr Surg*. 2018;142(1):17e-22e. doi:10.1097/PRS.0000000000004523.

12. Non-Invasive Laser Treatment - SculpSure®. Cynosure; April 23, 2021. Available at: https://www.cynosure.com/product/sculpsure/#popup-10.

13. Katz B, Doherty S. Safety and efficacy of a noninvasive 1,060-nm diode laser for fat reduction of the flanks. *Dermatol Surg*. doi:10.1097/DSS.0000000000001298.

14. Jewell ML, Solish NJ, Desilets CS. Noninvasive body sculpting technologies with emphasis on high-intensity focused ultrasound. *Aesthetic Plast Surg*. 2011;35:901-912. doi:10.1007/s00266-011-9700-5.

15. Teitelbaum SA, Burns JL, Kubota J, et al. Noninvasive body contouring by focused ultrasound: Safety and efficacy of the contour I device in a multicenter, controlled, clinical study. *Plast Reconstr Surg*. 2007;120(3):779-789. doi:10.1097/01.prs.0000270840.98133.c8.

16. Shek S, Yu C, Yeung CK, Kono T, Chan HH. The use of focused ultrasound for non-invasive body contouring in Asians. *Lasers Surg Med*. 2009;41(10):751-759. doi:10.1002/lsm.20875.

17. Fatemi A, Kane MAC. High-intensity focused ultrasound effectively reduces waist circumference by ablating adipose tissue from the abdomen and flanks: A retrospective case series. *Aesthet Plast Surg*. 2010;34(5):577-582. doi:10.1007/s00266-010-9503-0.

18. Jewell ML, Baxter RA, Cox SE, et al. Randomized sham-controlled trial to evaluate the safety and effectiveness of a high-intensity focused ultrasound device for noninvasive body sculpting. *Plast Reconstr Surg*. 2011;128(1):253-262. doi:10.1097/PRS.0b013e3182174278.

19. Alster TS, Lupton JR. Nonablative cutaneous remodeling using radiofrequency devices. *Clin Dermatol*. 2007;25(5):487-491. doi:10.1016/j.clindermatol.2007.05.005.

20. BTL Vanquish ME. April 23, 2021. Available at: https://btlexcellence.com/vanquish-me.php.

21. Hye Suh D, Min Kim C, Jun Lee S, Kim H, Keu Yeom S, Jung Ryu H. Safety and efficacy of a non-contact radiofrequency device for body contouring in Asians. *J Cosmet Laser Ther*. 2017;19(2):89-92. doi:10.1080/14764172.2016.1256486.

22. Weiss R, Weiss M, Beasley K, Vrba J, Bernardy J. Operator independent focused high frequency ISM band for fat reduction: Porcine model. *Lasers Surg Med*. 2013;45(4):235-239. doi:10.1002/lsm.22134.

23. VelaShape® - Circumferential & Cellulite Reduction Treatment | Candela Medical. April 23, 2021. Available at: https://candelamedical.com/int/patient/product/velashape.

24. Brightman L, Weiss E, Chapas AM, et al. Improvement in arm and post-partum abdominal and flank subcutaneous fat deposits and skin laxity using a bipolar radiofrequency, infrared, vacuum and mechanical massage device. *Lasers Surg Med*. 2009;41(10):791-798. doi:10.1002/lsm.20872.

17

Botulinum Toxins: Racial/Ethnic Considerations and Expert Techniques for Optimal Outcomes

Jasmine O. Obioha, Pearl E. Grimes

SUMMARY AND KEY FEATURES

- White populations show signs of aging decades earlier than other racial/ethnic groups.
- Botulinum toxin is a safe and effective treatment in Fitzpatrick skin types IV–VI.
- Commonly treated areas are glabellar and forehead lines.
- The aesthetic application of botulinum toxin is rapidly growing and may differ geographically, ethnically, and/or based on varying standards of beauty.

INTRODUCTION

Botulinum toxin leads as the most popular nonsurgical cosmetic procedure performed worldwide.[1] Until recent years, White consumers predominated as study subjects in the cosmetic literature, as well as the target consumers for antiaging procedures; however, the demographic trends in the aesthetic industry are changing. The rate of cosmetic procedures is growing among non-White racial and ethnic groups. According to the American Society of Aesthetic Plastic Surgery, 30% of the 16,349,031 nonsurgical cosmetic procedures performed in 2019 in the United States were performed on racial or ethnic minorities, with botulinum toxin remaining as the most frequent nonsurgical cosmetic procedure in African-Americans, Hispanics, and Asian-Americans.[1] As the non-Caucasian ethnic population grows rapidly, the demand for cosmetic procedures is expected to follow.

The US Census Bureau projects by the year 2056, greater than 50% of the US population will be of non-Caucasian descent.[2] With an increasingly diverse patient population, there is no longer a universal standard of beauty. Aesthetic ideals vary geographically as well as within and across different ethnic groups; however, the general principles of facial rejuvenation with wrinkle reduction often starts with botulinum toxin. As such, it is important to understand the safety, efficacy, and treatment approach to botulinum toxin in all racial/ethnic groups.

RACIAL/ETHNIC CONSIDERATIONS: THE AGING FACE

Skin aging occurs by both intrinsic and extrinsic pathways. Photoaging describes the influence of exposure to ultraviolet (UV) radiation on skin aging and manifests in the development of rhytids, lentigines, keratoses, mottled pigmentation, telangiectasias, decreased elasticity, and skin textural irregularities. Darker skin types exhibit fewer rhytids with photoaging but are more likely to develop mottled pigmentation, textural changes, and dermatosis papulosa nigra.[3] In general, as studies by Hexsel and Brunetto and Rossi and Alexis report, individuals with richly pigmented skin (i.e.,

Fitzpatrick skin types IV to VI) demonstrate less severe signs of photoaging, including rhytids, and at a later age than do individuals with fair skin (Fitzpatrick skin types I to III).[4,5] This is largely due to the photoprotective effect of increased epidermal melanin, which serves as an UV filter.[6] Kaidbey and colleagues demonstrated that the mean sun protective factor (SPF) from ultraviolet (UV) B in Black skin was found to be 13.4 as compared to 3.4 for White skin in a cadaveric skin study.[7] This difference in UV penetration thereby delays the onset and severity of photoaging in individuals with darker skin, as compared to lighter skin types.[3,5,6]

When comparing race/ethnicity, signs of photoaging in the White population occur 10 to 20 years earlier than in Black/African-American individuals, Asians, and Hispanics. In a comparative study by Nouveau-Richard et al., of Chinese and French women, the onset of facial wrinkles was found to be approximately 10 years later in Chinese versus French women.[8] In a multinational survey study by Alexis et al., most Asian and Hispanic women did not report moderate/severe facial aging until 50 to 69 years, as compared to 40 to 59 years in White women and 60 to 79 years in Black/African-American women.[9] Another study by Grimes found a much lower percentage of women of color perceived having wrinkles than did their White counterparts.[10]

Notwithstanding these differences in aging, facial rhytids remain a common concern across the racial and ethnic spectrum. Repetitive contraction of facial muscles result in hyperdynamic wrinkles and lines in all skin types. Ethnic populations are more likely to develop facial lines and wrinkles in the glabellar region, whereas perioral rhytids are uncommon (Fig. 17.1), and therefore the upper face is the primary site of wrinkle reduction with botulinum toxin in patients of color.[3,11]

SAFETY AND EFFICACY

Apart from the standard precautions to treatment, which are universal in all skin types, such as allergies to the formulation or neuromuscular diseases, the use of botulinum toxin is safe and effective in non-White patient populations.[12–23] Published data pertaining to the safety and efficacy of botulinum toxin to smooth hyperdynamic wrinkles in non-White patient populations are summarized herein (Table 17.1).[12–23]

A multicenter, double-blind, placebo-controlled study of onabotulinumtoxinA (OnaBoNT-A) (Botox Cosmetic®,

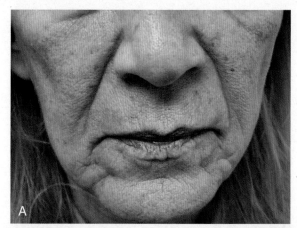
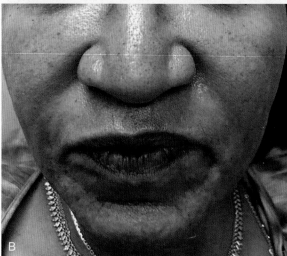

Fig. 17.1 Aging of the lower face in a 65-year-old (A) White woman and (B) Black/African-American woman. Note the significant fine and course wrinkles in the White patient, as compared to the texture irregularities and hyperpigmentation in the Black/African-American patient.

Allergan, Inc., Irvine, CA) by Carruthers et al., in 2002 investigated safety and efficacy in the treatment of glabellar lines in 409 patients. No appreciable differences were observed between various skin phototypes.[24]

In a post-hoc analysis of pooled safety and efficacy data from six clinical trials, Taylor et al. found a significantly greater clinical response among patients with skin of color than White patients at 30 days in the use of abobotulinumtoxinA (AboBoNT-A) (Dysport®, Galderma Laboratories, Fort Worth, TX) for the correction of glabellar lines. Pooled safety data demonstrated no significant differences in adverse effects.[25]

TABLE 17.1 Safety and Efficacy of Botulinum Toxin in Darker Skin Types

Study	Design	Cohort	Treatment (Serotype [Brand], Dose)	Site	Follow up (Month)	Outcome Measures (1—Primary; 2—Secondary)	Efficacy (Objective Assessment at Peak Response)	Adverse Events	Conclusions	Efficacy or Safety Differences in Race/Ethnicity	
										Efficacy	Safety
Jackson and Vogel	Open-label, postmarketing study; single site	29 subjects, Fitzpatrick skin types IV–VI, 86% female, ages 18–65	IncobotulinumtoxinA 4 U/0.1 cm³	Glabellar rhytids	3	1—Investigator's rating of glabellar line severity at maximum frown using a five-point scale; 2—Subjects' rating of glabellar severity at maximum frown using a five-point scale	Day 30 100%	Adverse events: Burning	IncobotulinumtoxinA has a similar safety and efficacy profile among patients with Fitzpatrick skin types IV–VI as in lighter skin types at 30 and 60 days after treatment for glabellar rhytids	None	None
Lee et al.	Prospective, split-face, evaluator-blinded; multicenter	25 Korean subjects, 96% female, ages 21–58, Fitzpatrick skin type IV	OnaBoNT-A: 24–46 U; AboBoNT-A: 61–117 U	Masseter muscle hypertrophy	3	1—Investigator's assessment of global improvement on a four-point graded scale by comparing pretreatment and posttreatment photos	Week 8 AboBoNT-A: mean grade of clinical improvement 2.8 points; OnaBoNT-A: mean grade of clinical improvement 2.7 points	No major complications reported	Abobotulinum toxin achieved more pronounced improvement at 8 and 12 weeks although not statistically significant. A conversion factor of 2.5:1 of AboBoNT-A to OnaBoNT-A is safe and effective in the treatment of masseter muscle hypertrophy	None	None
Grimes and Shabazz	Randomized, double-blind; single site	31 Black/African-American women, Fitzpatrick skin types V and VI, ages 18–65	OnaBoNT-A: 20 U, 30 U	Glabellar rhytids	4	1—Investigator's assessment on a facial wrinkle scale at maximum frown and repose; 2—Patient's assessment of rhytid severity at maximum frown and repose, patient satisfaction, and incidence of adverse events	Day 30 20 U: 92.4% 30 U: 100%	20 U: 13.3%, 30 U: 12.5%; 1. Mild tingling; 2. Headache; 3. Dull forehead sensation	Efficacious, safe, and well-tolerated at doses of 20 U and 30 U in Black/African-American women with skin types V and VI, with no statistical significant difference between dosage	None	None

Continued

TABLE 17.1   Safety and Efficacy of Botulinum Toxin in Darker Skin Types—cont'd

Study	Design	Cohort	Treatment (Serotype Brand, Dose)	Site	Follow up (Month)	Outcome Measures (1—Primary) (2—Secondary)	Efficacy (Objective Assessment at Peak Response)	Adverse Events	Conclusions	Efficacy or Safety Differences in Race/Ethnicity	
										Efficacy	Safety
Harii and Kawashima	Randomized, double-blind, placebo-controlled; multicenter	142 Japanese subjects, 90% female, ages 20–64	OnaBoNT-A: 10 U, 20 U	Glabellar rhytids	5	1—Physician-rated line severity at maximal contraction 4 weeks after treatment 2—Physician/subject ratings and estimates of the effect's duration	Week 4 10 U: 86.4% 20 U: 88.6%	*Adverse events* 10 U: 67.4%, 20 U: 75.0%. *Placebo:* 59.2% 1. Blepharoptosis 2. Heavy eyelids *Adverse drug reactions* 10 U: 32.6%, 20 U: 273%. Placebo: 22.4%	Doses of BoNT-A of 10 U and 20 U are effective and safe for treating glabellar lines in Japanese subjects 20 U dose provides greater efficacy and longer duration of effect	None	None
Kawashima and Harii	Randomized, open-labeled; multicenter	363 Japanese subjects, BoNT-A-naive, 95% female, ages 20–64 years	OnaBoNT-A: 10 U, 20 U	Glabellar rhytids	16	1—Physician-rated line severity at maximal contraction (used for the analysis of the duration of efficacy and responder rates) assessed at all posttreatment visits for each treatment cycle 2—Physician-rated line severity at rest and the subject-rated line improvement	Week 4 10 U: 92.2–97.6% 20 U: 91.5–98.7%	Adverse events 10 U: 86.7%, 20 U: 83.1% Adverse drug reactions 10 U: 30.6%, 20 U: 32.2% 1. Abnormal sensations in eye 2. Headache 3. Blepharoptosis 4. Pruritus (injection site) 5. Discomfort (injection site) 6. Pain (injection site)	Repeated treatments of glabellar lines with 10 U or 20 U of BoNT-A provided long-term safety and efficacy in Japanese subjects 20 U dose provided longer duration, greater subject satisfaction, and greater subject-rated improvement Repeated treatments with BoNT-A did not affect the duration and effectiveness, provided an unchanged safety profile, and was well tolerated	None	None

Kane et al.	Phase III, double-blind, placebo-controlled; multi-center	816 subjects, 80.6% BoNTA-naive, 88.1% female, 32% non-White, mean age = 49 years	AboBoNT-A: Female: 50, 60, and 70 U Male: 60, 70, and 80 U	Glabellar rhytids	5	1—Live assessment by a blinded evaluator and patient self-assessment at maximum frown using the Glabellar Line Severity Score	30 days	White: 84% Black/African-American: 89% Other race: 85%	Treatment-emergent adverse events and related-ness to study treatment Probable: 6% Possible: 3% 1. Eye disorders: Eyelid ptosis Blurred vision Asthenopia Eyelid edema Blepharo-spasm Dry eye Eyelid disorder 2. Administration-site conditions: Erythema Bruising Hemorrhage Pain/discomfort Irritation Edema 3. Nervous disorder; Headache Migraine Dizziness Facial paresis Hypoesthe-sia Parasthesia Tension headache	A single treatment with BoNTA, with the dose based on gender and muscle mass is well tolerated, efficacious, and long lasting in the treatment of moderate-to-severe glabellar lines Response rates were higher in Black/African-American patients than in White patients Although Black/African-American patients had an incidence of total treatment-emergent adverse events similar to other ethnic groups, BoNTA-treated Black/African-American had a slightly higher incidence of ocular adverse events in the treated group and a lower incidence of injection-site reactions	Yes / Yes

Continued

TABLE 17.1   Safety and Efficacy of Botulinum Toxin in Darker Skin Types—cont'd

Study	Design	Cohort	Treatment (Serotype Brand, Dose)	Site	Follow up (Month)	Outcome Measures (1—Primary) (2—Secondary)	Efficacy (Objective Assessment at Peak Response)	Adverse Events	Conclusions	Efficacy or Safety Differences in Race/Ethnicity — Efficacy	Safety
Farahvash and Arad	Retrospective, non-blinded; single site	108 Iranian subjects, 88% female, ages 20–79 years	AboBoNT-A: 76–90 U	Lateral canthal, frontal, glabellar rhytids	7	1—Investigator's assessment of dynamic (animation) lines on a wrinkle improvement scale	<1 month 97.2%	76–90 U: 1. Mild swelling: 13.9% 2. Ecchymosis: 9.2% 3. Eyelid ptosis: 15%	Safe and effective, providing good-to-excellent cosmetic results lasting at least 4 months in the majority of the Iranian patients	None	None
Ahn et al.	Retrospective, non-blinded; single site	32 Korean subjects, 86.8% female, ages 26–56 years	OnaBoNT-A: 5–10 U	Lateral canthal, frontal, nasal dorsum, glabellar rhytids	12	1—Patient satisfaction	4–5 months unsatisfied: 6.25% slightly improved: 15.6% slight line retained: 78.1%	5–10 U: 1. Altered facial appearance: 9.36% 2. Mild local swelling: 6.25% 3. Ecchymosis at injection site: 9.36%	BoNTA seems to be an effective method of eliminating wrinkle lines on the upper third of the face in Korean patients None of the patients experienced complete removal of wrinkle lines	None	None
Lew et al.	Randomized, non-blinded, nonplacebo-controlled; single site	20 Korean subjects, 80% female, ages 24–60 years	AboBoNT-A: 20 U/0.1 cm³ OnaBoNT-A: 5 U/0.1 cm³	Lateral canthal, frontal, nasal dorsum, nasolabial fold, glabellar rhytids	12	1—Investigator's assessment of changes in degree of facial wrinkles on a graded scale and a graded wrinkle spread test	3–5 months OnaBoNT-A: 72.7% AboBoNT-A: 64.3%	OnaBoNT-A: 35.7% AboBoNT-A: 100% 1. Lagophthalmos 2. Tingling 3. Temporary lid edema	Either preparation of BoNT-A seems to be a safe, simple, and effective nonsurgical method of eliminating periorbital wrinkles in Korean patients Mean corrective effect was better in OnaBoNT-A than AboBoNT-A although not statistically significant Complications occurred in all AboBoNT-A patients and in 35.7% of OnaBoNT-A patients and differences were statistically significant	None	None

Study	Study design	Subjects	BoNT-A/dose	Injection site	No.	Outcome measures	Efficacy	Adverse events	Comments		
Chang et al.	Randomized, double-blind, placebo-controlled, split-face study; single site	Nine BoNTA-naive Taiwanese subjects, 88.9% female, ages 35–55 years	OnaBoNT-A: 20–25 U	Bilateral temporal areas, bilateral cheeks from infraorbital to jaw line	4	1—The effect of face lift, skin tightness and wrinkles soothing on a graded scale evaluated subjectively by patients; the bilateral facial wrinkles and face-lifting effect of subjects evaluated objectively by a dermatologist 2—Evaluation of histologic changes of biopsy samples	Week 4 66.7%	20–25 U: 1. Periorbital muscle weakness: 11.1% 2. Mild/moderate stinging 3. Tolerable pain at injection site: 100%	Face-lifting effects of intradermal BoNTA injection in this study was not conclusive The technique demonstrated in this study, however, showed moderate but significant wrinkles soothing effect on the lower face for 8 weeks The use of BoNTA among this Asian cohort demonstrated moderate efficacy, tolerability and no severe adverse events	None	None
Kadunc et al.	Randomized, double-blind, placebo-controlled, intrapatient study; single site	12 women, Fitzpatrick skin types II–IV ages 47–69	OnaBoNT-A: 1.5 U	Unilateral vermillion border	36	1—Investigator's assessment of comparing pretreatment and posttreatment photographs on a facial wrinkle scale at maximum contraction	6 months 83.3%	1.5 U: 1. Edema: 100% 2. Erythema: 66.6% 3. PIH: 33.3% 4. Localized hypochromia: 8.3% 5. Mild herpes simplex virus eruption: 8.3% 6. Interference with eating/drinking: 33.3%	Pretreatment with BoNTA improves short- and long-term results of perioral chemabrasion in the treatment of severe vertical upper perioral rhytids Transient PIH was notably observed in 16.6% Fitzpatrick type III and 100% type IV patients. PIH was reported to be transient and amenable to bleaching creams	None	Yes

Continued

TABLE 17.1   Safety and Efficacy of Botulinum Toxin in Darker Skin Types—cont'd

Study	Design	Cohort	Treatment (Serotype Brand, Dose)	Site	Follow up (Month)	Outcome Measures (1—Primary 2—Secondary)	Efficacy (Objective Assessment at Peak Response)	Adverse Events	Conclusions	Efficacy or Safety Differences in Race/Ethnicity — Efficacy	Safety
Wu et al.	Prospective, double-blind, randomized, placebo-controlled, parallel-group comparative study	222 Chinese subjects, 83.5% female, mean age 42.3 years	OnaBoNT-A: 20 U	Glabellar rhytids	4	1—Investigator's rating of glabellar line severity at maximum frown on day 30 using a facial wrinkle scale 2—Subjects' global assessment of change in the appearance of glabellar lines graded on a nine-point scale	30 days BoNTA: 94.1% Placebo: 3.5%	*Adverse events* BoNTA: 32.3% *Placebo: 19.3%* 1. Headache BoNTA: 8.8%, Placebo: 1.7% 2. Abnormal eye sensation BoNTA: 5.3% 3. Ptosis BoNTA: 0.6% 4. Nasopharyngitis BoNTA:71%	The efficacy results showed highly statistically significant differences between the study drug and placebo groups at all time points, with 94.1% of subjects in the BoNTA group responding at maximum frown as rated at day 30 by investigators This response exceeded the results reported for US studies of 83.7% and 76.7% and is comparable with the Japanese response rate of 88.6% OnaBoNT-A administered intramuscularly at a total dose of 20 U in the corrugator and procerus muscles is an effective treatment for reducing the severity of glabellar lines for up to 120 days in Chinese people with moderate and severe glabellar lines who are younger than 65. Treatment is safe and well tolerated	None	None

AboBoNT-A, Abobotulinumtoxin-A; *BoNT-A*, botulinum toxin A; *OnaBoNT-A*, onabotulinumtoxinA; *PIH*, postinflammatory hyperpigmentation; *SOC*, skin of Color.

PrabotulinumtoxinA (PraBoNT-A) (Jeuveau®, Evolus, Inc., Newport Beach, CA) has also demonstrated to be safe and effective for glabellar lines in Fitzpatrick skin types IV–VI in a phase III clinical trial with 492 pooled subjects.[26]

EXPERT TECHNIQUES

In contrast to the previously accepted ideal that botulinum toxin alone was effective for the correction of hyperdynamic wrinkles, current guidelines promote the combination of treatment with botulinum toxin and hyaluronic acid fillers, if volume loss is a significant contributor to rhytids.[27]

Additionally, several Global Aesthetics Consensus Group recommendations describe lower toxin doses than in previous guidelines.[27] Lower dosing of botulinum toxin modulates the activity of the excessively contracting the muscle instead of paralyzing the muscle completely.

Upper Face

To optimize treatment outcomes, it is important to evaluate each unique individual's muscle contraction pattern, which may vary based on age-related muscle mass, ethnicity, or gender. The main muscles of the glabellar complex are the corrugators, orbicularis oculi, procerus, depressor supercilii, and frontalis muscles. The corrugators and orbicularis oculi muscles depress the eyebrows and pull the brows downward and toward center.[28] The procerus and depressor supercilii pull the medial eyebrow downward, and the lower fibers of the frontalis muscle elevates the eyebrows.[28] This muscle activity causes hyperkinetic lines in between the eyebrows (Fig. 17.2).

de Almeida and colleagues propose five glabellar contraction patterns.[29] A 2017 pilot study by Jiang et al., found that there was a statistically significant difference in the distribution of glabellar patterns between Chinese and Westerners when comparing the patterns proposed by de Almeida and colleagues.[29,30] Compared to Westerners, wherein a V-shaped pattern is the most common, Chinese subjects exhibit a significantly higher frequency of "Converging Arrows" pattern and a significantly lower frequency of "V" pattern, suggesting that the role of the procerus is less significant and thereby not necessary to inject the procerus with BoNT-A in almost half of the subjects for treatment of their glabellar lines.[30]

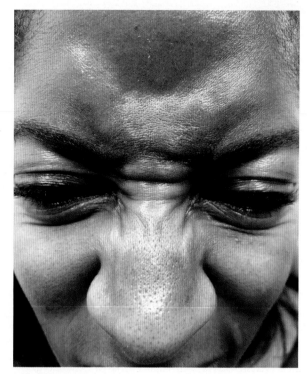

Fig. 17.2 Dynamic glabellar contraction lines in Black/African-American woman.

In contrast, glabellar injection technique has not been shown to vary in Black/African-Americans based on the limited research to date. In a study by Grimes and Shabazz, both 20 and 30 units (U) of OnaBoNT-A were found to be effective in the treatment of glabellar lines without a statistically significant difference in efficacy or safety between the two doses among a sample of 31 African American female subjects.[14] A maximal response was observed on day 30, with 92.4% and 100% response rates (i.e., a score of "none" or "mild" on the facial wrinkle scale) in the 20 U and 30 U groups, respectively.[14] Adverse events, including tingling, slight headaches, and dullness of the forehead, were mild and transient and did not differ between the dosing groups.[14]

There is also limited evidence highlighting that Black/African-Americans may have a longer duration of action and response rate with AboBoNT-A for glabellar lines. In a phase III study by Kane et al., of AboBoNT-A (Dysport®, Galderma Laboratories, Fort Worth, TX)Medicis Aesthetics, Phoenix, AZ) for the correction of moderate-to-severe glabellar lines, the response rates and duration of action of a single treatment with 50, 60, or 70 U of

AboBoNT-A for women and 60, 70, or 80 U for men in a single treatment were found to be slightly higher in Black/African-American subjects than the overall population.[17] The median duration of action was 117 days and 109 days, respectively.[17] However, AboBoNT-A-treated Black/African-American patients had a slightly higher rate of ocular adverse events (6% for Black/African-American patients vs. 4% for other ethnicities) and a lower rate of injection site reactions (3% vs. 5% for other ethnicities).[17]

Lower Face

The adjunctive use of OnaBoNT-A for the treatment of perioral vertical wrinkles in Brazilian subjects (Fitzpatrick skin types II to IV) was investigated in a randomized, double-blind, intrapatient controlled study by Kadunc et al. (n = 12).[22] Subjects with moderate-to-severe vertical rhytids of the upper lip were randomized to receive OnaBoNT-A or saline (control) at the vermilion border followed by chemabrasion with 35% trichloroacetic acid and manual dermabrasion 7 days post injection.[22] Transient postinflammatory hyperpigmentation occurred in 33% (4/12) of subjects, and this was observed in subjects with higher Fitzpatrick skin types—type III (n = 2) and type IV (n = 2). Significantly less wrinkling (on the Facial Wrinkle Severity scale) was seen from day 90 to year 3 in the OnaBoNT-A-treated sides than in placebo.[22]

In a prospective study of 19 female Brazilian subjects, the injection of 0.5U of AboBoNT-A in four points along the vermilion border of the upper lip resulted in a statistically significant change in lip volume (P = 0.002) and patient satisfaction with change in lip shape (P = 0.003).[31]

RACIAL-ETHNIC-SPECIFIC APPLICATIONS

As with any cosmetic procedure, approach to treatment should be unique. The perception of beauty and aesthetic ideals are constantly changing. There are certain aesthetic goals that may be observed more frequently in specific racial or ethnic groups and contribute to variations in the use of botulinum toxin in different populations.

In East Asian populations, a wider and rounder appearance of the eye is a widely accepted aesthetic ideal and botulinum toxin is a popular noninvasive option for widening the palpebral aperture. As reported by Flynn et al., treating the lower eyelid with 2 U of OnaBoNT-A (into the orbicularis oculi in the midpupillary line 3 mm below the ciliary margin) combined with 12 U in the crow's feet, can produce an approximately 3 mm widening of the palpebral aperture at full smile and is a useful approach in addressing this concern in East Asians.[32]

Compared to the White population, Asians have a wider lower third of the face due to a larger mandibular width and/or hypertrophy of the masseter muscle often resulting in a square-shaped face.[33–35] In Asian women, the use of botulinum toxin for masseter muscle hypertrophy is a popular procedure to reshape the undesired square shape into a more contoured, oval-shaped face that is considered more aesthetically pleasing. Studies by Kim and colleagues (n = 1021) and Yu and colleagues (n = 10) demonstrate a 22% to 30% reduction in masseter size 3 months after one treatment with BoNT-A.[34,36] Additional studies highlight that the masseter volume continues to decrease with increasing number of treatments and repeated treatments are needed to maintain this reduced volume.[13,34–37]

Before masseter muscle injection, it is important to ask the patient to clench their teeth to identify the borders of the safe injection zone within the muscle. The recommended safe injection borders are from the mouth corner to the earlobe (upper border), the anterior and posterior edges of the muscle (anterior and posterior borders, respectively), and the inferior edge of the mandible (inferior border)[34–38] (Fig. 17.3). The most common injection-based technique to avoid complications involves injecting BoNT-A deep into the lower

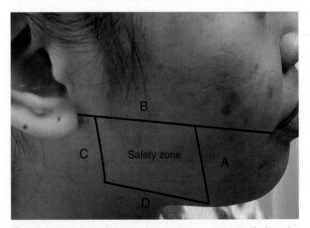

Fig. 17.3 Injection safe zone of the masseter muscle. (A) Anterior border: anterior edge of the masseter muscle. (B) Superior border: ear lobe–mouth corner line. (C) Posterior border: posterior edge of the masseter muscle. (D) Inferior border: inferior edge of the mandible.

third of the masseter muscle at three injection points within the safety zone, two points injected 5 to 10 mm apart in the lower third of the zone, and one point in the center of the middle third of the zone, 5 to 10 mm apart from the other injection points.[38] Data suggest a dose of 30 U onabotulinum toxin A per side significantly reduces masseter muscle size, but amount may vary based on masseter muscle size.[34–38]

Botulinum toxin also offers a nonsurgical alternative to reducing an oversized calf, which is a frequent cosmetic concern in Asian women.[39–41] Administration of 160 to 200 U of prabotulinumtoxinA to both the medial and lateral gastrocnemius muscles can safely and effectively decrease calf circumference without causing disturbance in gait.[40]

The practice of microbotox, defined as injecting multiple microdroplets of diluted OnaBoNT-A into the dermis or subdermal plane to target sweat glands, sebaceous glands, and superficial facial muscle fibers, is gaining popularity in Asia since its initial description in 2000. Wu documents the reduction of platysmal neck bands and a sharper cervicomental angle and jawline in Asian subjects with 1 ml of microbotox to each side with a concentration of 20 units per 1 ml (in patients with thin necks) and 28 units per 1 ml (for thicker necks or deep lines) delivered in 100 to 120 tiny blebs.[42]

CONCLUSIONS

Given extensive published data demonstrating similar safety and efficacy in darker skin populations as seen in Whites, individual variations in muscle anatomy are more important than skin type or racial or ethnic background in the context of treating patients with botulinum toxin for facial aesthetic concerns. As a general rule, tailoring each treatment to a given patient's individual anatomy and aesthetic goals (rather than relying on broad generalizations about racial or ethnic facial features) is the best strategy to use when injecting neurotoxins. However, some ethnic-specific variations in common aesthetic concerns exist, and these, in turn, contribute to unique applications for botulinum toxins in certain populations. Understanding these nuances in aesthetic ideals and the specific techniques to address them is increasingly important given the growing diversity of the patient population seeking cosmetic treatments with botulinum toxins.

REFERENCES

1. Available at: https://www.isaps.org/media/pubgf4jc/global-survey-full-report-2019-english.pdf.
2. US Census Bureau. *Population Projections of the US by Age, Sex, Race and Hispanic Origin: 1995-2050. Current Population Report: 25-1130*. Washington, DC: US Government Press, 2002
3. Davis EC, Callender VD. Aesthetic dermatology for aging ethnic skin. *Dermatol Surg.* 2011;37(7):901-917.
4. Hexsel DM, Hexsel CL, Brunetto LT. Botulinum toxin. In: Grimes PE, ed. *Aesthetics and Cosmetic Surgery for Darker Skin Types.* 1st ed. Philadelphia, PA: Lippincott Williams & Wilkins; 2008:214-215.
5. Rossi A, Alexis A. Cosmetic procedures in skin of color. *G Ital Dermatol Venereol.* 2011;146(4):265-272.
6. Yamaguchi Y, Beer JZ, Hearing VJ. Melanin mediated apoptosis of epidermal cells damaged by ultraviolet radiation: Factors influencing the incidence of skin cancer. *Arch Dermatol Res.* 2008;300(suppl 1):s43-s50.
7. Kaidbey KH, Agin PP, Sayre RM, Kligman AM. Photoprotection by melanin—a comparison of black and Caucasian skin. *J Am Acad Dermatol.* 1979;1(3):249-260.
8. Nouveau-Richard S, Yang Z, Mac-Mary S, et al. Skin ageing: A comparison between Chinese and European populations. A pilot study. *J Dermatol Sci.* 2005;40(3):187-193.
9. Alexis AF, Grimes P, Boyd C, et al. Racial and ethnic differences in self-assessed facial aging in women: Results from a multinational study. *Dermatol Surg.* 2019;45(12):1635-1648.
10. Grimes P. Skin of color. Diseases and cosmetic issues of major concern. *Cosmet Dermatol.* 2003;16:1-4.
11. Grimes PE, ed. *Aesthetics and Cosmetic Surgery for Darker Skin Types.* 1st ed. Philadelphia, PA: Lippincott Williams & Wilkins; 2004.
12. Jackson BA, Vogel MR. Efficacy and safety of incobotulinumtoxin A for the correction of glabellar lines among patients with skin types IV to VI. *J Drugs Dermatol.* 2015;14(4):350-353.
13. Lee SH, Wee SH, Kim HJ, et al. Abobotulinum toxin A and onabotulinum toxin A for masseteric hypertrophy: A split-face study in 25 Korean patients. *J Dermatol Treat.* 2013;24(2):133-136.
14. Grimes PE, Shabazz D. A four-month randomized, double-blind evaluation of the efficacy of botulinum toxin type A for the treatment of glabellar lines in women with skin types V and VI. *Dermatol Surg.* 2009;35(3):429-436.
15. Harii K, Kawashima M. A double-blind, randomized, placebo-controlled, two-dose comparative study of botulinum toxin type A for treating glabellar lines in Japanese subjects. *Aesthetic Plast Surg.* 2008;32(5):724-730.

16. Kawashima M, Harii K. An open-label, randomized, 64-week study repeating 10- and 20-U doses of botulinum toxin type A for treatment of glabellar lines in Japanese subjects. *Int J Dermatol*. 2009;48(7):768-776.

17. Kane MA, Brandt F, Rohrich RJ, et al. Evaluation of variable-dose treatment with a new U.S. botulinum toxin type A (Dysport) for correction of moderate to severe glabellar lines: Results from a phase III, randomized, double-blind, placebo-controlled study. *Plast Reconstr Surg*. 2009;124(5):1619-1629.

18. Farahvash MR, Arad S. Clostridium botulinum type A toxin for the treatment of upper face animation lines: An Iranian experience. *J Cosmet Dermatol*. 2007;6(3):152-158.

19. Ahn KY, Park MY, Park DH, Han DG. Botulinum toxin A for the treatment of facial hyperkinetic wrinkle lines in Koreans. *Plast Reconstr Surg*. 2000;105(2):778-784.

20. Lew H, Yun YS, Lee SY, Kim SJ. Effect of botulinum toxin A on facial wrinkle lines in Koreans. *Ophthalmologica*. 2002;216(1):50-54.

21. Chang SP, Tsai HH, Chen WY, et al. The wrinkles soothing effect on the middle and lower face by intradermal injection of botulinum toxin type A. *Int J Dermatol*. 2008; 47:1287-1294.

22. Kadunc BV, Trindade DE, Almeida AR, Vanti AA, Di Chiacchio N. Botulinum toxin A adjunctive use in manual chemabrasion: controlled long-term study for treatment of upper perioral vertical wrinkles. *Dermatol Surg*. 2007;33(9):1066-1072, discussion 1072.

23. Wu Y, Zhao G, Li H, et al. Botulinum toxin type A for the treatment of glabellar lines in Chinese: a double-blind, randomized, placebo-controlled study. *Dermatol Surg*. 2010;36(1):102-108.

24. Carruthers JA, Lowe NJ, Menter MA, et al. A multicenter, double-blind, randomized, placebo-controlled study of the efficacy and safety of botulinum toxin type A in the treatment of glabellar lines. *J Am Acad Dermatol*. 2002; 46(6):840-849.

25. Taylor SC, Callender VD, Albright CD, et al. AbobotulinumtoxinA for reduction of glabellar lines in patients with skin of color: Post hoc analysis of pooled clinical trial data. *Dermatol Surg*. 2012;38(11):1804-1811.

26. Taylor SC, Grimes PE, Joseph JH, Jonker A, Avelar RL. PrabotulinumtoxinA for the treatment of moderate-to-severe glabellar lines in adult patients with skin of color: Post hoc analyses of the US phase III clinical study data. *Dermatol Surg*. 2021;47(4):516-521.

27. Carruthers JD, Glogau RG, Blitzer A. Facial Aesthetics Consensus Group Faculty. Advances in facial rejuvenation: botulinum toxin type A, hyaluronic acid dermal fillers, and combination therapies—consensus recommendations. *Plast Reconstr Surg*. 2008;121(suppl 5): s5-s30, quiz s31-s36.

28. Casabona G, Kaye K, Barreto Marchese P, Boggio R, Cotofana S. Six years of experience using an advanced algorithm for botulinum toxin application. *J Cosmet Dermatol*. 2019;18(1):21-35.

29. de Almeida AR, da Costa Marques ER, Banegas R, Kadunc BV. Glabellar contraction patterns: A tool to optimize botulinum toxin treatment. *Dermatol Surg*. 2012;38(9): 1506-1515.

30. Jiang H, Zhou J, Chen S. Different glabellar contraction patterns in Chinese and efficacy of botulinum toxin type A for treating glabellar lines: A pilot study. *Dermatol Surg*. 2017;43(5):692-697.

31. Pinto C, Rebellato P, Schmitt J, de Torre D. Lip volumization using botulinum toxin. *Surg Cosmet Dermatol*. 2017; 9(1):24-28.

32. Flynn TC, Carruthers JA. Botulinum-A toxin treatment of the lower eyelid improves infraorbital rhytids and widens the eye. *Dermatol Surg*. 2001;27(8):703-708.

33. McKnight A, Momoh AO, Bullocks JM. Variations of structural components: Specific intercultural differences in facial morphology, skin type, and structures. *Semin Plast Surg*. 2009;23(3):163-167.

34. Kim NH, Chung JH, Park RH, Park JB. The use of botulinum toxin type A in aesthetic mandibular contouring. *Plast Reconstr Surg*. 2005;115:919-930.

35. Kim NH, Park RH, Park JB. Botulinum toxin type A for the treatment of hypertrophy of the masseter muscle. *Plast Reconstr Surg*. 2010;125(6):1693-1705.

36. Yu CC, Chen PK, Chen YR. Botulinum toxin A for lower facial contouring: A prospective study. *Aesthetic Plast Surg*. 2007;31:445-451.

37. Ahn J, Horn C, Blitzer A. Botulinum toxin for masseter reduction in Asian patients. *Arch Facial Plast Surg*. 2004; 6(3):188-191.

38. Peng HP, Peng JH. Complications of botulinum toxin injection for masseter hypertrophy: Incidence rate from 2036 treatments and summary of causes and preventions. *J Cosmet Dermatol*. 2018;17(1):33-38.

39. Lee HJ, Lee DW, Park YH, et al. Botulinum toxin a for aesthetic contouring of enlarged medial gastrocnemius muscle. *Dermatol Surg*. 2004;30(6):867-871, discussion 871.

40. Suh Y, Jeong GJ, Noh H, et al. A multicenter, randomized, open-label comparative study of prabotulinumtoxinA with two different dosages and diverse proportional injection styles for the reduction of gastrocnemius muscle hypertrophy in Asian women. *Dermatol Ther*. 2019;32(5):e13009.

41. Han KH, Joo YH, Moon SE, Kim KH. Botulinum toxin A treatment for contouring of the lower leg. *J Dermatol Treat*. 2006;17(4):250-254.

42. Wu WT. Microbotox of the lower face and neck: Evolution of a personal technique and its clinical effects. *Plast Reconstr Surg*. 2015;136(suppl 5):s92-s100.

18

Soft Tissue Fillers in Skin of Color

Malika A. Ladha, Hassan Galadari, Cheryl Burgess

SUMMARY AND KEY FEATURES

- There is an ongoing increase in soft tissue filler procedures by populations with skin of color (SOC).
- There are important inter- and intraracial anatomical variations, as well as differences in aesthetic preferences.
- While limited in nature, the current body of evidence demonstrates that SOC patients can safely undergo soft tissue filler.

Demographic trends, in conjunction with increased awareness and availability of minimally invasive treatments, have led to a more diverse patient population in the aesthetic industry. The American Society of Aesthetic Plastic Surgery reports a 50% increase, over the last 12 years, in the uptake of aesthetic procedures by patients with skin of color in the United States of America.[1,2] In 2017, approximately 32% of cosmetic procedures were performed on racial/ethnic minorities.[3] In 2019, Hispanics were the largest ethnic population with SOC to undergo minimally invasive aesthetic procedures (14%), followed by Black/African-Americans (10%) and Asians (6%).[2]

With this increased uptake, practitioners must have a deep understanding of anatomical variations, aesthetic preferences, and evidence for cosmetic treatments for patients of SOC. This chapter defines patients of *SOC* as individuals with darker skin tones, in the range of Fitzpatrick IV–VI phototypes. This includes but is not limited to those of Asian, African, Hispanic/Latino, Middle Eastern, and mixed racial (bi- and multiracial) backgrounds. The descriptions and comparisons herein involve White populations of European descent as the comparative group.

CHARACTERISTICS OF AGING

Signs of facial aging tend to be delayed in patients of *SOC* due to the photoprotective properties of increased eumelanin. However, cultural and geographic variations in sun-exposure behavior may also contribute to observed racial/ethnic differences in photoaging. Patients with SOC generally experience age-related changes 10 to 20 years after their White counterparts.[4–6] White patients tend to experience more rhytids. In contrast, patients with SOC more prominently exhibit gravity-induced descent of soft tissue and atrophy of the underlying bone structure, leading to midface laxity.[7]

Aging in the Black/African-American population tends to be characterized by malar fat pad sagging, tear-trough deformity, deepening of the nasolabial folds, jowl formation, and loss of upper lip volume with preservation of the lower lip volume (Figs. 18.1–18.3).[4,8,9] For East Asians, the aging pattern typically includes soft-tissue laxity of the midface and tear trough formation due to a weaker skeletal framework and thicker skin.[8,10] South Asians frequently experience more facial fullness and descent of the mid-face tissue with aging.[11] For Hispanics, aging most commonly includes eyebrow and eyelid drooping, infra-orbital

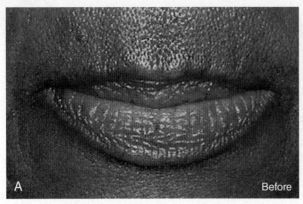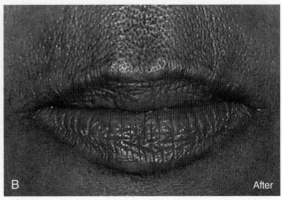

Fig. 18.1 (A) The lips of a 70-year-old Black female prior to filler treatment. Note the loss of volume in the upper lip. (B) The lips of a 70-year-old Black female after hyaluronic acid filler treatment. The goal of the treatment was to restore the 1:1 upper to lower lip ratio for this patient.

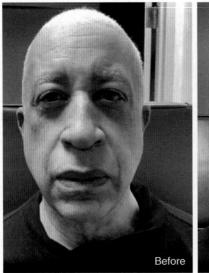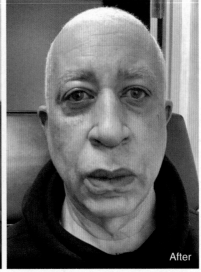

Fig. 18.2 Before and after images of a 68-year-old Black/African-American male who underwent midface voluminization with hyaluronic acid fillers.

hollowing, and thickening of the nasolabial folds (Fig. 18.4).[8,10,12] Aging in Middle Eastern patients commonly presents as mid-face sagging and jowl formation.[13]

SOFT TISSUE FILLERS—THE EVIDENCE

At present, there are 13 soft tissue fillers approved by the Food and Drug Agency (FDA) for treatment of the cheeks, nasolabial folds, chin, lips, and dorsal hands. Soft tissue fillers provide facial volumization, contouring, and definition. Currently available soft tissue fillers can be considered in two categories: hyaluronic acid and biostimulatory fillers. The former is the most injected type of filler. The latter, which includes calcium hydroxyapatite and poly-L-lactic acid, stimulates a gradual, progressive fibroplasia leading to increased collagen and elastin formation, and ultimately dermal remodeling.[14]

To date, there are five clinical studies on the use of soft tissue fillers in Fitzpatrick IV–VI phototype patients (Table 18.1).

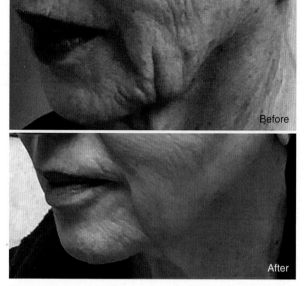

Fig. 18.3 Before and after images of a Black/African-American female treated with hyaluronic acid fillers, calcium hydroxyapatite fillers, and polydioxanone threads to the lower face.

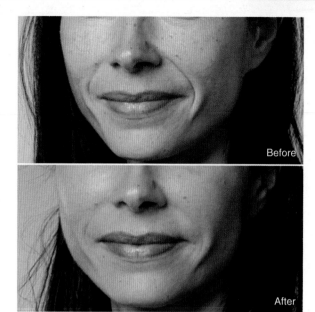

Fig. 18.4 Before and after images of a 24 year old Middle Eastern woman who has HA fillers in the cheeks and nasolabial folds.

TABLE 18.1	**Summary of Soft Tissue Filler Studies in Fitzpatrick IV–VI Patients**				
Author	**Study Details**	**Number of Participants**	**Filler Type**	**Location**	**Adverse Effects**
Downie et al.[16]	Open-label, nonrandomized trial	93	Hyaluronic acid	Nasolabial fold	Temporary injection site bruising, discoloration
Grimes et al.[17]	Double-blind, randomized trial	160	High-concentration hyaluronic acid	Nasolabial fold	None reported
	Open-label, randomized trial	119	Low-concentration hyaluronic acid	Nasolabial fold	Mild hyperpigmentation
Marmur et al.[21]	Open-label, nonrandomized, prospective trial	100	Calcium hydroxyapatite	Nasolabial fold	None reported
Taylor et al.[15]	Randomized, evaluator-blinded trial	150	Nonanimal stabilized hyaluronic acid	Nasolabial fold	Temporary bruising, tenderness, edema, redness, itching, and changes in pigmentation
Taylor et al.[20]	Pooled data from two randomized trials	72 included in evaluation	Hyaluronic acid	Lip and perioral	Temporary swelling, firmness, tenderness, and pigment changes

In a prospective, multicentered, randomized, evaluator-blinded study, Taylor et al. used nonanimal stabilized hyaluronic acid filler to correct moderate to severe nasolabial folds in Fitzpatrick skin types IV–VI.[15] Investigators injected large-particle gel hyaluronic acid filler into the deep dermis to the superficial subcutaneous tissue and small particle-gel hyaluronic acid filler into the mid- to deep dermis using a fan, linear-threading approach, or droplet with serial puncture technique. Less than a mean of 2 mL of filler was required to achieve correction of the nasolabial fold, and efficacy was maintained at 24 weeks. Mild pigmentation changes occurred in 6% and 9% of patients treated with large-particle gel and small-particle gel, respectively. The majority resolved in 12 weeks except for three patients with postinflammatory hyperpigmentation. Most hyperpigmentation cases were associated with multiple or serial puncture sites.

In an open-label, multicenter trial, 93 patients of Fitzpatrick skin types IV–VI had correction of their nasolabial folds with a cohesive, polydensified hyaluronic acid filler.[16] The mean initial volume used was 1.46 mL and 1.47 mL in the left and right nasolabial fold, respectively. This led to an improvement in the Wrinkle Severity Rating Scale and the Global Aesthetic Improvement Scale. At 2 weeks, 72% of patients required a touch up. One patient developed mild hypopigmentation and two others developed mild hyperpigmentation.

In two prospective studies, a total of 160 subjects had one of three high-concentration fillers injected while 119 subjects were treated with one of three low-concentration fillers for their nasolabial folds.[17] At 24 weeks, all had maintained a one-or-more-point improvement in their Nasolabial Fold Score. Near 8% of subjects developed transient discoloration.

Two pivotal prospective clinical trials assessing the effectiveness and safety of two hyaluronic acid fillers for lip and perioral enhancement included patients of all Fitzpatrick skin types.[18,19] Taylor et al. pooled the data for Fitzpatrick phototype IV–VI patients from these trials. The effectiveness of hyaluronic acid dermal fillers for lip and perioral enhancement was similar for all phototypes in the original studies.[20] The mean initial filler used was 1.58 mL and 55.8% required a touch up. At 3 months, mean lip fullness improved by 1.1 on the Lip Fullness Scale; this was sustained at 6 months. In addition, the types and incidence of side effects such as bruising, redness, and discoloration in patients of Fitzpatrick IV–VI phototypes were lower than those of lighter-skinned counterparts.[20]

Through an open-label, nonrandomized prospective trial, Marmur et al. demonstrated the safety of calcium hydroxyapatite filler for nasolabial fold treatment in 100 patients.[21] In this postmarket study, a mean of 1.24 mL of calcium hydroxyapatite was injected subdermally with a linear threading and fanning technique. No adverse outcomes were reported. At 6 months, no patient sustained keloid formation, hypertrophic scarring, or pigment changes. The authors postulated that the lack of pigmentation side effects may be due to the deeper injections used for calcium hydroxyapatite.

There are no controlled studies on poly-L-lactic acid in patients with SOC.

CLINICAL APPROACH

The first step for soft tissue filler use in populations with skin of color is to appropriately identify and classify patients. A potential pitfall is to assume a patient's racial or ethnic background solely based on skin color. At the first consultation, physicians should review the patient's racial background (Table 18.2). Bi- or multiracial patients should be asked with which race they physically identify.

Specific description terminology, as opposed to labeling by Fitzpatrick phototype only, should be used. The Fitzpatrick phototype system is based on an individual's

TABLE 18.2   **Examples of Specific Questions to Ask About Race and Ethnicity**
• What is your racial/ethnic background(s)? (Alternative approaches: With what racial/ethnic background do you identify?; How would you describe your racial/ethnic background?)
• What is your mother's racial/ethnic background?
• What is your father's racial/ethnic background?
• If you are bi- or multiracial, with which group do you physically identify?
• What facial features of your race/ethnicity do you like?
• What facial features of your face/ethnicity do you not prefer?
• Which facial features do you wish to maintain, enhance, and change?

response to ultraviolet exposure;[22] however, it does not consider anatomic differences or age-related changes.[23] For example, Latino and Middle Eastern patients can both be Fitzpatrick phototypes IV and yet have very different facial anatomy. Specific description terms should thus be identified in conjunction with the patient.

Aesthetic preferences are informed by culture and race, and as such, will differ from Westernized beauty standards.[8] Patients with SOC come from diverse backgrounds and beauty standards vary across the globe. Practitioners should thus develop strong cultural awareness to understand and meet the aesthetic goals of patients with skin of color. To avoid broad generalizations, patients should be consulted on their individual goals. Some patients may wish to deviate from standards of beauty inherent to their race.

In addition, there are morphological differences between various races and within races. A deep understanding of these anatomic variations is required to

identify what is aesthetically pleasing and how to achieve optimal cosmetic outcomes. For example, East Asians seek hyaluronic acid filler treatments to address midface structural retrusion (Fig. 18.5). However, practitioners must also consider the increased bizygomatic width of East Asians. Soft tissue fillers should be placed in the central face to provide anterior projection while also not widening the face.[24]

Another example is lip enhancement in Black/African-American patients (Fig. 18.1 A and B). There is a common misconception that Black/African-American patients do not seek lip filler treatments. In contrast to White patients who aim to increase the size of their lips, Black/African-American patients tend to restore the 50:50 lip proportion from their youth.[9] Black/African-American patients present later in life for soft tissue filler enhancements of their lips compared to White patients.[25]

Filler type should also be considered. For example, patients with SOC may have compact and increased

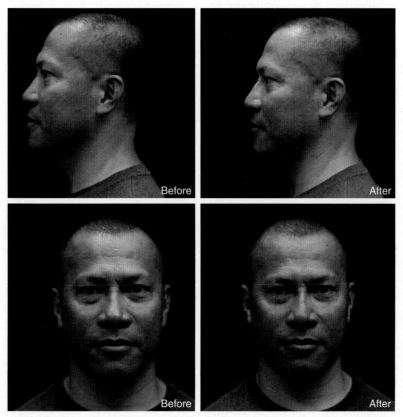

Fig. 18.5 Before and after image images of a 45-year-old Filipino male who underwent hyaluronic acid filler injections of the nose.

collagen bundles (e.g., as shown in studies involving Black subjects); this provides a scaffold for volumization. Stimulatory soft tissue fillers, including calcium hydroxyapatite and poly-L-lactic acid, thus may be preferred.[9] Overall, patients with SOC achieve the desired outcome after fewer treatments; this results in a longer interval between treatments to avoid overcorrection.[26,27]

Overall, all patients of all ethnic groups can benefit from soft tissue filler treatments (Figs. 18.1–18.6).

COMPLICATIONS & BEST PRACTICES

Awareness and application of safety data are imperative for successful and safe soft tissue filler injections. The current literature demonstrates that patients with SOC can safely undergo filler treatments.

In general, patients of all skin tones are at risk of bruising, edema, tenderness, and erythema—these tend to be mild and transient. A case review of 60 patients demonstrated no difference in complication rates for hyaluronic acid filler treatments between Fitzpatrick I–III phototype patients and IV–VI patients.[28]

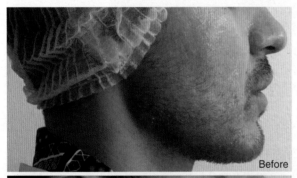
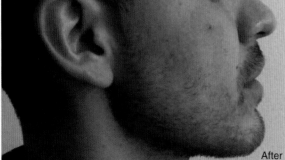

Fig. 18.6 Before and after images of a 36-year-old Middle Eastern male who had calcium hydroxyapatite injections to his jawline.

A frequently shared myth is that patients with SOC specifically should not undergo soft tissue filler treatments due to the increased risk of hyperpigmentation and keloid scar formation. While transient hyperpigmentation has been described in small numbers, no studies have reported an increased risk of permanent discoloration or scarring for patients with SOC. Two techniques can reduce these risks: 1) minimize the total number of punctures to the skin and 2) place fillers in the mid-dermis to avoid direct disruption of the epidermal–dermal junction.[15,21]

The Tyndall effect—blue discoloration due to light scattering—can occur if fillers are placed too superficially.[29] This most often occurs in an area with thin skin, such as the periorbital area. The risk of the Tyndall effect may be minimized in some patients with SOC due to thicker skin properties.[30] Nonetheless, superficial placement of hyaluronic acid fillers in the periorbital area should be avoided.

Inadvertent intraarterial injections result in the most dangerous complications, including tissue necrosis or embolism that can cause stroke or blindness. A review of the cases with this feared complication revealed the most commonly injected locations leading to blindness are the nose (55%), glabella (35%), and forehead (11%).[31]

Interestingly, a higher incidence of this complication occurs in East Asian countries, such as Korea (40%) and China (19%).[31,32] Asians have a relatively flat central facial profile, and nonsurgical rhinoplasties and other techniques utilize fillers to increase three-dimensionality of the central face (Fig. 18.5).[24] The uptake of these techniques likely contributes to the higher incidence. Anatomic variations may also play a role. As the dorsal nasal artery directly feeds into the ophthalmic artery, inadvertent injection to the dorsal nasal artery can cause blindness. In an anatomic study, 60% of East Asian cadavers had a single oblique vessel for the dorsal nasal artery, in contrast to bilateral vessels.[33] Direct injections to higher-risk areas such as the glabella and nasal tip should be avoided, and filler placement should be at the periosteal layer.[34] Given the complexity of anatomical considerations and the associated risks, only highly experienced physician injectors should complete such an advanced technique.

COMBINATION TREATMENTS

Soft tissue fillers are a single tool in the aesthetic physician's armamentarium. To achieve the best clinical outcomes, a global assessment and multi-modal approach must be utilized (Figs. 18.3 and 18.7).

Neurotoxins are the mainstay of dynamic wrinkle treatment and often the "gateway" treatment for comprehensive facial rejuvenation. The combination of hyaluronic acid and botulinum toxin A treatment is superior to hyaluronic acid treatment alone.[35,36] In addition to superior results, the duration of general effect can be increased by 14 weeks with combination treatment.[36] Hyaluronic acid fillers and neurotoxins work synergistically to reduce skin rhytids: hyaluronic acid fillers provide a more natural return to baseline as the toxin loses efficacy, and the toxin's muscle-relaxing effect slows the breakdown of the hyaluronic acid (Fig. 18.7).

As with soft tissue filler, differences in facial anatomy and cultural preferences will determine the placement and dosage of botulinum toxin A. For example, the corrugator muscles of East Asians tend to be shorter and narrower. Therefore, a lower dosage of botulinum toxin A is typically recommended for the East Asian glabella complex.[37] In contrast, East Asians are more likely to have increased masseter muscle mass. As such, off-label botulinum toxin A injections are more commonly utilized by East Asians for shaping the lower face.[37]

Lasers and energy-based treatments are gaining popularity to improve skin quality, texture, and color, while soft tissue fillers provide volumization, contouring, and

definition. Radiofrequency devices tighten the skin. It has been suggested that same-day treatment of both modalities may provide synergistic long-term effects for volume loss.[37] Goldman et al. have demonstrated that hyaluronic acid fillers can be combined with 1320-nm Nd:YAG laser or 1450-nm diode laser without impacting effect or safety.[38] Of note, long-pulsed 1064-nm Nd:YAG is the preferred device for hair reduction in patients with SOC.[39]

FUTURE DIRECTIONS

The future direction of soft tissue augmentation in SOC populations comprises three important components: research, classification, and education.

SOC patients are underrepresented in premarket clinical studies and very few post-approval studies have assessed safety.[40] Premarket trials must incorporate SOC patients in larger numbers.

The Fitzpatrick scale is currently used to identify subjects in clinical trials. Multiple other classifications have been proposed, such as the Goldman World Classification of Skin Type, the Taylor Hyperpigmentation Scale, and the Roberts Hyperpigmentation Scale.[41–43] The latter enables practitioners to rate a patient's phototype, hyperpigmentation, photoaging, and scarring capability and thus enables physicians to anticipate some of the short- and long-term effects of cosmetic procedures.

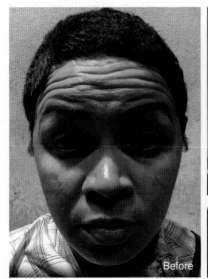
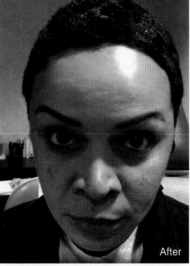

Fig. 18.7 Before and after images of a 43-year-old Black/African-American female who had the following combination treatment: mid-face hyaluronic acid fillers and botulinum toxin-A to the glabellar and forehead areas.

However, no scale captures the nuances of underlying facial morphology variation.[23,43] A more comprehensive and encompassing classification system for patients with SOC is thus required.

Regarding education, Rodrigues et al. completed a national survey of Australian dermatologists that found that 85% were not confident in undertaking cosmetic treatments in patients with SPC.[44] This survey also indicated a strong desire for more education regarding SOC cosmetic issues. Racial or ethnic concordance between patients and physicians may contribute to increased cultural understanding but is not a prerequisite for successful outcomes; an individual dermatologist's broad training, clinical expertise, and general cultural competence are paramount.[45] Thus training on SOC cosmetics should encompass all dermatologists.

REFERENCES

1. The American Society for Aesthetic Plastic Surgery. *ASAPS 1997 Statistics on Cosmetic Surgery.* Available at: https://cdn.theaestheticsociety.org/media/statistics/1997-TheAestheticSocietyStatistics.pdf.
2. Surgery. *Aesthetics Plastic Surgery National Databank Statistics 2019.* ASfAP. 2019.
3. *Procedural Statistics.* The American Society for Aesthetic Plastic Surgery; 2017.
4. Alexis, Boyd C, Callender V, Downie J, Sangha S. Understanding the female African American facial aesthetic patient. *J Drugs Dermatol.* 2019;18(9):858-866.
5. Borda LJ, Ross A, Villada G, Milikowski C. Acute mucocutaneous methotrexate toxicity with marked tissue eosinophilia. *BMJ Case Rep.* 2018;2018:bcr2017221489. doi:10.1136/bcr-2017-221489.
6. Nouveau-Richard S, Yang Z, Mac-Mary S, et al. Skin ageing: A comparison between Chinese and European populations. A pilot study. *J Dermatol Sci.* 2005;40(3):187-193. doi:10.1016/j.jdermsci.2005.06.006.
7. Quiñonez RL, Agbai ON, Burgess CM, Taylor SC. An update on cosmetic procedures in people of color. Part 2: Neuromodulators, soft tissue augmentation, chemexfoliating agents, and laser hair reduction. *J Am Acad Dermatol.* 2022;86(4):729-739. doi:10.1016/j.jaad.2021.07.080.
8. Talakoub L, Wesley NO. Differences in perceptions of beauty and cosmetic procedures performed in ethnic patients. *Semin Cutan Med Surg.* 2009;28(2):115-129. doi:10.1016/j.sder.2009.05.001.
9. Burgess C, Awosika O. Ethnic and gender considerations in the use of facial injectables: African-American patients. *Plast Reconstr Surg.* 2015;136(suppl 5):28S-31S. doi:10.1097/PRS.0000000000001813.
10. Vashi NA, de Castro Maymone MB, Kundu RV. Aging differences in ethnic skin. *J Clin Aesthet Dermatol.* 2016;9(1):31-38.
11. Shetty R. Outer circle versus inner circle: Special considerations while rejuvenating an Indian face using fillers. *J Cutan Aesthet Surg.* 2015;8(3):169-172. doi:10.4103/0974-2077.167281.
12. Grimes P. Beauty: A historical and societal perspective. In: Grimes P, Kim J, Hexsel D, Soriano T, eds. *Aesthetics and Cosmetic Surgery for Darker Skin Types.* Lippincott Williams & Wilkins; 2007:chap 9–10.
13. Kashmar M, Alsufyani MA, Ghalamkarpour F, et al. Consensus opinions on facial beauty and implications for aesthetic treatment in Middle Eastern women. *Plast Reconstr Surg Glob Open.* 2019;7(4):e2220. doi:10.1097/GOX.0000000000002220.
14. Berlin A, Cohen JL, Goldberg DJ. Calcium hydroxylapatite for facial rejuvenation. *Semin Cutan Med Surg.* 2006;25(3):132-137. doi:10.1016/j.sder.2006.06.005.
15. Taylor SC, Burgess CM, Callender VD. Safety of nonanimal stabilized hyaluronic acid dermal fillers in patients with skin of color: A randomized, evaluator-blinded comparative trial. *Dermatol Surg.* 2009;35 suppl 2:1653-1660. doi:10.1111/j.1524-4725.2009.01344.x.
16. Downie JB, Grimes PE, Callender VD. A multicenter study of the safety and effectiveness of hyaluronic acid with a cohesive polydensified matrix for treatment of nasolabial folds in subjects with Fitzpatrick skin types IV, V, and VI. *Plast Reconstr Surg.* 2013;132(4 suppl 2):41S-47S. doi:10.1097/PRS.0b013e318299ff53.
17. Grimes PE, Thomas JA, Murphy DK. Safety and effectiveness of hyaluronic acid fillers in skin of color. *J Cosmet Dermatol.* 2009;8(3):162-168. doi:10.1111/j.1473-2165.2009.00457.x.
18. Dayan S, Bruce S, Kilmer S, et al. Safety and effectiveness of the hyaluronic acid filler, HYC-24L, for lip and perioral augmentation. *Dermatol Surg.* 2015;41 suppl 1:S293-S301. doi:10.1097/dss.0000000000000540.
19. Geronemus RG, Bank DE, Hardas B, Shamban A, Weichman BM, Murphy DK. Safety and effectiveness of VYC-15L, a hyaluronic acid filler for lip and perioral enhancement: One-year results from a randomized, controlled study. *Dermatol Surg.* 2017;43(3):396-404. doi:10.1097/dss.0000000000001035.
20. Taylor SC, Downie JB, Shamban A, et al. Lip and perioral enhancement with hyaluronic acid dermal fillers in individuals with skin of color. *Dermatol Surg.* 2019;45(7):959-967. doi:10.1097/dss.0000000000001842.
21. Marmur ES, Taylor SC, Grimes PE, Boyd CM, Porter JP, Yoo JY. Six-month safety results of calcium hydroxylapatite

for treatment of nasolabial folds in Fitzpatrick skin types IV to VI. *Dermatol Surg.* 2009;35 suppl 2:1641-1645. doi:10.1111/j.1524-4725.2009.01311.x.

22. Fitzpatrick TB. The validity and practicality of sun-reactive skin types I through VI. *Arch Dermatol.* 1988;124(6):869-871. doi:10.1001/archderm.124.6.869.

23. Ware OR, Dawson JE, Shinohara MM, Taylor SC. Racial limitations of Fitzpatrick skin type. *Cutis.* 2020;105(2): 77-80.

24. Liew S. Ethnic and gender considerations in the use of facial injectables: Asian patients. *Plast Reconstr Surg.* 2015;136(suppl 5):22S-27S. doi:10.1097/PRS.000000000 0001728.

25. Burgess CM. Dermal fillers in ethnic skin. In: Alexis AF BV, eds. *Skin of Color: A Practical Guide to Dermatologic Diagnosis and Treatment.* New York: Springer; 2013:247-262.

26. Burgess CM. Special considerations in African American skin. In: Alam M BA, Kundu R, et al., eds. *Cosmetic Dermatology for Skin of Color.* McGraw-Hill Companies; 2008:163-167.

27. Hamilton TK, Burgess CM. Considerations for the use of injectable poly-L-lactic acid in people of color. *J Drugs Dermatol.* 2010;9(5):451-456.

28. Odunze M, Cohn A, Few JW. Restylane and people of color. *Plast Reconstr Surg.* 2007;120(7):2011-2016. doi:10.1097/01.prs.0000287330.94038.63.

29. King M. Management of Tyndall effect. *J Clin Aesthet Dermatol.* 2016;9(11):E6-E8.

30. Choi HS, Whipple KM, Oh SR, et al. Modifying the upper eyelid crease in Asian patients with hyaluronic acid fillers. *Plast Reconstr Surg.* 2011;127(2):844-849. doi:10.1097/ PRS.0b013e3181fed6cb.

31. Sorensen EP, Council ML. Update in soft-tissue filler-associated blindness. *Dermatol Surg.* 2020;46(5):671-677. doi:10.1097/dss.0000000000002108.

32. Beleznay K, Carruthers JDA, Humphrey S, Carruthers A, Jones D. Update on avoiding and treating blindness from fillers: A recent review of the world literature. *Aesthet Surg J.* 2019;39(6):662-674. doi:10.1093/asj/sjz053.

33. Tansatit T, Apinuntrum P, Phetudom T. Facing the worst risk: Confronting the dorsal nasal artery, implication for non-surgical procedures of nasal augmentation. *Aesthetic Plast Surg.* 2017;41(1):191-198. doi:10.1007/s00266-016-0756-0.

34. Liew S, Scamp T, de Maio M, et al. Efficacy and safety of a hyaluronic acid filler to correct aesthetically detracting or deficient features of the Asian nose: A prospective, open-label, long-term study. *Aesthet Surg J.* 2016;36(7): 760-772. doi:10.1093/asj/sjw079.

35. Dubina M, Tung R, Bolotin D, et al. Treatment of forehead/glabellar rhytide complex with combination botulinum toxin a and hyaluronic acid versus botulinum toxin A injection alone: A split-face, rater-blinded, randomized control trial. *J Cosmet Dermatol.* 2013;12(4):261-266. doi:10.1111/jocd.12059.

36. Carruthers J, Carruthers A. A prospective, randomized, parallel group study analyzing the effect of BTX-A (Botox) and nonanimal sourced hyaluronic acid (NASHA, Restylane) in combination compared with NASHA (Restylane) alone in severe glabellar rhytides in adult female subjects: Treatment of severe glabellar rhytides with a hyaluronic acid derivative compared with the derivative and BTX-A. *Dermatol Surg.* 2003;29(8): 802-809. doi:10.1046/j.1524-4725.2003.29212.x.

37. Jiang H, Zhou J, Chen S. Different glabellar contraction patterns in Chinese and efficacy of botulinum toxin type A for treating glabellar lines: A pilot study. *Dermatol Surg.* 2017;43(5):692-697. doi:10.1097/DSS.0000000000001045.

38. Goldman MP, Alster TS, Weiss R. A randomized trial to determine the influence of laser therapy, monopolar radiofrequency treatment, and intense pulsed light therapy administered immediately after hyaluronic acid gel implantation. *Dermatol Surg.* 2007;33(5):535-542. doi:10.1111/j.1524-4725.2007.33111.x.

39. Woolery-Lloyd H, Viera MH, Valins W. Laser therapy in Black skin. *Facial Plast Surg Clin North Am.* 2011;19(2):405-416. doi:10.1016/j.fsc.2011.05.007.

40. Heath CR, Taylor SC. Fillers in the skin of color population. *J Drugs Dermatol.* 2011;10(5):494-498.

41. Goldman MP. Universal classification of skin type. In: Shiffman MA, Mirrafati SJ, Lam SM, Cueteaux CG, eds. *Simplified Facial Rejuvenation.* Springer Berlin Heidelberg; 2008:47-50.

42. Taylor S, Westerhof W, Im S, Lim J. Noninvasive techniques for the evaluation of skin color. *J Am Acad Dermatol.* 2006;54(5 suppl 2):S282-S290. doi:10.1016/j. jaad.2005.12.041.

43. Roberts WE. Skin type classification systems old and new. *Dermatol Clin.* 2009;27(4):529-533, viii. doi:10.1016/ j.det.2009.08.006.

44. Rodrigues MA, Ross AL, Gilmore S, Daniel BS. Australian dermatologists' perspective on skin of colour: Results of a national survey. *Australas J Dermatol.* 2018;59(1):e23-e30. doi:10.1111/ajd.12556.

45. Harvey VM, Ozoemena U, Paul J, Beydoun HA, Clemetson NN, Okoye GA. Patient-provider communication, concordance, and ratings of care in dermatology: Results of a cross-sectional study. *Dermatol Online J.* 2016;22(11):13030/qt06j6p7gh.

19

Periorbital Rejuvenation: Racial/Ethnic Considerations and Expert Techniques

Abigail I Franco, Sherrif F. Ibrahim, Mara Weinstein Velez

SUMMARY AND KEY FEATURES

- This chapter discusses the structural and functional differences in the periorbital region of patients with skin of color and how these differences manifest through the aging process.
- The chapter describes a variety of modalities that may be employed to address aesthetic concerns in the periorbital region.

- Modalities reviewed include: topical agents, fillers, neuromodulators, lasers/energy devices, and surgical procedures.

IMPORTANT ETHNIC CONSIDERATIONS

Anatomic and Structural Considerations in the Periorbital Region

With any procedure, it is important to have an understanding of the anatomic structures in the region being treated. For a detailed anatomic review of the periorbital region, please refer to "Periorbital facial rejuvenation; applied anatomy and pre-operative assessment" in the reading list.[1] There are certain anatomic differences in the periorbital region that must be considered by gender and ethnicity.

The most prominent gender-based difference in the periorbital region is the structure of the eyebrow. In youthful women, the eyebrow extends above the orbital rim and is arched, with its apex lateral to the lateral limbus. Over time this lateral arch can flatten, resulting in an aged appearance. In youthful men, the brow is flatter and runs more horizontally over the orbital rim. Over time the brow–eyelid complex descends and can

result in impairment in the upper visual field, which may result in compensatory eyebrow elevation via chronic frontalis activation.[1] This can be demonstrated by asking a patient to close their eyes and then open them, observing the patient's need to activate frontalis to raise the brows in the process.

African Ancestry

There are anthropometric differences that have been described in the eye and periorbital region. Data pertaining to populations of African ancestry are largely derived from US studies involving Black/African-American. Compared with the White population, African Americans have been shown to have greater palpebral fissure width (distance between medial and lateral canthus) and greater pretarsal show (the distance between superior lid margin and the upper eyelid crease, superior to the pupil).[2] African Americans also tend to have a greater upward slant of the eye, with an increased vertical height between the medial and lateral commissures (resulting in a greater lateral canthal angle of inclination). The lateral canthal angle of inclination refers to the angle between two imaginary lines, one extending from the medial canthus horizontally, and the other extending from the medial canthus through the lateral canthus. Over time, this angle has also been found to decrease more dramatically in the Black/African-American population compared to the White population, which contributes to an aging appearance.[3] African Americans also have greater orbital proptosis, which can contribute to infraorbital shadowing.[4]

Asian Ancestry

Facial structure and aging is more well studied in East Asians (patients of Chinese, Japanese, and Korean descent), with limited evidence evaluating Southeast Asians, and thus the use of the word "Asian" in this chapter generally refers to East Asians.

Asians are reported to have weaker facial skeletal framework allowing for greater descent of soft tissue, tear-trough formation, and fat pad ptosis with aging.[4] Approximately 50% of Asians have no eyelid crease, and those who do have an eyelid crease may have the crease located closer to the eyelid margin than other ethnicities.[1] Thicker eyelid skin, higher eyebrows, and increased size of the fat pads above and below the eye have been reported in Asians and this can result in a fuller upper eyelid and "puffy eye" appearance in some individuals.[1,4] Middle Eastern and Asian groups both show increased intercanthal widths and smaller eye openings.[4] Asians also have increased lateral canthal angle of inclination.[5] Another unique consideration is that Asians have variable degrees of epicanthal folds (skin of the upper eyelid that covers the corner of the medial canthus).[1] Different Asian cultures have varied ideals regarding the degree of epicanthal fold and the desire for eyelid creases, so clarifying the patient's goals is important.[6,7]

Hispanic/Latino Ancestry

There are a broad range of ethnicities considered "Hispanic," including all people who originate from Spanish-speaking countries. Some of these ethnicities have facial features more similar to White people, while others may exhibit features more similar to those of African ancestry.[6] Anthropometric measurements in Central and South American women are similar to those in White women, whereas measurements in Caribbean women are more similar to Africans. In general, Hispanic populations may have increased bizygomatic distance, bimaxillary protrusion, and heavier fat pads that can produce eyebrow and eyelid drooping and fat pad herniation.[4] Eyelid features are variable, but some may have features similar to Asian eyelids (such as increased lateral canthal angle of inclination, or the presence of a medial canthal fold).[5]

Aging in Ethnic Skin

Structural and functional differences in skin of color have a unique impact on aging (see Chapter 1 for further details). Common signs of aging include dark spots, loss of volume, loss of elasticity, and rhytids. Skin of color has increased epidermal melanin and may have a thicker/more compact dermis with increased numbers and size of fibroblasts. Increased melanin results in greater protection from photodamage, and as a result, some aspects of aging (such as rhytids) are less severe and occur 10 to 20 years later as compared with age-matched Caucasians. However, the increased melanin concentration also makes people with darker skin more vulnerable to problems of dyspigmentation and uneven skin tone, thus hypo- and hyperpigmentation are more frequent signs of photoaging. Thicker dermis and increased fibroblasts preserve skin elasticity longer but may contribute to an increased prevalence of keloids and hypertrophic scarring.[4,6]

In general, aging in the periorbital region occurs due to both intrinsic and extrinsic factors. Intrinsic factors include maxillary resorption, increased orbital size, and displacement of the malar fat pad. This results in a sunken appearance to the eyes and accentuated nasolabial folds. Rhytids develop in part due to repetitive muscle action, but extrinsic factors play a significant role as well. Extrinsic factors, including UV exposure, visible light, air pollutants, and tobacco smoke, upregulate matrix metalloproteases resulting in elastic fiber cleavage, thus decreasing the skin's tensile strength. This leads to course wrinkles, loss of elasticity, and skin atrophy. UV-induced damage (photoaging) is responsible for much of these consequences and additionally contributes to hyperpigmentation, xerosis, telangiectasias, and keratosis development.[6] These intrinsic and extrinsic factors affect skin of color in different ways.

African Ancestry

The periorbital mid-face region is an important focus for aging in patients of African ancestry. Intrinsic aging can manifest as laxity of the eyelids and descent of malar fat pads, resulting in a double convexity. Hypoplastic malar eminence and ocular proptosis result in scleral show and shadowing under the eye. UV-induced damage results in mottled pigmentation, fine wrinkles, and dermatosis papulose nigra (a variant of seborrheic keratoses that present as numerous small papules around the eyelids and malar cheeks).[6] An online study conducted to survey facial concerns and treatment priorities among Black/African-American women reported that of the 401 patients who responded, the most frequently reported concerns were uneven skin tone/color (57%) and dark circles under the eyes (48%).[8] For more details on aging in patients of African ancestry, see Chapter 3.

Asian Ancestry

Intrinsic aging in East Asians typically manifests with soft tissue descent of the midface, malar fat pads, and tear troughs as well as with significant pigmentary changes. Rhytids are not usually present until the fifth decade (10 years later than in the White population). Pigmented growths such as ephelides, melasma, lentigines, and seborrheic keratoses are common aesthetic concerns in Asian patients. An online study conducted to survey facial concerns and treatment priorities among Asian American women reported that of the 403 patients who responded, the most frequently reported concerns were uneven skin tone (64%), wrinkles (50%), and sun damage (48%), with the single most bothersome facial area being the under-eye/tear-trough region (32%), followed closely by crow's feet lines (29%) and forehead lines (29%).[9] For more details on aging in populations of Asian ancestry see Chapters 4 and 7.

Hispanic/Latino Ancestry

Latino/Hispanic populations encompass diverse populations with varying facial structures. In general, intrinsic aging in Hispanic patients results in increased eyelid hooding, drooping of the brows, and fat pad accumulation/descent in the midface. Photoaging varies significantly given the wide range of skin colors seen in patients of Hispanic ancestry.[6] An online study conducted to survey facial concerns and treatment priorities among Hispanic/Latin American women reported that of the 401 patients who responded, the most frequently reported concerns were facial wrinkles (56%), dark circles under the eyes (55%), uneven skin tone (47%), and bags under the eyes (45%). The most

bothersome facial area was sagging under chin (41%), followed by the under-eye/tear-trough (37%) and crow's feet (37%) areas.[10] For more details on aging in populations of Hispanic/Latino ancestry, see Chapter 5.

PERIORBITAL HYPERPIGMENTATION

Periorbital hyperpigmentation (POH), or "dark circles" under the eyes, is a common aesthetic concern in ethnic patients. There are several different causative factors that must be considered to guide treatment options. Causes for POH include excess pigmentation (including postinflammatory hyperpigmentation [PIH], often secondary to allergic or atopic diseases), periorbital edema, excessive vascularity, and shadowing secondary to aging-related structural changes.[11]

Vascular etiologies often have a blue/pink/purple hue and can contribute to periorbital puffiness. Structural etiologies can be related to infraorbital bags, infraorbital grooves, and blepharoptosis, and result in "dark circles" secondary to shadowing. Pigmentary types can have a brown hue, and there may be other signs of inflammation such as eczematous dermatitis or lichenification from chronic rubbing. Mixed types are most frequent, encompassing some combination of vascular, structural, and/or pigmentary etiologies.

Clinical exam can help differentiate the above types, and the addition of wood's lamp and ultrasonography can also be used to help with classification.[12] Simply stretching the skin under the eye can help elucidate if there is true pigment (which remains present with stretching), shadowing effect (in which dark coloration disappears with stretching), or if the discoloration is due to thin skin/hypervascularity (in which stretching will result in increased violaceous discoloration).[11] Wood's lamp can cause epidermal pigmentation to become more prominent, and ultrasound can differentiate causes of puffiness/bags, with vascular causes showing an increased preseptal thickness (from venous congestion), and structural causes showing protruded retroseptal fat pads.[12]

Considering the cause of dark eye circles is helpful in guiding treatment. When pigmented types are present, treatment with bleaching agents, chemical peels, and light-source devices are considered. With vascular types, vascular lasers and intense pulsed light can be considered. Additionally, resurfacing lasers and the addition of topical vitamin C and retinoids may promote collagen production and increase dermal thickness to conceal congested blood. For structural types, fillers and surgical modalities (such as blepharoplasty and autologous fat transplantation) may be employed to improve tear-trough deformities, eye bags, and blepharoptosis.[11,12] Resurfacing lasers may also be used for skin tightening to improve the shadows and "bags" from lax skin.

TOPICAL AGENTS AND CHEMICAL PEELS

Topical treatments are an important component of periorbital rejuvenation. They may be aimed at moisturizing, increasing collagen, improving wrinkles/skin tightness, evening skin tone, and decreasing hyperpigmentation. There are numerous available products, but the key ingredients with the most evidence are reviewed below.

Lightening agents can act by decreasing melanin synthesis, decreasing melanosome transfer to keratinocytes, or increasing skin turnover. Hydroquinone is a lightening agent used for hyperpigmentation, which acts by inhibiting tyrosinase and thus inhibiting melanin synthesis. It should not be used long term as it can result in exogenous ochronosis. Treatment periods tend to be around 3 to 7 months.[11] Kojic acid, azelaic acid, arbutin, and cysteamine also have activity against tyrosinase and can be beneficial for hyperpigmentation. Niacinamide improves epidermal barrier, increases collagen production, and prevents melanosome transfer to keratinocytes. Hydroxy acids (i.e., glycolic acid) and retinoids increase skin shedding. Glycolic acids also increase epidermal thickness, improve synthesis of collagen and glycosaminoglycans, and disperse melanin pigment.[13]

Retinoids also improve dyschromia through inhibitions of tyrosinase activity.[14] While retinoids are well known to improve skin thickness/texture/fine lines, increasing dermal collagen synthesis, and improve hyperpigmentation, the side effects of irritation is a limitation for use on the thin/sensitive skin in the periorbital area. Retinol and retinaldehyde, which can be found in numerous cosmeceutical agents, may result in less skin irritation.[13]

Antioxidants such as vitamins C and E scavenge free radicals to prevent cellular and DNA damage.[14] Vitamin C is also a co-factor for collagen syntheses, stimulates collagen gene expression and syntheses, and also inhibits the enzymes responsible for collagen degradation. It

inhibits tyrosinase resulting in a lightening/brightening effect and has antiinflammatory properties as well that can promote healing and prevent PIH. Vitamin C is most effective/stable when formulated at pH <3.5. Efficacy is proportional to concentration, up 20%. And the stability can be improved through use of esterified derivatives such as magnesium ascorbyl phosphate and ascorbyl-6-palmitate.[13,15]

Sunscreen is an essential component of the antiaging regimen to prevent photodamage and reduce after-procedure PIH. While physical blockers (zinc and titanium) provide more complete photoprotection, they can often leave an unsightly residue on dark-skinned patients. As a result, chemical sunscreens may be more appropriate for patients with darker skin. Finding a sunscreen that the patient feels comfortable using is essential.

Chemical peels can also be used for treatment of hyperpigmentation, with glycolic acid 20% peels being the most commonly used. Lactic acid 15% in combination with trichloroacetic acid (TCA) 3.75% have also been used. Of note, to avoid abnormal demarcation between the treated and untreated areas, it is best to treat the entire face in ethnic patients (Video 19.1). Additionally, pretreatment with tretinoin and hydroquinone for 2 to 4 weeks can decrease the risk of PIH.[11] For further details regarding prevention and treatment for hyperpigmentation, see Chapters 8, 9, 10, and 15.

FILLERS

With aging, one of the most prominent features seen in the periorbital area is loss of volume (in collagen, fat pads, and bony support), which can have numerous consequences including a hollow/sunken appearance to the eye, a deepened superior sulcus, prominence of the infraorbital rim, and under-eye bags/circles). It is important to recognize that volume depletion plays such a prominent role in the aging eye because the traditional surgical modalities used to remove fat can accentuate loss of volume and result in increased hallowing. Thus, the use of fillers to replace volume is a key aspect in periorbital rejuvenation.[16]

Fillers can be particularly helpful in correcting prominent tear troughs. The tear trough represents a crease or depression that occurs over the inferiomedial orbital rim with age. It develops as a result of loss of subcutaneous fat and thinning of the overlying skin, with descent of the cheek and pseudoherniation of the infraorbital fat pad.[11] Fillers can also be used to support the brow apex and lift the lateral brow.[17]

Types of Fillers

Various fillers have been used in the periorbital region. Hyaluronic acid (HA) fillers are the workhorse due to their relative safety and efficacy. They can be molded and spread after injection for a smooth appearance, and they can be reversed with hyaluronidase if needed. Additionally HA is a glycosaminoglycan whose structure is uniform across species, decreasing the chance of immunogenicity/reactivity.[16] When choosing a filler in a patient with skin of color, it is important to choose a filler with minimal reactivity. Those that are less reactive are less likely to cause inflammation and PIH.[18] Clinical data support the efficacy and safety of HA fillers in people of color.[19]

Injection Technique

General considerations with regard to injection technique in patients with skin of color include minimization of needle punctures and bruising. The use of cannulas, threading, and fanning techniques are preferred to decrease puncture wounds and bruising. Avoidance of bruising is important to prevent hemosiderin deposition. Additionally, the Tyndall effect can result in more prominent discoloration in patients with skin of color so avoiding placement of filler too superficially is important.[18]

Fillers injected into the preperiosteal plane along the orbitomental ligament are recommended to be of low to mid G' and low hydrophilicity (hydrophilic fillers can result in lower eyelid edema). Usually, 0.2 to 0.3 cc are recommended per tear trough; larger amounts have increased risk of edema.[20]

Injections are best done with the patient looking straight ahead (neutral gaze), as other positions can change to location of the fat pads. The lower lid is gently stretched to reveal the underlying vertically running veins to avoid. The filler can then be directly injected into the preperiosteal plane. Alternatively, some prefer to place the injection below the infraorbital rim and fan the product vertically.[20]

A 30-gauge needle can be used to puncture the skin down into the suborbicularis plane in the hallowed areas over the infraorbital rim and then filler is deposited in a linear, feathered fashion, often via a cannula

(Videos 19.2 and 19.3). After deposition, the fingers can be used to apply pressure and mold the filler.[16] The orbital rim may also be filled superiorly and laterally, if desired.

NEUROMODULATORS

Rhytids on average occur, 10 years later in darker skin types as compared to lighter skin types, and as such may be a lower priority than dark/uneven skin tone or under-eye bags in skin of color. However, in patients of Asian and Hispanic decent, more so than those of African descent, crow's feet area/lines are a leading concern.[8–10]

Clinical data support the safety and efficacy of botulinum toxin (BoNT) in populations with skin of color.[19] BoNT can be used to eliminate dynamic rhytids and additionally can be used to nonsurgically lift the brow–eyelid complex. To accomplish a brow lift, targeted muscles include the brow depressors. Treating the lateral/superior aspect of the orbicularis oculi can result in lifting of the lateral and midbrow, with lateral placement also targeting crow's feet. To lift the medial brow, the glabellar complex is injected, targeting the procerus, corrugators, and depressor supercilii. Suppressing activity in these muscles will also reduce glabellar lines (i.e., "11s" or "frown lines"). A microdroplet technique has also been described with subdermal injections around the rim of the orbicularis oculi muscle for lifting the eyebrow/eyelid.[21] For patients who suffer from brow ptosis at baseline, BoTN should be avoided in the frontalis muscle (especially the inferior aspect) due to risk for exacerbate of ptosis. Targeting the nasalis can also provide reduction of dynamic horizontal lower eyelid lines and bulking of the lower eyelid tissue.[21]

Additionally, in the infraorbital region, orbicularis oculi contraction and hypertrophy can result in an infraorbital bulge that is colloquially referred to as the "jelly roll" and can be treated with small aliquots of subcutaneous BoNT. However, caution is recommended in populations of Asian descent. While individuals of White descent often interpret this bulge as something that results in a "dull" appearance, in some Asian cultures the bulge is *desired* and referred to as the "charming roll." At times, patient's may even seek filler to increase the size of this bulge. After a discussion of patient goals, injection points may need to be altered for infraorbital rhytids: for example, 1 to 2 mm below the ciliary margin in White people (which will minimize the bulge), versus 1 cm below the ciliary margin in Asians (in order to preserve the infraorbital bulge). It is also important to note that these infraorbital injections should be avoided in patients with poor skin elasticity due to risk of scleral show.[22,23]

There is significant variation in concentrations of BoNT used in these areas. In general, lower concentrations will allow for more natural movement but with shorter duration of effect, whereas higher concentrations may risk a "frozen" appearance but last longer.[14,24] A global aesthetics consensus for HA filler and BoTN in diverse populations (including people of ethnic descent) recommended combined treatment for optimizing outcomes. Typical doses of BoNT and preferred fillers were identified for each facial region. Ranges of neurotoxin were typically 12 to 40 Units (U) for the glabellar area, 6 to 15 U per side for the lateral periorbital area, and 0.1 to 2 U per side for the lower eyelid (infraorbital rhytids).[19] For a more in-depth review on botulinum toxins please refer to Chapter 17.

LASERS AND ENERGY DEVICES

Laser and light therapies have increased in popularity; however, in patients with skin of color, there are some safety limitations due to the risk of PIH. The degree of pigmentation in the palmar creases may be a useful indicator of risk of hyperpigmentation.[25] In general, ablative devices (which might be used for rejuvenation in White skin) have the potential to produce significant hyperpigmentation in skin of color and should be approached with caution. However, with appropriate adjustments to laser settings, laser and energy devices can be used safely in skin of color and should be considered for periorbital rejuvenation.

In general, when treating patients with darker skin types, it is safest to use conservative settings to avoid complications.[26] Conservative settings include choosing longer wavelengths, longer pulse durations, lower fluence, a smaller spot size, and lower densities of microthermal zones.[25,27] Other potential preventive measures include pretreatment with topical lightening agents for 6 weeks prior to using a laser/energy device, performing a "test spot" prior to treating an entire area, with 2- to 4-week follow up to observe safety and patient compliance, and using efficient cooling measures to the epidermis. After treatment with laser/energy devices, strict photoprotection (including frequent use of sunscreen

SPF >60) is required, and a short pulse of potent topical steroids can also be used to decrease inflammation.[25,27]

Lasers

In the periorbital region, lasers can be used for treatment of pigmented and vascular types of POH, resurfacing, and skin tightening. For epidermal or dermal pigment, Q-switched Ruby, Q-switched Alexandrite, and Nd:Yag have been used successfully in some populations. For hyperpigmentation secondary to vascularity, Nd:Yag can also be effective.[11] In 2008 Momosawa et al. published a paper with a regimen for POH in Japanese patients that combined 6 weeks of pretreatment with a bleaching cream (hydroquinone and tretinoin) followed by use of Q-switched Ruby laser and found that 15/18 subjects had good to excellent results after three to four treatments. PIH was only observed in two patients.[11,28]

Resurfacing lasers (fractionally and fully ablative/nonablative lasers) can be used in the periorbital region for overall rejuvenation, to increase dermal thickness and elasticity, decrease rhytids, and remove surface abnormalities such as seborrheic keratoses and syringomas. In the author's experience, these resurfacing lasers can be used safely in people of color by employing the general conservative laser principles previously discussed. Of note, a corneal shield must be employed to protect the patient's eyes when using lasers on eyelids. Despite the author's success with these resurfacing lasers, great caution should be employed with the use of ablative resurfacing lasers (especially fully ablative resurfacing lasers) in skin types V and VI.

Permanent hypopigmentation and scarring is possible due to the violation of the epidermal layer. Nonablative resurfacing lasers are safer because they avoid the disruption of the epidermis, though they may require an increased number of treatment sessions to achieve the desired outcome.[27]

In 2017, Kaushik and Alexis published an evidence-based review on nonablative fractional laser resurfacing in skin of color. Only a handful of studies have been done to assess fractional laser resurfacing for rejuvenation in patients with skin types IV–VI, but the evidence suggested safety and efficacy of nonablated fractional resurfacing for skin rejuvenation in patients with skin of color. PIH was observed in 0% to 25% depending on the study.[29] See Chapters 10 and 14 for further details regarding resurfacing in skin of color patients.

Radiofrequency, Infrared, and Ultrasound Devices

There are few studies that demonstrate efficacy of these energy devices in patients with skin of color, and even less that specifically discuss the periorbital region. These devices do not target melanin and thus may be safe in darker skin types. Radiofrequency energy devices induce dermal heating, collagen denaturation, and remodeling. Studies in Asians using radiofrequency demonstrate safety with minimal to no PIH, and though data are lacking, others have reported similar safety in Black/ African-American.[26,30] Infrared tightening devices thermally induce collagen contraction, remodeling, and synthesis, and ultrasound devices vibrate tissue resulting in heating of the reticular dermis/subcutis, immediate tissue contraction, and delayed remodeling. These devices appear safe in Black/African-American patients and can be used to address lax skin or treat the forehead to produce tightening and eyebrow elevation.[26]

SURGICAL PROCEDURES

Blepharoplasty and Brow-lifting Procedures

Increased laxity of upper eyelid skin results in sagging of this skin, also known as dermatochalasis. This loss of elasticity results in the eyelid skin folding over the lid crease (hooding) and can sometimes even impair vision (especially in Asians). Excess skin can be excised via a blepharoplasty. Blepharoplasty is the third most common plastic surgery procedure performed in the United States. Upper blepharoplasty can be performed under local anesthesia and is safer and more common than lower-eyelid blepharoplasty, which must be done under general anesthesia and carries a higher complication rate.[31]

Eyelid and eyebrow ptosis are often seen together, and addressing the sagging eyelid skin without addressing the brows is inadequate in some patients.[32,33] In fact, at times a brow lift alone may result in sufficient eyelid lifting and can be performed in lieu of a blepharoplasty.[33]

Surgical Procedures in Asian Patients

Ethnic variations should be considered when planning surgeries in the periorbital area, with the greatest differences noted in the Asian eye. The "Asian blepharoplasty," or "double eyelid," operation was first reported in 1896. This usually involves the creation of an eyelid crease (which is absent in 50% of Asians), and there are numerous methods reported for optimizing this procedure. The double eyelid operation is the most commonly performed cosmetic procedure in Asia, and it is felt that the addition of an eyelid crease results in more expressive appearances. It is important to note that the procedure is not intended to "Westernize" the Asian eye. Amongst Asians who do have an eyelid crease, the pretarsal show is generally smaller, and there is great variability in size, shape, and height of the crease amongst different Asian populations. Thus, before creating this crease, it is important to have a discussion with the patient about their specific desires.[7]

While White eyelid creases tend to be semilunar shaped (crease is closer to the eyelid margin medially/ laterally and farther centrally), Asian eyelid creases tend to be either parallel (distance from crease to eyelid margin remains similar along entire length) or nasally tapered (crease converges medially with the lid margin, but not laterally). In the White eyelid there is a fibrous attachment that spans from the levator aponeurosis through the orbicularis to the skin, which results in a crease upon contraction/retraction of the levator. In Asians, this fibrous attachment is absent, or only minimally present, which is the main reason for the lack of an eyelid crease, and also the target for surgical correction. The crease can be created by surgically fixing two structures together (skin to levator aponeurosis, skin to tarsus, or orbicularis to aponeurosis). There are various methods for fixing these structures together, including external incision techniques, and suture ligation techniques, the details of which are beyond the scope of this chapter. One should generally avoid creating a semilunar crease (which is the most frequent complaint from Asians who have blepharoplasties done in the United States), and the double eyelid should be smaller than that seen in White individuals. The height and shape of the crease should be discussed with the patient and is usually created between 6 to 8 mm above the lid margin. If the crease is created too high, it can result in a "startled" appearance.[7] Please refer to the reading list for more detailed procedural considerations.

The Asian blepharoplasty may occur with a brow-lifting procedure given their weaker structural framework and the relationship of brow-lid continuum. The blepharoplasty may (or may not) also involve removing some of the orbital fat (given the increased quantity of periorbital fat in Asians).[7,33] Removing orbital fat should be done conservatively to prevent periorbital hallowing that can exacerbate an aged appearance. Fat grafting (injecting centrifuged fat) can be performed to combat hallowing, and fat repositioning (transposition of fat pads with securement of pads up onto the orbital margin) can correct pseudoherniation while simultaneously preventing the sunken appearance that may have occurred with fat removal.[33]

Finally, there are newer procedures that focus on the elimination of the epicanthal fold. There are four different types of epicanthal folds described, with varying origin and insertion. The epicanthal fold is present in 60% to 90% of Asians (and only 2% of non-Asian populations overall). Since the epicanthal fold is considered a natural feature on the Asian face, its elimination is controversial. During creation of the eyelid crease, increased tension may form on the epicanthal fold resulting in its accentuation (which is why some opt to eliminate the epicanthal fold). However, others argue that simply creating a nasally tapered eyelid crease will result in the crease merging with the origin of the epicanthal fold, creating a more natural look and avoiding potential complications.[7]

SURGICAL PROCEDURES IN PATIENTS OF AFRICAN ANCESTRY

As in Asian patients, nuances exist in the approach to aesthetic surgical procedures in patients of African descent and having a conversation about their goals and fears regarding surgery is a key first step in the consultation. Studies have indicated that Black/African-American individuals in particular fear overcorrection and loss of facial features associated with their ancestry. Black/African-American patients often feel their eyes are more similar to Asians than White people. An important focus in Black/African-American patients is the naturally elevated lateral canthus seen in youth (increased lateral canthal angle of inclination, i.e., positive canthal tilt). Treating other periorbital concerns without addressing the descent of the lateral canthus will often result in dissatisfaction, even if the patient is unable to voice why. Reviewing patient photos from youth is helpful in general and particularly important in patients of African ancestry given the more pronounced descent of the lateral canthus with aging. Canthopexy, which involves placement of sutures to stabilize and support the lateral canthal tendon, is an important aspect of surgical rejuvenation of

the African eye.[17] Canthoplasty, which is a more invasive procedure involving detachment, shortening, and reattachment of the lateral canthal tendon, can also result in a positive lateral canthal tilt.

Patients of African ancestry have relatively less upper-face aging (forehead/brow) with less brow ptosis, and thus may not need brow lifting procedures as often. Aging in the African face is most prominent in the periorbital area and midface. Like Asians, those of African ancestry have a shorter distance between the upper-eyelid margin and the eyelid crease (6–8 mm, as compared with 8–10 mm in White individuals). As a result, pseudoherniation of fat pads, coupled with ptosis of lacrimal glands, results in prominent upper eyelid fullness.[34]

Another important difference is that those of African descent tend to have hypoplastic malar eminences and increased eye proptosis compared to White individuals, which increases scleral show and infraorbital shadowing. The changes seen in the lower-lid area are also affected by age-related changes of the midface. Selective hypertrophy of the malar fat pads and thicker/heavier skin results in earlier descent of the melolabial mounds, hollowing and accentuating the tear trough and resulting in prominent nasolabial folds. Surgery in the lower lid should be done with great caution to prevent exacerbation of scleral show. A better approach may be repositioning of malar fat pad, autologous fat transfer, and use of fillers to restore mid face volume.[34]

Finally, general considerations when planning surgical correction in Black/African-American patients includes minimizing skin incisions and using noninflammatory suture material. The upper eyelid can be used as an access point for lateral canthopexy. The midface and lower lid can be accessed through a transconjunctival approach to minimize scar formation. The use of nonabsorbable sutures is generally preferred to decrease the inflammatory response that occurs with absorbable suture materials.[17]

SURGICAL PROCEDURES IN HISPANIC PATIENTS

Hispanic patients have varied eyelid features, which tend to span between White and Asian features. For example, one anthropometric analysis found that on average, Hispanic eyelids had increased lateral canthal angle of inclination (6.0°) as compared with White eyelids (2.5°), which was closer to the measurements seen in Asians

(8.0°). Additionally, 50% of Hispanic patients had some degree of an epicanthal fold, again more closely mirroring features seen in Asian eyes. In Hispanics, both the distance between their medial canthi, and the distance from upper-eyelid margin to eyelid crease fell between the measurements seen in Asians and Whites.[5] Additionally, as discussed earlier, Hispanics generally have heavier fat pads that can produce eyebrow and eyelid drooping and fat pad herniation. Since Hispanic eyes have such great variability, it is important to request photos from the patient's youth and have a clear discussion on goals prior to planning surgical treatment. A combination of the approaches discussed in the sections above may be utilized depending on said goals.

REFERENCES

1. Kashkouli MB, Abdolalizadeh P, Abolfathzadeh N, Sianati H, Sharepour M , Hadi Y. Periorbital facial rejuvenation; applied anatomy and pre-operative assessment. *J Curr Ophthalmol.* 2017;29:154-168.
2. Price KM, Gupta PK, Woodward JA, Stinnett SS, Murchison AP. Eyebrow and eyelid dimensions: an anthropometric analysis of African Americans and Caucasians. *Plast Reconstr Surg.* 2009;124:615-623.
3. Odunze M, Rosenberg DS , Few JW. Periorbital aging and ethnic considerations: A focus on the lateral canthal complex. *Plast Reconstr Surg.* 2008;121:1002-1008.
4. Vashi NA, de Castro Maymone MB, Kundu RV. Aging differences in ethnic skin. *J Clin Aesthet Dermatol.* 2016;9:31-38.
5. Fry CL, Naugle Jr TC, Cole SA, et al. The Latino eyelid: Anthropometric analysis of a spectrum of findings. *Ophthalmic Plast Reconstr Surg.* 2017;33:440-445.
6. Venkatesh S, Maymone MBC, Vashi NA. Aging in skin of color. *Clin Dermatol.* 2019;37:351-357.
7. Nguyen MQ, Hsu PW, Dinh TA. Asian blepharoplasty. *Semin Plast Surg.* 2009;23:185-197.
8. Alexis A, Boyd C, Callender V, Downie J , Sangha S. Understanding the female African American facial aesthetic patient. *J Drugs Dermatol.* 2019;18:858-866.
9. Chiu A, Mariwalla K, Hui-Austin A, Narurkar V, de la Guardia C. Understanding the female Asian American facial aesthetic patient. *J Drugs Dermatol.* 2019;18:633-641.
10. Fabi S, Montes JR, Aguilera SB, Bucay V, Brown SM, Ashourian N. Understanding the female Hispanic and Latino American facial aesthetic patient. *J Drugs Dermatol.* 2019;18:623-632.
11. Sarkar R, Ranjan R, Garg S, Garg VK, Sonthalia S, Bansal S. Periorbital hyperpigmentation: A comprehensive review. *J Clin Aesthet Dermatol.* 2016;9:49-55.
12. Huang YL, Chang SL, Ma L, Lee MC, Hu S. Clinical analysis and classification of dark eye circle. *Int J Dermatol.* 2014;53:164-170.
13. Pilkington SJ, Belden S , Miller RA. The tricky tear trough: A review of topical cosmeceuticals for periorbital skin rejuvenation. *J Clin Aesthet Dermatol.* 2015;8:39-47.
14. Glaser DA , Kurta A. Periorbital rejuvenation: Overview of nonsurgical treatment options. *Facial Plast Surg Clin North Am.* 2016;24:145-152.
15. Telang PS. Vitamin C in dermatology. *Indian Dermatol Online J.* 2013;4:143-146.
16. Lee S, Yen MT. Nonsurgical rejuvenation of the eyelids with hyaluronic acid gel injections. *Semin Plast Surg.* 2017;31:17-21.
17. Few JW. Rejuvenation of the African American periorbital area: Dynamic considerations. *Semin Plast Surg.* 2009;23:198-206.
18. Alexis AF, Alam M. Racial and ethnic differences in skin aging: Implications for treatment with soft tissue fillers. *J Drugs Dermatol.* 2012;11:s30-s32; discussion s32.
19. Sundaram H, Liew S, Signorini M, et al. Global Aesthetics Consensus: Hyaluronic acid fillers and botulinum toxin type A-recommendations for combined treatment and optimizing outcomes in diverse patient populations. *Plast Reconstr Surg.* 2016;137:1410-1423.
20. Woodward J. Review of periorbital and upper face: Pertinent anatomy, aging, injection techniques, prevention, and management of complications of facial fillers. *J Drugs Dermatol.* 2016;15:1524-1531.
21. Varga R. Providing optimal rejuvenation to the periocular area using botulinum toxin A neuromodulators and hyaluronic acid dermal fillers. *Plast Surg Nurs.* 2019;39: 119-124.
22. Ahn BK, Kim YS, Kim HJ, Rho NK, Kim HS. Consensus recommendations on the aesthetic usage of botulinum toxin type A in Asians. *Dermatol Surg.* 2013;39: 1843-1860.
23. Sundaram H, Huang PH, Hsu NJ, et al. Aesthetic applications of botulinum toxin A in Asians: An international, multidisciplinary, Pan-Asian consensus. *Plast Reconstr Surg Glob Open.* 2016;4:e872.
24. Beer KR, Bayers S, Beer J. Aesthetic treatment considerations for the eyebrows and periorbital complex. *J Drugs Dermatol.* 2014;13:s17-s20.
25. Jalalat S, Weiss E. Cosmetic laser procedures in Latin skin. *J Drugs Dermatol.* 2019;18:s127-s131.
26. Woolery-Lloyd H, Viera MH, Valins W. Laser therapy in Black skin. *Facial Plast Surg Clin North Am.* 2011;19: 405-416.
27. Richter AL, Barrera J, Markus RF, Brissett A. Laser skin treatment in non-Caucasian patients. *Facial Plast Surg Clin North Am.* 2014;22:439-446.

28. Momosawa A, Kurita M, Ozaki M, et al. Combined therapy using Q-switched Ruby laser and bleaching treatment with tretinoin and hydroquinone for periorbital skin hyperpigmentation in Asians. *Plast Reconstr Surg.* 2008;121:282-288.

29. Kaushik SB, Alexis AF. Nonablative fractional laser resurfacing in skin of color: Evidence-based review. *J Clin Aesthet Dermatol.* 2017;10:51-67.

30. Tan MG, Jo CE, Chapas A, Khetarpal S, Dover JS. Radiofrequency microneedling: A comprehensive and critical review. *Dermatol Surg.* 2021;47:755-761.

31. Zoumalan CI, Roostaeian J. Simplifying blepharoplasty. *Plast Reconstr Surg.* 2016;137:196e-213e.

32. Karimi N, Kashkouli MB, Sianati H, Khademi B. Techniques of eyebrow lifting: A narrative review. *J Ophthalmic Vis Res.* 2020;15:218-235.

33. Park DD. Aging Asian upper blepharoplasty and brow. *Semin Plast Surg.* 2015;29:188-200.

34. Brissett AE, Naylor MC. The aging African-American face. *Facial Plast Surg.* 2010;26:154-163.

READING LIST

1. Sarkar R, Ranjan R, Garg S, Garg VK, Sonthalia S, Bansal S. Periorbital hyperpigmentation: A comprehensive review. *J Clin Aesthet Dermatol.* 2016;9:49-55.

2. Huang YL, Chang SL, Ma L, Lee MC, Hu S. Clinical analysis and classification of dark eye circle. *Int J Dermatol.* 2014;53:164-170.

3. Kashkouli MB, Abdolalizadeh P, Abolfathzadeh N, Sianati H, Sharepour M, Hadi Y. Periorbital facial rejuvenation; applied anatomy and pre-operative assessment. *J Curr Ophthalmol.* 2017;29:154-168.

4. Nguyen MQ, Hsu PW, Dinh TA. Asian blepharoplasty. *Semin Plast Surg.* 2009;23:185-197.

20

Hair Disorders: Aesthetic Approaches for Patients of African Ancestry

Taylor A. Jamerson, Achiamah Osei-Tutu, Crystal Aguh

SUMMARY AND KEY FEATURES

- Aesthetic approaches to restoring hair loss in patients of African descent encompass several important factors. Consideration of the unique properties of the hair and cultural hair practices is critical in achieving optimal therapeutic outcomes
- Early identification of harmful hair practices and review of healthy hair-care practices are fundamental

- in properly managing hair loss in patients of African descent.
- While some forms of alopecia will respond well to medical therapies with improved aesthetic appearance of hair loss, advanced presentations of alopecia warrant more aggressive approaches with systemic agents or procedural techniques.

INTRODUCTION

Hair loss in patients of African descent presents unique challenges to dermatologists and requires basic knowledge of hair properties and cultural hair practices. Recent estimates indicate that more than 50% of Black women will experience hair loss at some point throughout their lifetime.[1] Hair loss can often be frustrating and lead to a disfiguring appearance, causing significant psychosocial impact in these patients, most pronounced in younger women.[2,3] In this chapter, we will cover the most common forms of hair loss that present in patients of African descent and focus on the medical, procedural, and special treatment considerations required in the proper management of these conditions.

HAIR PROPERTIES IN PATIENTS OF AFRICAN DESCENT

The hair shaft is an epidermally derived unit that consists of three layers: the cuticle, cortex, and medulla.[4]

The cuticle is the outermost layer of the hair shaft and is made up of keratin, a structural fibrous protein that provides protection from water and chemicals to the underlying cortex of the hair shaft.[4] The cuticle is relatively thin in individuals with tightly curled or coiled hair when compared to White or Asian hair strands and contributes to a higher susceptibility for hair shaft breakage in individuals of African descent.[5] The middle layer of the hair shaft is called the cortex and is responsible for the mechanical properties of the hair.[6] Within this part of the hair shaft, there is an adhesive layer of cells referred to as the cell membrane complex (CMC).[7] The CMC is particularly sensitive to disruption from thermal straightening, chemical straighteners, bleaching, or dyeing of the hair.[5] Finally, the medulla is the porous center of the hair strand and is variably present within the hair shaft but is more likely to be identified in coarser hair fibers.[8]

Afro-textured hair is characterized by tightly coiled or kinky strands.[5] The helical shape of the coils creates geometric points of weakness across the hair strand and leads to a higher incidence of hair-shaft breakage and knotting. Cross-sectional images of tightly curled or coiled hair strands reveal an elliptical asymmetric shape that causes additional points of weakness where breakage can occur.[9] As a result, the hairstyling and grooming practices that straight hair strands of most White and Asian individuals can withstand often lead to mechanical trauma in those with curlier hair types of African descent.[10] While sebum, an oily substance excreted by the sebaceous glands in the scalp, serves to provide an added layer of protection by coating the hair shaft, in tightly curled or coiled hair it is unable to make its way down the hair shaft due to the helical nature of the hair strand.[11] This further contributes to the dry and brittle nature of tightly curled or coiled hair.

EVALUATION OF HAIR LOSS

Patients of African descent are susceptible to all forms of nonscarring or scarring alopecia. The threshold for a punch biopsy in patients presenting with clinical signs and symptoms concerning for a cicatricial process should remain low, as pathology examination allows for a more definitive identification of inflammatory infiltrates. Often, two areas of the scalp are biopsied, both taken from the edge of an area of active inflammation to identify predominant cell types and provide possible insight on the underlying pathology.[12] However, biopsy alone may be nondiagnostic and insufficient in making an accurate diagnosis.[13] A thorough patient history and clinical examination are key to establish onset, disease course, family history, medication history, associated symptoms, and hairstyling and hair care practices.

This chapter will focus primarily on the four subtypes of hair loss that Black women are particularly prone to experiencing: androgenetic alopecia, traction alopecia, acquired trichorrhexis nodosa, and cicatricial alopecia called central centrifugal cicatricial alopecia.

Androgenetic Alopecia

Androgenetic alopecia (AGA) is a form of nonscarring hair loss that increases in prevalence with age.[14] Though AGA does not have a higher prevalence in patients of African descent compared to other ethnic and racial groups, AGA is the most common form of progressive hair loss in all patients, thought to affect at least 50% of women and 70% of men by the age of 50.[15] It is a polygenetic condition that leads to

increased 5-alpha-reductase activity, elevated dihydrotestosterone levels, and subsequently a shortened anagen phase (growth phase) in the hair cycle and miniaturization of hair follicles.[14,16]

AGA has distinct clinical manifestations in male and female patients. In males, AGA primarily involves the gradual recession of the bitemporal and frontal hairline with sparing of the occipital scalp.[17] As the disease progresses to more advanced stages, complete loss of the frontal and crown of the scalp can occur in men, leaving a shiny appearance that can mimic fibrosis. It is rare for women to experience this complete hair loss. Instead, women develop characteristic thinning along the frontal scalp, appearing as widening of the frontal part and described to resemble the pattern of a Christmas tree though bitemporal involvement can occur as well.[18]

Acquired Trichorrhexis Nodosa

Acquired trichorrhexis nodosa (ATN) refers to hair breakage that occurs along the hair shaft from extrinsic factors.[19] While this form of hair loss can occur in any patient, it is more common in patients of African descent, as tightly curled or coiled hair is more susceptible to damage and breakage.[20] Patients may present with the concern that their hair does not grow past a particular length, reporting short hair despite not trimming the hair. Often, the extrinsic factors contributing to the onset of ATN are frequent use of damaging hairstyling practices such as thermal straightening with flat irons, hot combs, and blow dryers and chemical processing.[20]

ATN can be classified as proximal or distal depending on the point of breakage along the hair shaft.[19] On clinical examination, shortened terminal hairs of unequal length are usually evident. While the occipital scalp is the most common area of involvement, in more severe cases, hair breakage is noted throughout the scalp.[21] The fragility of the hair shafts can be assessed on examination by performing a tug test where the distal ends of the hair strands are gently pulled.[21] The breakage of small fragments of the hair strands is considered a positive result and should further raise clinical suspicion for ATN. Thorough examination of the scalp using a dermatoscope will reveal multiple sites of swelling along the hair strands, indicating potential sites of future breakage.[22] A 4-mm punch biopsy is often unrevealing, as there are no associated findings of inflammation or scarring that contribute to the hair loss and breakage.[23] Careful attention should be placed to avoid the misdiagnosis of other conditions with similar presentations such as tinea capitis, which has peak incidence in Black children or the early presentation of a cicatricial alopecia.[24,25]

Traction Alopecia

Traction alopecia (TA) is a highly prevalent form of hair loss among women of African descent.[26] Hairstyling practices among Black patients are widely variable. These hairstyling practices include different types of braiding, installation of weaves, tight ponytails with extensions to increase the length and fullness of the hair, and different types of wigs often secured in place with an adhesive glue or combs sewn into the wig unit. These styles provide increased ease in the manageability of the hair and allow for little to no manipulation of the hair in its natural state. Unfortunately, these styles are also associated with increased risk of TA due to the resulting tension they place on the hair follicles causing inflammation and dormancy of the hair follicles.[27] Added with chemical straighteners such as lye relaxers containing sodium hydroxide or no-lye relaxers containing guanidine hydroxide that increase the brittleness of the hair shaft, the risk for resulting TA is further amplified.[23]

The affected area of the scalp in TA is highly dependent on the hairstyle inflicting mechanical stress on the hair follicles. In women who detail history of wearing tight braids or cornrows, thinning and hair loss often occurs along the frontal and bi-frontotemporal margin of the hairline.[28] Signs of impending TA include papules, stinging, pain, crusting, and erythema occurring within days of the hairstyle installation.[27,29] If the traction-inducing hairstyle remains in place over an extended period of time, eventually characteristic features of TA such as the "fringe sign" or the retention of vellus hairs on the anterior margin of the hairline and loss of hair posterior to the fringe may develop.[27] A close examination of the scalp will reveal preservation of the follicular ostia with variable presence of vellus hairs. With repeated trauma however, end-stage traction alopecia can present with loss of the follicular ostia secondary to irreversible damage from persistent inflammation.[30] At this stage, fibrous tracts replace terminal hair follicles and patients have permanent, scarring hair loss.

Central Centrifugal Cicatricial Alopecia

Central centrifugal cicatricial alopecia (CCCA) is a scarring alopecia that almost exclusively affects women of

African descent with an average age of onset between the third and fourth decades of life.[31,32] When first described in the literature, CCCA was referred to as "hot comb" alopecia due to the theory that disease onset was linked to hairstyling practices and later, to chemical relaxants.[33] Subsequent studies disputed any link to hot combing or chemical relaxers and suggested instead a link to use of extensions as this hairstyling practice became more popular.[34] There has since been no substantial evidence that links any one hairstyling practice to the onset of CCCA, casting this hypothesis into doubt. Recent evidence instead suggests that CCCA is an autosomal dominant condition with incomplete penetrance and is associated with variance in the peptidyl arginine deiminase 3 gene (PADI3) in 24% of patients.[35] Additionally, this condition has been connected to higher prevalence of uterine leiomyomas and type II diabetes, indicating potential contribution of metabolic factors in disease pathogenesis.[36,37]

CCCA presents with an insidious, centrifugal pattern of permanent hair loss beginning in the scalp vertex.[38] In the early stages of disease, the hair loss may present as hair breakage and thinning at the crown of the scalp and progressively expands to involve the surrounding areas with permanent hair loss. Some patients may experience symptoms secondary to inflammation in the affected scalp including tenderness, pruritis, scale, pustules, and papules, while others have no symptoms outside of progressive hair loss.[38]

TREATMENT APPROACHES

The treatment of hair loss differs for each subtype of alopecia and importantly, each patient. While AGA and TA usually respond well to medical therapies with improved aesthetic appearance of hair loss, advanced presentations of these conditions warrant more aggressive approaches with systemic agents or procedural techniques. For conditions like CCCA, medical therapy is fundamental in halting progressive hair loss.[39] In some cases, early initiation of medical treatment can result in regeneration of hair follicles that were once under inflammatory attack but have yet to fully succumb to fibrosis. This is important, as patients may experience hair regrowth in areas previously thought to represent end-stage scarring.[40] This may be evidenced by some improvement in follicular density with treatment.

Topical and Intralesional Therapies

Topical minoxidil is a readily available over-the-counter medication with a mechanism of action that requires further study. It is thought to work by reversing miniaturization of the hair follicles and prolonging the anagen phase (growth phase) of the hair cycle. It is considered a first-line therapy in the treatment of AGA in both men and women, as well as in early TA to promote hair regrowth.[41] Topical minoxidil is available as a foam or solution in two concentrations, 2% (primarily for women) and 5% (primarily for men), though the 5% concentration is more efficacious in both men and women.[42] For patients who require more aggressive therapy, compounding minoxidil preparations up to 10% can be effective. This can be combined with retinoic acid for enhanced penetration into the scalp and topical steroids to minimize irritant contact reactions. In women of African descent who have tightly curled or coiled hair that requires less frequent washing, the topical minoxidil solution is preferred to reduce product buildup within the hair. The solution can cause an irritant contact dermatitis due to its alcohol base (propylene glycol) and to minimize the risk of a contact reaction, the use of a light oil or moisturizer following application of topical minoxidil solution is advised.[43]

Topical potent corticosteroids, often combined with intralesional corticosteroid injections to the scalp, are generally considered a first-line therapeutic option for cicatricial alopecia and can also be used in TA when there is evidence of active inflammation on examination.[44] Intralesional corticosteroids can be given at a concentration of 5 to 10 mg/cc every 6 to 8 weeks until clinical evidence of active inflammation has resolved.[45] For patients with CCCA, measurement of disease activity is difficult, as many women present with absence of overt inflammation. In these patients, a series of 5 to 8 sessions followed by a 6 to 9 month treatment-free period is common. For recalcitrant CCCA, positive outcomes have been demonstrated with topical metformin cream 10% compounded in Lipoderm, showing evidence of hair regrowth.[46] No side effects have been reported outside of dryness and irritation at the site of application in the scalp that improved with use of a topical moisturizer, and it is thought to be well tolerated due to topical therapeutic concentrations being below the threshold of systemic absorption.

Steroid-induced atrophy, a well-known adverse effect associated with intralesional corticosteroid injections, poses an even higher risk of occurrence in patients concurrently using potent topical steroids.[47] Spacing out injections is essential to avoid this complication. As described above, intralesional steroid injections are generally recommended at 6 to 8 week intervals to reduce risk of atrophy, and potent topical corticosteroids should be used for a maximum of 2-week intervals if applied daily, with a 1-week break in between.[48] In patients who ultimately develop pale, atrophied skin at the site of injection or topical application, further injection to the area should be avoided. Steroid-induced atrophy is typically self-limited and resolves in 1 to 2 years; however, several methods have been described to improve the appearance of atrophic areas including the use of serial saline injections, pulsed-dye laser, and fat grafting.[49,50]

Systemic Therapies

Oral agents are alternative treatment options for patients who fail or are unable to tolerate topical therapies. In patients with cicatricial alopecia such as CCCA, systemic therapies can allow for better control of inflammation through use of hydroxychloroquine, oral antibiotics such as doxycycline, and mycophenolate mofetil.[39,51,52] Oral antibiotics can also be appropriate in patients with TA who are experiencing active inflammation.[53]

Oral anti-androgens, such as finasteride for men and off-label use of spironolactone in women, are also useful alternative or adjunct treatment options to topical therapies proven to enhance cosmesis. When initiated early at 1 mg daily, finasteride is highly effective in increasing hair regrowth and follicular density.[54] However, a principal limitation of finasteride is its associated side effects including sexual dysfunction, impotence, and the rare development of post-finasteride syndrome where sexual, physical, and psychological adverse effects from finasteride persist even following discontinuation of the drug. In women, oral spironolactone can be a beneficial adjunct to topical minoxidil given its anti-androgen effects on the hair follicles in the scalp.[55,56] It is generally recommended to initiate therapy at 50 mg daily titrated up to a therapeutic range between 100 and 200 mg as tolerated.[57] Spironolactone causes feminization of male fetal genitalia and is contraindicated in women who are pregnant or intend on becoming pregnant during the projected course of treatment.[58]

Autologous Platelet-rich Plasma

Studied since the 1970s primarily for applications in the stimulation of wound healing, platelet-rich plasma (PRP) has recently gained traction in its aesthetic use in dermatology for the treatment of hair loss.[59] PRP works by enhancing cells involved in tissue regeneration such as adipose-derived stem cells and dermal fibroblasts.[60] The proposed mechanism of PRP stimulation of hair growth is thought to involve platelet activation that leads to a cascade of reactions and ultimately the secretion of cytokines and growth factors essential in the process of wound healing.[61] These growth factors then act on stem cells within the bulge region of the hair follicle, promoting neovascularization and follicular regeneration. In addition, beta-catenin and fibroblast growth factor-7 (FGF-7) activity have been found to be upregulated in patients following PRP treatment. The increased beta-catenin activity further induces proliferation of follicular stem cells, while upregulation of FGF-7 activity prolongs the anagen phase of the hair cycle to further stimulate growth.[61]

Most studies, including randomized controlled trials examining the efficacy of PRP for the treatment of AGA, have reported positive results, with significant increase in follicular density, normalization of hair loss, and patient satisfaction following treatment.[62] Poorer results are expected in patients with more advanced AGA (Norwood VI–VII classifications) and are instead more promising in patients with earlier stages of disease.[63] Fewer studies exist on the use of PRP in the treatment of cicatricial alopecia; however, one study found 50% improvement in the hair density at the scalp vertex in a woman of African descent with CCCA following three sessions of PRP spaced 4 weeks apart (Figs. 20.1A and B).[40]

An important pretreatment recommendation all providers should consider prior to initiating PRP treatment is the concurrent use of topical minoxidil formulations. Topical minoxidil should not be initiated within 3 months of starting PRP sessions due to terminal hair shedding at the start of topical minoxidil application experienced by some patients.[64] This could potentially compromise PRP results. If patients have been on long-term topical minoxidil therapy initiated more than 3 months prior to the start of PRP, patients can be continued on this therapy throughout PRP sessions.

PRP is usually a well-tolerated treatment with very minimal side effects with the exception of discomfort during the treatment. Patients can expect edema or

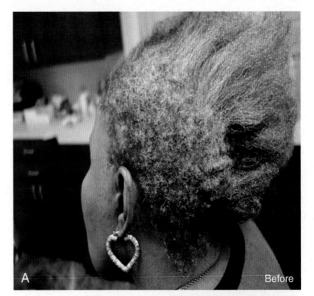
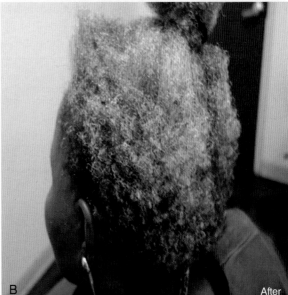

Fig. 20.1 (A) Patient with CCCA prior to PRP treatment. (B) Patient with CCCA 18 months following three sessions of PRP treatment

erythema of the injection sites, pain, and headache immediately following treatment.[58] These symptoms usually resolve within hours of treatment. The use of analgesics with antiplatelet activity such as Nonsteroidal anti-inflammatory drugs (NSAIDs) should be avoided to prevent counteracting the effects of treatment. A cold pack applied before and after a PRP session can be helpful in tempering pain.[59] In addition, koebernization, or the induction of new areas of disease, is a theoretical concern with PRP treatment; however, this has yet to be reported in the literature.[65] Lastly, patients should be counseled that the results achieved with PRP sessions are not indefinite. Evidence of disease reactivation has been reported in patients as soon as 6 months following their last PRP session.[40] Therefore, the need for continued, longitudinal treatment with repeat PRP sessions if desired should be expected and discussed with patients.

Hair Transplantation

Surgical hair restoration is a safe and effective option for patients looking to achieve more permanent hair restoration. The consultation visit is key in establishing candidacy for surgical hair restoration. A thorough examination of the scalp is important in patients with cicatricial alopecia, as any evidence of inflammation is an absolute contraindication to hair transplantation. It is generally recommended patients undergo aggressive medical management with antiinflammatory agents and show disease stability with no clinical signs of active inflammation for at least 12 months prior to considering surgical hair restoration.[66] A punch biopsy of the recipient site can aid in preventing transplantation of active areas of disease by ensuring there is no subclinical evidence of inflammation. The intended donor site should also be identified and examined at this time to ensure an adequate number of follicular units are present (at least 40 follicular units/cm²).[67]

A detailed medical and dermatologic history can aid in identification of conditions, such as seborrheic dermatitis, that can affect hair growth without treatment.[68] Obtaining an in-depth history of hairstyling and hair-care practices is also fundamental in providing early guidance to correct harmful practices that can later compromise graft survival. This should also involve a discussion of postprocedural hairstyling plans to aid in selection of the appropriate donor harvesting technique and allow adequate time for the patient to coordinate with their hairstylist if necessary, especially in women of African descent who often have their hair routinely styled in a salon. All patients with scarring hair loss should be counseled on the possibility of disease reactivation and lower rate of graft survival in the fibrotic scalp tissue.[69]

Once a patient has been deemed an appropriate candidate for hair transplantation, a test session is recommended to observe if the sample graft will take prior to pursuing full transplantation. This consists of harvesting 5 to 6 round, 4-mm grafts from the donor scalp and transplanting the grafts into corresponding 3.5-mm recipient sites located in the scarred, alopecic area (Figs. 20.2A–C).[69] A window of 3 to 6 months should be allotted to monitor for proper hair growth and disease stability at the test site. Patients should be advised that hair regrowth at the grafted sites is expected to be relatively slow compared to areas of unaffected, healthy scalp.[70] Once graft survival and hair regrowth of the test sites has been documented, patients can then proceed with full hair transplantation.

Hair transplantation in tightly curled or coiled hair poses several challenges that must be considered in advance to achieve satisfactory results. Patients of African descent have below the average follicular density, requiring careful planning of harvesting the donor hairs in transplantation to prevent significant reduction in follicular density that would result in notable thinning. The best surgical technique for hair transplantation depends on several factors such as the location and extent of hair loss, expected surgical scarring, vascular supply, texture of hair, and preferred patient hairstyling.[71] Linear strip excision (LSE) and follicular unit extraction (FUE) are the two main donor harvesting techniques used in surgical hair restoration.[72] LSE involves harvesting a 1-cm single strip from the donor region above the occipital protuberance extending from helix to helix.[73] This region is generally less affected by traction alopecia, AGA, and CCCA.[73,74] LSE is the preferred method of transplantation in patients with traction alopecia due to the ability to conceal the scar and the lower risk of transection (graft failure).[75] FUE is instead the preferred technique for hair transplantation in patients with CCCA and requires the use of larger grafts and larger recipient sites to decrease the risk of transection and offer more scalp coverage.[69] This technique involves harvesting follicular units with 0.9- to 1.25-mm punch excisions made from the safe donor area (region of the scalp expected to be spared from disease involvement in the occipital scalp) and offers less visible scarring compared to LSE.[76] The FUE technique results in less visible scarring, which is particularly beneficial in Black males who often prefer short, tapered haircuts.[73] However, FUE does come with potential disadvantages such as extended time required to harvest donor hairs, higher transection rate, and a larger

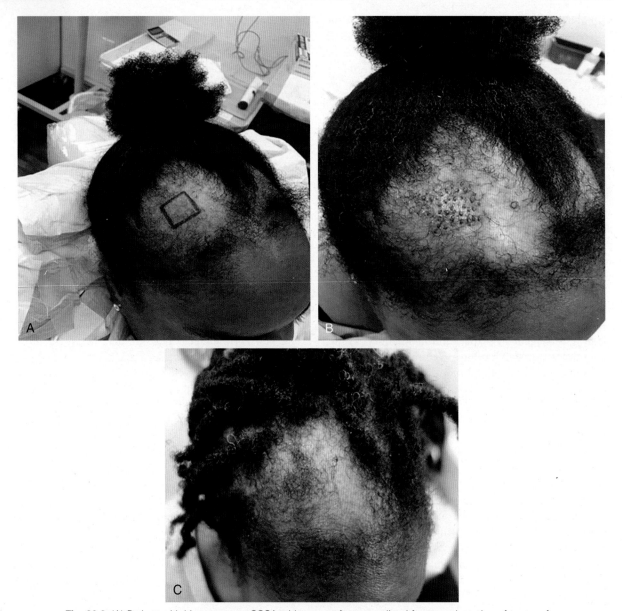

Fig. 20.2 (A) Patient with biopsy-proven CCCA with test graft area outlined for transplantation of test grafts. (B) Patient with biopsy-proven CCCA immediately following transplantation of test grafts in the scarred, fibrotic scalp. (C) Patient with biopsy-proven CCCA with demonstrated growth and take of test grafts in the recipient's, affected scalp. This patient would be considered a candidate for hair transplantation.

donor area that requires shaving, which poses concern for some female patients (Fig. 20.3).[73]

Following hair transplantation, patients are recommended to follow up in 10 days to 2 weeks to examine the surgical sites for proper wound healing or signs of infection. Potential postoperative complications include hypertrophic scarring, keloid formation, hyper- or hypopigmentation of the donor area, folliculitis, depletion of donor site hair density, and potential slower hair growth in patients of African descent compared to other

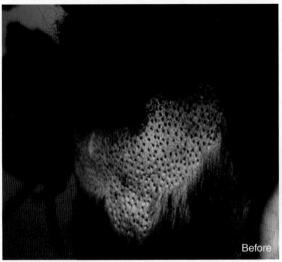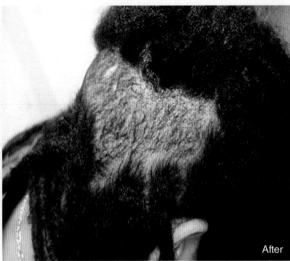

Before

After

Fig. 20.3 The shaved donor site of a patient undergoing follicular unit extraction (left) and the same patient 15 days postprocedurally with a well-healing donor area (right).

ethnic groups.[77] A timeframe of 12 to 15 months postoperation is typically adequate time to assess the need for additional hair transplantation. Following hair transplantation, it is important to emphasize daily washing and care of the donor and recipient area to prevent infection and crusting of the area until the site has completely healed, especially in Black women who often wash their hair in 1- to 4-week intervals.

Low-level Light Therapy

Low-level light therapy (LLLT) is an expanding technology discovered in the 1960s and has since been used in medical applications for the reduction of pain and inflammation, prevention of tissue damage, and stimulation of tissue repair and regeneration.[78] LLLT consists of exposing tissue to low levels of near-infrared and red light at energy levels less than those used in other forms of laser therapy such as ablation, of near-infrared and red light.[79] The mechanism of action of LLLT is unknown but is thought to involve accelerated mitosis of fibroblasts and keratinocytes through the production of antioxidants and reactive oxygen species.[78]

For dermatologic use in hair loss, LLLT is currently approved by the US Food and Drug Administration (FDA) for the treatment of AGA.[80] LLLT home devices include the TOPHAT 665®, the HairMax Lasercomb®, and the Capillus® laser cap, and the Revian® hair cap. The efficacy of LLLT alone appears to be comparable to

that of conventional medical therapies in AGA when used for similar durations, though direct comparisons of efficacy have not been extensively studied.[80] It is generally considered as a second-line therapy if no response is seen with the use of minoxidil or oral antiandrogens and can also be used in combination with these therapies. More studies are needed to determine the optimal settings for power, wavelength, and frequency of therapy in the treatment of AGA, especially as a monotherapy. Scalp paresthesias, pruritis, headache, acne, and urticarial dry skin were notable adverse effects reported across clinical trials and only affected a small percentage of study participants.[80] There are no known studies on the use of LLLT in CCCA patients, though limited data exist on the use for treatment of other scarring alopecias such as LPP and FFA where LLLT was noted to markedly reduce inflammation in these patients.[81,82]

ADDITIONAL CONSIDERATIONS

For patients of African descent, almost any discussion of the treatment and management of hair loss requires additional counseling on hairstyling practices, regardless of alopecia subtype. Patients often attempt to camouflage their hair loss through wear of extensions and wigs, which can paradoxically lead to more breakage and hair loss, confounding any expected improvement with initiation of treatment. Early identification of harmful hair practices and review of healthy hair-care practices are fundamental in properly managing hair loss in patients of African descent. Proper hair care is the treatment of choice for ATN but is also critical for Black women suffering from all types of hair loss, as maintaining hair fullness is key to camouflaging hair loss due to other reasons. Key recommendations in building a healthy hair-care routine include the use of sulfate-free shampoos (or those containing mild sulfates such as sodium C14-C16 olefin sulfonate), conditioning with every wash, deep conditioning once weekly for at least 10 minutes (with optional application of heat from a warm towel or dryer to maximize penetration of the deep conditioner), use of a leave-in conditioner three to five times each week, and application of carrier oils such as jojoba oil, grapeseed oil, or argan oil to the hair shaft (Table 20.1).[5] The process of applying a conditioner and a light oil to wet hair is akin the "soak and smear" approach commonly recommended for those with severe dry skin and serves a similar purpose in dry hair. Protein treatments are also beneficial in patients with significant hair damage and can be applied once weekly for the first 3 months of hair health restoration. These treatments contain one of several forms of hydrolyzed proteins to provide conditioning and added strength to the hair and can be applied in a salon or at home. After several months of consistent healthy hair practices, complete reversal of hair loss and breakage is expected in conditions such as ATN and early TA.[83]

Importantly, advising of hair practices is even essential in hair transplantation patients to increase graft survival and reduce postprocedural complications in patients of African descent. Patients are encouraged to avoid high-tension hairstyles including weaves, braids, and ponytails. Acceptable hairstyling options include wigs worn with silk or satin lining underneath, natural hair worn down to cover the growing grafts, or a silk scarf lightly wrapped around the hairline.

SUMMARY

Aesthetic approaches to restoring hair loss in patients of African descent encompasses several important factors. As with all patients independent of ethnicity, adequate medical management and treatment of hair loss is important in helping patients achieve restoration of hair growth. However, this also includes consideration of the unique properties of the hair and cultural hair practices. Medical or procedural measures alone can prove futile and ineffective without first addressing how the hair is cared for by patients. Furthermore, hair loss conditions are not exclusive of one another and it is possible for more than one subtype of hair loss to contribute to a patient's presentation, especially in patients of African descent where the hair is more prone to breakage and damage. Having a basic understanding of the unique considerations in treating hair loss in patients of African descent is fundamental to the ability to offer optimal aesthetic results.

REFERENCES

1. Tolliver S, Shipp D, Alexis A, Kaffenberger BH. A descriptive study of black women with and without hair loss and their perception of dermatologists. *Int J Dermatol.* 2019; 58(9):e182-e184.
2. Malkud S. A hospital-based study to determine causes of diffuse hair loss in women. *J Clin Diagn Res.* 2015;9(8): WC01-WC04.
3. Koo JY, Shellow WV, Hallman CP, Edwards JE. Alopecia areata and increased prevalence of psychiatric disorders. *Int J Dermatol.* 1994;33:849-850.
4. Harrison S, Sinclair R. Hair colouring, permanent styling and hair structure. *J Cosmet Dermatol.* 2003;2(3-4): 180-185. doi:10.1111/j.1473-2130.2004.00064.x.
5. Aguh C, Okoye GA, eds. *Fundamentals of Ethnic Hair: The Dermatologist's Perspective.* Cham, Switzerland: Springer International Publishing; 2017.
6. Dawber RPR, Messenger AG. Hair follicle structure, keratinization and the physical properties of hair. In: Dawber R, ed. *Diseases of the Hair and Scalp.* 3rd ed. Oxford: Blackwell Science; 1997:23-50.
7. Robbins C. The cell membrane complex: Three related but different cellular cohesion components of mammalian hair fibers. *J Cosmet Sci.* 2009;60(4):437-465.

TABLE 20.1 Sample Hair-Care Regimen for Damaged Curly Hair
• Apply protein treatment to dry or damp hair. Cover with shower cap or heating source for 30 minutes.
• Wash hair once weekly with sulfate-free shampoo.
• Deep condition with every shampoo. Follow deep conditioning with moisturizing rinse-out conditioner.
• Add leave-in conditioner after washing, at least 3x/week. Heavy glycerin-based leave-in conditioners are especially effective for very dry hair.
• End washing session with light oil.

8. Gavazzoni Dias MF. Hair cosmetics: An overview. *Int J Trichology*. 2015;7(1):2-15.

9. Herskovitz I, Miteva M. Central centrifugal cicatricial alopecia: Challenges and solutions. *Clin Cosmet Investig Dermatol*. 2016;9:175-181. doi:10.2147/CCID.S100816.

10. Bernard BA. Hair shape of curly hair. *J Am Acad Dermatol*. 2003;48(suppl 6):S120-S126. doi:10.1067/mjd.2003.279.

11. Tanus A, Oliveira CC, Villarreal DJ, Sanchez FA, Dias MF. Black women's hair: The main scalp dermatoses and aesthetic practices in women of African ethnicity. *An Bras Dermatol*. 2015;90(4):450-465. doi:10.1590/abd1806-4841.20152845.

12. Shapiro J. Cicatricial alopecias. *Dermatol Ther*. 2008;21:211.

13. Mirmirani P, Willey A, Headington JT, Stenn K, McCalmont TH, Price VH. Primary cicatricial alopecia: Histopathologic findings do not distinguish clinical variants. *J Am Acad Dermatol*. 2005;52:637-643.

14. Gan DC, Sinclair RD. Prevalence of male and female pattern hair loss in Maryborough. *J Investig Dermatol Symp Proc*. 2005;10:184-189.

15. Ho CH, Sood T, Zito PM. *Androgenetic Alopecia*. IStatPearls Publishing; 2020. Available at: https://www.ncbi.nlm.nih.gov/books/NBK430924.

16. Sadick NS, Callender VD, Kircik LH, Kogan S. New insight into the pathophysiology of hair loss trigger a paradigm shift in the treatment approach. *J Drugs Dermatol*. 2017;16(11):s135-s140.

17. Hamilton JB. Patterned hair loss in men: Types and incidence. *Ann N Y Acad Sci*. 1951;53:708-714.

18. Olsen EA. Female pattern hair loss. *J Am Acad Dermatol*. 2001;45:S70-S80.

19. Halder RM, Roberts CI, Nootheti PK. Cutaneous diseases in the Black races. *Dermatol Clin*. 2003;21(4):679-687, ix. doi:10.1016/s0733-8635(03)00084-6.

20. McMichael AJ. Hair breakage in normal and weathered hair: Focus on the Black patient. *J Investig Dermatol Symp Proc*. 2007;12(2):6-9. doi:10.1038/sj.jidsymp.5650047.

21. Mirmirani P. Ceramic flat irons: Improper use leading to acquired trichorrhexis nodosa. *J Am Acad Dermatol*. 2010;62(1):145-147. doi:10.1016/j.jaad.2009.01.048.

22. Tosti A. Hair weathering. In: Tosti A, ed. *Dermoscopy of the Hair and Nails*. 2nd ed. Boca Raton, FL: CRC Press; 2016:98-100.

23. Haskin A, Kwatra SG, Aguh C. Breaking the cycle of hair breakage: Pearls for the management of acquired trichorrhexis nodosa. *J Dermatolog Treat*. 2017;28(4):322-326. doi:10.1080/09546634.2016.1246704.

24. Woodard A, Le TK, DiBiagio J, Goldenberg NA, Cohen BA. A retrospective study of tinea capitis management in general pediatric clinics and pediatric emergency departments at two U.S. centers. *J Pediatr*. 2021;234:269-272. doi:10.1016/j.jpeds.2021.03.051.

25. Gomez-Zubiaur A, Saceda-Corralo D, Velez-Velázquez MD, Lario AR, Trasobares-Marugan L. Central centrifugal cicatricial alopecia following a patchy pattern: A new form of clinical presentation and a challenging diagnosis for the dermatologist. *Int J Trichology*. 2019;11(5):216-218. doi:10.4103/ijt.ijt_11_19.

26. Alexis AF, Sergay AB, Taylor SC. Common dermatologic disorders in skin of color: A comparative practice survey. *Cutis*. 2007;80(5):387-394.

27. Samrao A, Price VH, Zedek D, Mirmirani P. The "fringe sign" - a useful clinical finding in traction alopecia of the marginal hair line. *Dermatol Online J*. 2011;17(11):1.

28. Haskin A, Aguh C. All hairstyles are not created equal: What the dermatologist needs to know about Black hairstyling practices and the risk of traction alopecia (TA). *J Am Acad Dermatol*. 2016;75(3):606-611. doi:10.1016/j.jaad.2016.02.1162.

29. Khumalo NP, Jessop S, Gumedze F, Ehrlich R. Hairdressing and the prevalence of scalp disease in African adults. *Br J Dermatol*. 2007;157(5):981-988.

30. Billero V, Miteva M. Traction alopecia: The root of the problem. *Clin Cosmet Investig Dermatol*. 2018;11:149-159. doi:10.2147/CCID.S137296.

31. Dlova NC, Salkey KS, Callender VD, McMichael AJ. Central centrifugal cicatricial alopecia: New insights and a call for action. *J Investig Dermatol Symp Proc*. 2017;18:S54-S56.

32. Shah SK, Alexis AF. Central centrifugal cicatricial alopecia: retrospective chart review. *J Cutan Med Surg*. 2010;14(5):212-222. doi:10.2310/7750.2010.09055.

33. LoPresti P, Papa CM, Kligman AM. Hot comb alopecia. *Arch Dermatol*. 1968;98(3):234-238. doi:10.1001/archderm.1968.01610150020003.

34. Gathers RC, Jankowski M, Eide M, Lim HW. Hair grooming practices and central centrifugal cicatricial alopecia. *J Am Acad Dermatol*. 2009;60(4):574-578.

35. Malki L, Sarig O, Romano MT, et al. Variant PADI3 in central centrifugal cicatricial alopecia. *N Engl J Med*. 2019;380(9):833-841.

36. Dina Y, Okoye GA, Aguh C. Association of uterine leiomyomas with central centrifugal cicatricial alopecia. *JAMA Dermatol*. 2018;154(2):213-214.

37. Coogan PF, Bethea TN, Cozier YC, et al. Association of type 2 diabetes with central-scalp hair loss in a large cohort study of African American women. *Int J Womens Dermatol*. 2019;5(4):261-266.

38. Callender VD, Wright DR, Davis EC, Sperling LC. Hair breakage as a presenting sign of early or occult central centrifugal cicatricial alopecia: Clinicopathologic findings in 9 patients. *Arch Dermatol*. 2012;148:1047-1052.

39. Harries MJ, Sinclair RD, Macdonald-Hull S, et al. Management of primary cicatricial alopecias: Options for treatment. *Br J Dermatol*. 2008;159:1-22.

40. Dina Y, Aguh C. Use of platelet-rich plasma in cicatricial alopecia. *Dermatol Surg.* 2019;45(7):979-981.

41. Tsuboi R, Itami S, Inui S, et al. Guidelines for the management of androgenetic alopecia (2010). *J Dermatol.* 2012;39(2):113-120.

42. Roberts JL. Androgenetic alopecia: Treatment results with topical minoxidil. *J Am Acad Dermatol.* 1987;16:705-710.

43. Olsen EA, Whiting D, Bergfeld W, et al. A multicenter, randomized, placebo-controlled, double-blind clinical trial of a novel formulation of 5% minoxidil topical foam versus placebo in the treatment of androgenetic alopecia in men. *J Am Acad Dermatol.* 2007;57(5):767-774.

44. Filbrandt R, Rufaut N, Jones L, Sinclair R. Primary cicatricial alopecia: Diagnosis and treatment. *CMAJ.* 2013;185(18):1579-1585. doi:10.1503/cmaj.111570.

45. Tan E, Martinka M, Ball N, et al. Primary cicatricial alopecias: Clinicopathology of 112 cases. *J Am Acad Dermatol.* 2004;50:25-32.

46. Araoye EF, Thomas JAL, Aguh CU. Hair regrowth in 2 patients with recalcitrant central centrifugal cicatricial alopecia after use of topical metformin. *JAAD Case Rep.* 2020;6(2):106-108. doi:10.1016/j.jdcr.2019.12.008.

47. Firooz A, Tehranchi-Nia Z, Ahmed AR. Benefits and risks of intralesional corticosteroid injection in the treatment of dermatological diseases. *Clin Exp Dermatol.* 1995;20:363-370.

48. Drake LA, Dinehart SM, Farmer ER, et al. Guidelines of care for the use of topical glucocorticosteroids. *J Am Acad Dermatol.* 1996;35(4):615-619.

49. Shumaker PR, Rao J, Goldman MP. Treatment of local, persistent cutaneous atrophy following corticosteroid injection with normal saline infiltration. *Dermatol Surg.* 2005;31:1340-1343.

50. Mansouri P, Ranibar M, Abolhasani E, Chalangari R, Martits-Chalangari R, Hejazi S. Pulsed dye laser in treatment of steroid-induced atrophy. *J Cosmet Dermatol.* 2015;14:E15-E20.

51. Lyakhovitsky A, Amichai B, Sizopoulou C, Barzilai A. A case series of 46 patients with lichen planopilaris: Demographics, clinical evaluation, and treatment experience. *J Dermatolog Treat.* 2015;26(3):275-279.

52. Price VH. The medical treatment of cicatricial alopecia. *Semin Cutan Med Surg.* 2006;25:56-59.

53. McMichael AJ. Hair and scalp disorders in ethnic populations. *Dermatol Clin.* 2003;21(4):629-644. doi:10.1016/s0733-8635(03)00077-9.

54. Okereke UR, Simmons A, Callender VD. Current and emerging treatment strategies for hair loss in women of color. *Int J Womens Dermatol.* 2019;5:37-45.

55. Burns LJ, De Souza B, Flynn E, Hagigeorges D, Senna MM. Spironolactone for treatment of female pattern hair loss. *J Am Acad Dermatol.* 2020;83(1):276-278.

56. Sinclair RD. Female pattern hair loss: A pilot study investigating combination therapy with low-dose oral minoxidil and spironolactone. *Int J Dermatol.* 2017;57(1):104-109.

57. Camacho-Martínez FM. Hair loss in women. *Semin Cutan Med Surg.* 2009;28(1):19-32.

58. Dinh QQ, Sinclair R. Female pattern hair loss: Current treatment concepts. *Clin Interv Aging.* 2007;2(2):189-199.

59. Andia I. Platelet-rich plasma biology. In: Alves R, Grimalt R, eds. *Clinical Indications and Treatment Protocols with Platelet-Rich Plasma in Dermatology.* Barcelona: Ediciones Mayo; 2016:3-15.

60. Sclafani AP, Azzi J. Platelet preparations for use in facial rejuvenation and wound healing: A critical review of current literature. *Aesthetic Plast Surg.* 2015;39:495-505.

61. Li ZJ, Choi HI, Choi DK, et al. Autologous platelet-rich plasma: A potential therapeutic tool for promoting hair growth. *Dermatol Surg.* 2012;38(7 Pt 1):1040-1046.

62. Chen JX, Justicz N, Lee LN. Platelet-rich plasma for the treatment of androgenic alopecia: A systematic review. *Facial Plast Surg.* 2018;34(6):631-640. doi:10.1055/s-0038-1660845.

63. Gkini MA, Kouskoukis AE, Tripsianis G, Rigopoulos D, Kouskoukis K. Study of platelet-rich plasma injections in the treatment of androgenetic alopecia through an one-year period. *J Cutan Aesthet Surg.* 2014;7(4):213-219. doi:10.4103/0974-2077.150743.

64. Sinclair RD. Female pattern hair loss: A pilot study investigating combination therapy with low-dose oral minoxidil and spironolactone. *Int J Dermatol.* 2018;57(1):104-109.

65. Tawfik AA, Osman MAR. The effect of autologous activated platelet-rich plasma injection on female pattern hair loss: A randomized placebo-controlled study. *J Cosmet Dermatol.* 2018;17(1):47-53.

66. Rose P, Shapiro R. Transplanting into scar tissue and areas of cicatricial alopecia. In: Unger WP, Shapiro R, eds. *Hair Transplantation.* 4th ed. New York: Marcel Dekker; 2004:606-609.

67. Olsen EA, Messenger AG, Shapiro J, et al. Evaluation and treatment of male and female pattern hair loss. *J Am Acad Dermatol.* 2005;52:301-311.

68. Kristine Bunagan MJ. Diseases of the hair and scalp in Asians that are of interest to hair surgeons. In: Pathomvanich D, Imagawa K, eds. *Practical Aspects of Hair Transplantation in Asians.* Tokyo: Springer; 2018. Available at: https://doi.org/10.1007/978-4-431-56547-5_6.

69. Callender VD, Lawson CN, Onwudiwe OC. Hair transplantation in the surgical treatment of central centrifugal cicatricial alopecia. *Dermatol Surg.* 2014;40:1125-1131.

70. Salanitri S, Gonçalves AJ, Helene Jr A, Lopes FHJ. Surgical complications in hair transplantation: a series of 533 procedures. *Aesthetic Surg J.* 2009;29(1):72-76.

71. Dahdah MJ, Iorizzo M. The role of hair restoration surgery in primary cicatricial alopecia. *Skin Appendage Disord*. 2016;2(1-2):57-60. doi:10.1159/000448104.

72. Rogers NE, Callender VD. Advances and challenges in hair restoration of curly Afrocentric hair. *Dermatol Clin*. 2014;32:163-171.

73. Avram M, Rogers N. Contemporary hair transplantation. *Dermatol Surg*. 2009;35:1705-1719.

74. Lee TS, Minton TJ. An update on hair restoration therapy. *Curr Opin Otolaryngol Head Neck Surg*. 2009;17:287-294.

75. Dua A, Dua K. Follicular unit extraction hair transplant. *J Cutan Aesthet Surg*. 2010;3(2):76-81.

76. Rassman WR, Bernstein RM, McClellan R, et al. Follicular unit extraction: minimally invasive surgery in hair transplantation. *Dermatol Surg*. 2002;28:720-728.

77. Kerure AS, Patwardhan N. Complications in hair transplantation. *J Cutan Aesthet Surg*. 2018;11(4):182-189. doi:10.4103/JCAS.JCAS_125_18.

78. Avci P, Gupta GK, Clark J, Wikonkal N, Hamblin MR. Low-level laser (light) therapy (LLLT) for treatment of hair loss. *Lasers Surg Med*. 2014;46:144-151.

79. Avci P, Gupta A, Sadasivam M, et al. Low-level laser (light) therapy (LLLT) in skin: stimulating, healing, restoring. *Semin Cutan Med Surg*. 2013;32(1):41-52.

80. Darwin E, Heyes A, Hirt PA, Wikramanayake TC, Jimenez JJ. Low-level laser therapy for the treatment of androgenic alopecia: A review. *Lasers Med Sci*. 2018;33(2):425-434. doi:10.1007/s10103-017-2385-5.

81. Randolph MJ, Salhi WA, Tosti A. Lichen planopilaris and low-level light therapy: Four case reports and review of the literature about low-level light therapy and lichenoid dermatosis. *Dermatol Ther (Heidelb)*. 2020;10:311-319.

82. Fonda-Pascual P, Moreno-Arrones OM, Saceda-Corralo D, et al. Effectiveness of low-level laser therapy in lichen planopilaris. *J Am Acad Dermatol*. 2018;78(5):1020-1023.

83. Callender VD, McMichael AJ, Cohen GF. Medical and surgical therapies for alopecias in Black women. *Dermatol Ther*. 2004;17(2):164-176. doi:10.1111/j.1396-0296.2004.04017.x.

INDEX

Page numbers followed by '*b*' indicate boxes, '*f*' indicate figures, and '*t*' indicate tables.